The Vitamix Cookbook

Over 200 Delicious Whole Food Recipes
to Make in Your Blender

Jodi Berg

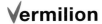
ermilion

1 3 5 7 9 10 8 6 4 2

Ebury Press, an imprint of Ebury Publishing,
20 Vauxhall Bridge Road,
London SW1V 2SA

Ebury Press is part of the Penguin Random House group of companies
whose addresses can be found at global.penguinrandomhouse.com

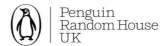

Copyright © Jodi Berg 2015

First published by Ebury Press in 2015

The information on p.23 is taken from www.ft.com 'The Healing Power of Gardens'; information on p.25 is taken from
www.gov.uk 'National Diet and Nutrition Survey'

This edition published by arrangement with Harlequin, a division of HarperCollins Publishers,
195 Broadway, New York, NY 10007. All rights reserved.

www.eburypublishing.co.uk

A CIP catalogue record for this book is available from the British Library

Anglicised by Clare Sayer
Design: Paula Russell Szafranski
Original photography by Allen Owens/Limoncello Productions

ISBN 9781785040375

Printed and bound in Italy by Printer Trento

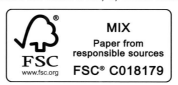

To our dedicated and committed Vitamix team, who work tirelessly to help make the world a healthier place, and to our loyal fans. Thank you for making a difference.

Vitamix was founded in 1921 by William G. Barnard. This fourth-generation family owned and operated company continues to manufacture superior blending and mixing products used by professional chefs and home cooks alike. Nestled in the valley of picturesque Olmsted Falls, Ohio, the company employs more than 600 people, has a global presence in more than 80 countries, and continues to win awards for product innovation.

Jodi Berg, the great-granddaughter of William G. Barnard, is the President and CEO of Vitamix.

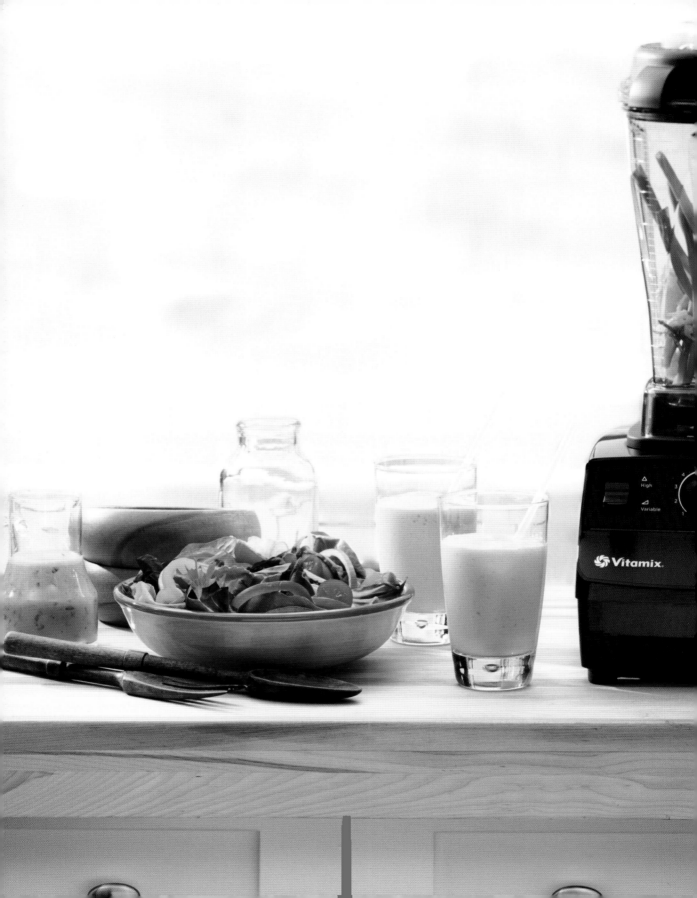

CONTENTS

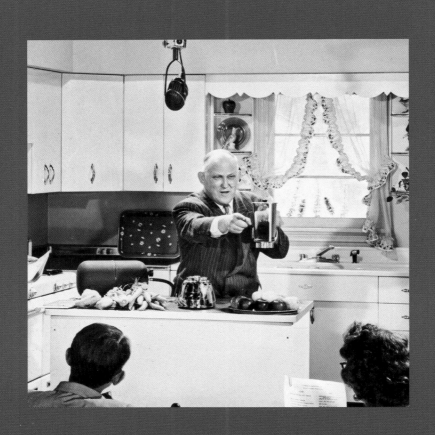

Introduction

If you have ever had the opportunity to experience a Vitamix demonstration, you may not be surprised to know that demonstration has been the backbone of our company for generations. Our dedicated demonstrators whipping up smoothies, soups and frozen dessert samples are both an iconic part of our brand and a tremendous teaching tool to help people successfully adopt a healthier lifestyle – a role that we have taken very seriously for over 90 years. In the 1940s, shortly after the first blender was invented, my great-grandfather was demonstrating the magic of blended whole foods in front of an audience equally eager to taste the rich flavours produced in mere moments. Hard to believe, right? My great-grandfather – our company's founder – had an incredible passion for whole foods, health, and wellness, as do our hundreds of Vitamix demonstrators in multiple countries around the world, that carry on this tradition today.

I, Jodi Berg, am the current president and CEO of Vitamix, a fourth-generation family business. As a family entity, Vitamix can continue to focus on a purpose greater and more encompassing than the almighty sale; it is not just about the bottom line, but about making a difference in improving the vitality of people's lives. We get to invite every employee and every customer to be a member of the

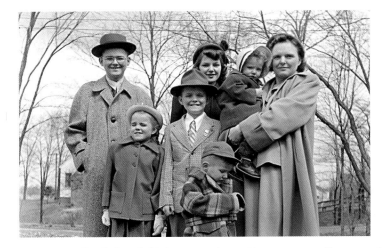

Vitamix family and an advocate for healthy change. If you are already part of our family, you know that Vitamix is more than just a company, and more than a life-changing appliance. If you are just joining us, then welcome!

Prior to talking about the importance of whole foods, and before you start looking at all of the delicious recipes, I want to tell you a bit of 'our' family's story, because when you adopt a Vitamix lifestyle, this becomes your story, too. And it's a good one! Full of laughter, hard work, a little log cabin and a cast of wonderful characters, all deeply devoted to one another and to the business they were building together – all of them passionate about helping people increase their vitality. And it all started with a tin opener.

Yes, a tin opener and one skilled, charismatic and resourceful salesman named William Grover Barnard. Living in Westpoint, Illinois, my great-grandfather, known affectionately to all as Papa Barnard, was a successful, ambitious jack-of-all-trades. Back in the early 1900s, Papa was mayor, undertaker, railroad station agent, banker and property investor to boot. He was the horse in a one-horse town, his son Bill once said. A workhorse, I would venture to say. But then his family, like many others, hit hard times around 1921. Papa had invested heavily in real estate, so when the land values plummeted, he had to reinvent himself. After all, he had a family to support, and he wasn't about to

> Back in the early 1900s, Papa was mayor, undertaker, railroad station agent, banker and property investor to boot. He was the horse in a one-horse town, his son Bill once said.

let them down. Papa tackled this challenge like many others: with tenacity, a twinkle in his eye and a big dose of perseverance. For a natural showman like Papa, being a travelling salesman was a perfect fit. He got his start demonstrating small housewares like the tin opener long before the blender was even invented.

Papa was a gregarious, fun-loving man, and he always drew a crowd. He was a lot more than an entertainer – he was passionate about the value of his products. To Papa, the value to the customer had to be greater than the price paid. It had to. Twenty-five cents for a tin opener was a lot of money in those days. Still, opening tinned goods with a knife was dangerous. Unlike many tin openers available in the late 1920s and early 1930s, the model Papa demonstrated had a small wheel to protect your fingers. Even in tight times, my great-grandfather was able to demonstrate that the value was well worth what one would spend on it. This cornerstone is foundational still to this day.

As the country slid towards the Great Depression, Papa Barnard built up a successful business. Before too long, Papa's one-man show became a multi-generational business when his sons William Grove Jr. (Grandpa Bill) and Great Uncle Louie came on board. Papa christened his growing business the Barnard Sales Company, and the three men took to the road in a Model-T Ford, demonstrating in small towns across the United States to sell their wares.

Exploring Health and Whole Foods

In 1934, my grandpa Bill married his college sweetheart, Ruth. Her father, Frank C. Pellett, a well-respected naturalist and bee expert, was quite accomplished in his own right. As fate would have it, it was not Frank's strengths but his weaknesses that changed our family's history. You see, Frank had long suffered from digestive problems. Both the Barnard and the Pellett families rallied together to help him regain his health, and it was this quest that lead them to wellness through whole foods. It was then that the Barnard family first became interested in health through diet, and Papa, Grandpa and Grandma wanted very much to learn all they could.

Papa and my grandpa became interested in the writings of Dr John Harvey Kellogg, an early health food advocate, who later went on to found what would become the Kellogg's cereal company, and a health lecturer by the name of Dr Bush. After a talk by Dr Bush, Grandma wrote that Papa and Grandpa were inspired. 'The philosophy of the thing got them, and Bill has refused to eat white flour, white sugar and meat ever since.' My grandpa hoped to eventually know enough about achieving wellness through a healthy diet to be able to lecture on it, but meanwhile, as Grandma wrote to her Aunt Milly, 'we live it'.

The 1930s ended up being a very significant decade for our family. First, Papa and his sons demonstrated for two summers at the Great Lakes Exposition in Cleveland. During their time at the Expo, the Barnard family fell in love with the hardworking people of northeast Ohio. Deciding it was the best place to grow their families and their business, they moved to this great city in 1937, just after the Expo finished.

The second big event also happened around the hundred-day Expo. The Barnard family became aware of yet another new product, a blender. Many salesmen saw no use for the blender beyond bars and mixed drinks. But Papa saw the blender as the perfect tool to help himself, his family and his customers add more whole food to their diets. Not only could you add more fruits and vegetables, but the foods you could make would be varied and delicious, too. It was truly an 'Aha' moment for Papa. Grandpa Pellett christened the new blender the 'Vita-Mix', because *vita* in Latin means life. The Barnards were then, as we are today, great livers of life, and the name fit perfectly with the product, the business and the family, too.

As you surely know, feeling good is an adrenaline rush that keeps you coming back for more. Papa and my grandparents were hooked on their new whole-food diet. They wanted to share their discoveries with others. In 1939, they opened a health food store where they sold bulk food, supplements and vitamins, quickly adding the blender to their product mix. This store evolved into a growing direct mail business. Little did any of them know how iconic their blender would become in both residential and commercial kitchens all over the world.

As my grandparents and Papa continued to explore whole foods and learn about health, they came across the work of Bernarr Macfadden. Macfadden, a passionate advocate for exercise and nutrition, held week-long hikes. Grandpa had written away for information about the walks, but, as Grandma wrote in a letter later:

I was the one who read the literature and decided it was just what I needed to make me strong and well again. Probably my future life depended on this. After two weeks of walking 265 miles from Cleveland to Dansville, New York, I was as fit and healthy and full of vim and vigor such as I had never before in my life experienced.

Grandma, who was then the mother of a three-year-old boy, Grove, and an eight-month-old baby, Ginny, recalled that the beginning of the walk was the most exciting day of her life. Papa, ever up for an adventure, came along to see her off and ended up walking right along with her – all the way to the Physical Culture Hotel in Danville, New York. Grandma and Papa found a wonderful community on that walk. And since I get to tell you this story, I must tell you my favourite part: some of the friends they made on that trip would one day introduce my dad, John, to my mum, Linda. Thank you, Bernarr Macfadden!

The House That Bill Built

In 1942, the country was emerging from the Great Depression and immersed in the war. Grandpa, tiring of city life, bought twelve acres in Olmsted Township, Ohio, a little over 18 miles from Cleveland. Today, the Olmsted community is bustling, but back in the early 1940s, it was little more than scattered farms and quite a few cows. The move was motivated, in part, by a desire to be outside. 'We were never city people', my grandpa later recalled in an interview. To Grandpa and Papa, it was a beautiful oasis in the woods. Our family still loves being in nature.

My grandpa, like his father, had big dreams and boundless enthusiasm. Grandpa was a tall man with a booming voice, a terrific sense of humour and a work ethic like no other. While my grandma and their three children lived in a tiny trailer, he set about building a house, growing the business and contributing to the war efforts. Grandpa was a talented salesman like his father, but he was not particularly good with his hands. Not one to let this limitation be an obstacle, he tackled the house-building project with good cheer. My uncle Grove always laughed when he reminisced that his dad, 'didn't have any plans. He was just going to build the house'. Grandma wisely insisted that there be plans. She had a real gift

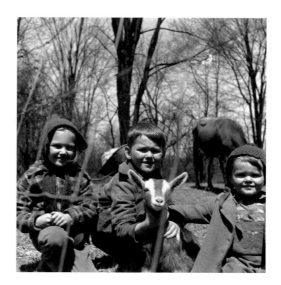

for giving Grandpa's dreams a solid foundation. It took some years, but the homestead was eventually finished. 'The house that Bill built' as I call it, still stands today. A simple house with knotty pine walls, rather like a rustic cabin, sits at the entrance to our corporate headquarters. This simple home, along with another building Bill built that housed the first Vitamix offices, remind us daily of our family roots, our focus on whole foods and wellness, and our purpose to help customers achieve greater vitality.

The Balancing Act

Balancing work and family is challenging at the best of times. My grandparents had their fair share of struggles: raising six children, growing a business and trying to change the way their fellow Americans thought about whole foods wasn't easy. Grandpa expected all family to be hands on deck. As my Aunt Ginny recalls, 'Mom and Dad maybe sat down and played a game with us once or twice in our life. If we were with them, it was because we were working'. All of my aunts and uncles were put to work in the family business, stuffing envelopes, packing mail-order boxes or working in the office.

Vitamix continued to grow, and Grandpa made sure it continued to be a family venture, a family adventure in many cases. And oh, were there ever a lot of adventures! My grandparents loved children, laughter, nature and hard work, and often there was some hilarious combination of these things all happening at once. For example, my aunts and uncles grew up with a whole menagerie of animals, including chickens, some rather unruly goats, a cow, ducks and a horse. And of course, the house that Grandpa built was right next door to the Vitamix offices. My aunt Patty laughs remembering how the goats caused trouble for the Vitamix employees:

> I remember watching her [one of the goats, Bootsie] chase women around the property. The women that used to work at Vitamix . . . would be screaming and running down the driveway with their hands in the air, and the goat would be behind them, butting them.

My aunts and uncles say that Grandpa left most of the discipline to Grandma and focussed, when he could, on the fun. He loved children and he loved to make them laugh. After the family moved to the Olmsted community, once a year he would clear a path to a place he called Mount Tooska-Ooska-Wooska-Choo. (A name he chose because it got the most giggles from the kids.) He would tromp his kids through the woods on the long, winding path to a clearing where they would have a picnic. When I think about these treks – to a destination that was probably not more than 350 feet away from the house – it reminds me that fun can be simple: as simple as packing so much silliness and wonder into a short walk in the woods!

The programme really put the company on the map, and gave them a bigger stage for their whole-foods message.

In the summer, when other kids were lounging about, Grandpa and Grandma took to the road with all the kids in tow. While my grandpa may have been a fun-loving man, these trips were not a family vacation. Nope. They piled five of the six kids in the back of a big farm truck (the youngest got to ride up front) and travelled to shows and fairs around the country. My dad remembers sleeping on top of the Vitamix boxes in the back of the truck with all of his siblings, packed together like a row of logs. If one kid wanted to roll over, they all had to roll over.

Some years my grandparents were able to tow a little camper along behind their truck. Once they parked overnight in a public park – a fairly common practice at the time – and awoke to find a parade lining up around them. Grandpa, ever a showman, managed to time their departure so they were the first vehicle in the parade – hardly a coincidence, I am sure. He honked and smiled, while my aunts and uncles all waved. Poor Grandma was so embarrassed; she giggled as she told us how she willed herself to be invisible! Riding home to Ohio at the end of the summer, Aunt Ginny recalls, was a bit more comfortable since many of the Vitamix boxes had been sold, so the kids had a little more space.

A New Stage for Papa

Another big year for the Barnard family was 1949. Grandpa, always looking for new ways to share his whole-foods message and the wonderful Vitamix with more people, got the idea that Papa should do his demonstration on television. Papa didn't agree. He was just as suspicious of this newfangled medium as Grandpa was passionate about its potential. After much coaxing, my grandpa convinced

Papa to rent a studio to do a live demonstration. The programme, considered the first infomercial, was an important move for the business. The phones started ringing about halfway through the segment, and the operator kept patching calls through until the middle of the night when she announced that she was going home. Grandpa remembers that 'now we knew we had something big'. The programme really put the company on the map, and gave them a bigger stage for their whole-foods message.

Marching to the Beat of a Different Drum

Committed to healthy living, Grandpa and Grandma raised their children as vegetarians, an unconventional decision at the time. My aunt Ginny says her friends didn't often know what being vegetarian meant, and my dad recalls being teased about the contents of his lunch box. My grandparents were dedicated to teaching others about whole foods and health, no matter how unfashionable it might be. They were definitely ahead of their time.

Grandpa continued to talk about health and how people could use the Vitamix to eat more whole food and set them on a path to vitality. Grandma was the glue that held it all together behind the scenes. For every ounce of passion and exuberance that Grandpa had, Grandma had a pound of common sense. She was also committed to developing new recipes and preparation techniques for the Vitamix.

While Grandpa was on the road, Grandma was learning a lot about what the machine could do. She was the one who discovered that you could grind wheat berries and other ingredients into flour. She figured out how to knead bread dough in the Vitamix, so you could go from fresh whole wheat berries to bread rising in a tin in just three minutes. Grandma taught herself how to make frozen treats in the Vitamix, and she figured out that you could make hot soup without adding a heating element, just with the speed and friction from the blades. She taught us all of the different, tasty and amazing ways we could use the machine to create nutritious and delicious food. We have carried on this tradition to today – with a state-of-the-art recipe development kitchen and a staff of talented chefs.

Both in the test kitchen and on the road, my grandparents were passionate about wellness – through whole foods. The Vitamix was an amazing kitchen tool but their goals were bigger – they wanted to make the world a healthier place. Even when it would have been easier to embrace the processed foods that were beginning to dominate the American diet, their commitment to healthy foods remained strong. They were not the first people to make the connection between diet and health, of course, but their dedication to healthy eating continues to inspire our family, our company and tens of thousands of dedicated Vitamix owners around the world today.

It's All About Family

My own memories of my grandparents are strongly tied to family reunions, because my dad had ventured out on his own and raised his family in Erie, Pennsylvania. For a long time, family reunions were held in the house that Bill built. When we would pull up to the house that Bill built, all five of us kids would pile out of the car after the long trip, and my grandparents, aunts, uncles, over a dozen cousins and all the family dogs would greet us at the door! If I shut my eyes, I can still hear the distinct clickity-clack of doggy feet, friendly barks and all of those voices, talking and laughing. It was a boisterous, chaotic scene, not so different in spirit from the house my dad grew up in.

After our reunions outgrew my grandparents' home in the 1970s, we held our ever-growing family get-togethers at the Vitamix offices. One of my most meaningful memories of Grandpa Bill happened at one of these gatherings. Like Papa, Grandpa believed passionately that our customers were the reason that we existed and we were here for them. When the phones at Vitamix rang, they rang throughout the building, so that Grandpa could be sure that the calls would be answered quickly. During one of these weekend reunions, Grandpa answered the phone. Being curious, I slipped into his office and listened as he spoke. He was patiently explaining, step-by-step, how to make bread in a Vitamix. A typically self-centred tween at the time, I was pretty riled that my beloved grandpa was working and not paying attention to us. When the call ended, I gave him a hard time for leaving the party. And this part I remember very clearly. My grandpa, not a bit angry, looked straight at me and said, 'Jodi, some day you will understand'. He went on to say that we were not in the business to sell machines. We were changing the way people thought about food and how they ate. We're not successful, he told me, until our customers are successfully using their Vitamix. We want to help them use it or we want to take it back, so we can put it in the hands of someone that will. His commitment to our customers, to really making people's lives better, helping them be healthier, has really stuck with me.

While Vitamix is definitely more than just the Barnards now, it has remained an unwaveringly family-run and family-involved business. As my mother, Linda, says, 'You cannot separate Vitamix from the [Barnard] family'. In the 1960s, my uncle William Grover III ('Grove') left his dream of pursuing a master's degree in statistics to come back to the family business. Grandpa had got his pilot's licence when he was in his forties and this new passion became a bit of a distraction. Grove persuaded the company to give up selling products as diverse as airplanes and cuckoo clocks and to refocus on the original core message of improving people's health and vitality. Once he came back, he stayed; the company transferred to the third generation when Grove took on the role of President and CEO after Grandpa retired in 1985.

Over the years, several of my aunts and uncles came back into the business. In the early 1980s, my dad, John, returned to Ohio after years away. He brought a strong engineering background and years of different business experience. He worked with his brother Frank to bring first-class research and development to the company. My dad knew that when the opportunity came to enter the commercial food service market, Vitamix needed to prepare itself to become an international company, assuring the customers that they would be cared for. We continue this commitment of being a global company with a local feel to this day.

My father was also instrumental in introducing a blender to the food service industry that was truly a reliable, lasting piece of equipment versus the disposable version that needed to be replaced every couple of months. Our goal was, and continues to be, to allow our food service customers to focus on expanding their brand and enhancing their experience, rather than worrying about their blending equipment. This revolutionised the blending industry. Vitamix flourished under my father's leadership after Uncle Grove retired in 1999.

The Fourth Generation

Being a part of a family business wasn't much more glamorous for my generation than it was for my father's. Thankfully we didn't spend our summers bouncing around in the back of a farm truck. Instead we painted walls, cleaned toilets and sorted post. Because I had heard so much about the company as a child, it felt very familiar when I began working here myself after dad moved the family to Ohio. Believe it or not, my favourite afterschool job ended up being answering phones! I discovered that I loved talking with our customers, answering their questions and even helping people learn to make Vitamix bread.

Like my dad before me, I started my professional life without any intention of working in the family business long term. And also like my dad, my work and my travels ultimately brought me home to Vitamix. When I came back several years into a different, yet successful, career, I transitioned from a minor character in the Vitamix story to one of the authors of its history. At that time, Vitamix was already a staple in many homes across the country, and we were really mixing it up in the food-service industry. I had the pleasure of setting up our international department, and I loved it. After several years, my father asked me to head up our household division too and I fell in love with that as well. This is where the story really gets interesting for me. As I dug in and did research in 2003, I started hearing a lot about whole foods, organics and health. People were talking about natural, fresh whole foods. Real food. People were starting to talk more about the ideas that we, here at Vitamix, had been talking about for decades. I could almost see the early generations of Barnards smiling down on all of us. At last it seemed people were ready to embrace whole food as a path to good health, and we here at Vitamix were ready to help them. It was time to take generations of passion and commitment to whole-food health and use it to help make the world a healthier place for generations to come. We simply needed to make sure our voice was heard.

The Road Ahead

I have given you a glimpse of the people and the philosophies that have shaped our family's past. But what of our future? The Barnard family directory is now more like a book, and our work family has grown significantly, too.

While we are a larger and even more diverse group now, our commitment to helping people lead healthier lives has never been stronger. We honour the memory of my grandparents by continuing to share a passion for health and nutrition. I have the honour and pleasure of working closely with my father and my cousin Loree Connors (our CFO), and we are both thrilled when members of the next generation join Vitamix, whether they are Barnards or the children of our employees. We have found that our passion for wellness and our values of family, customer, quality, integrity and teamwork are often carried down through the generations of our employees' families as well. With such a committed team behind us, we will continue talking about whole foods, advocating for better health through diet whenever and wherever we can. We will proudly carry on with the work that Papa, Grandma and Grandpa started so many years ago.

Part of the Barnard legacy is a healthy diet, of course. The Vitamix gives you hundreds of different ways to enjoy whole foods, many of which are highlighted in the following recipes. While green smoothies seem to be all the craze today, we've had a recipe for a Green Elixir, as it was called, from 1940. I actually crave this delightfully sweet and silky smooth beverage; there is no better way to start my day. My daughters and I are blessed to start our day with one made by my husband, Frank, our own personal 'Green Smoothie Extraordinaire'. Whatever you make in your Vitamix, we Barnards and the rest of the Vitamix family raise a glass of a delicious, whole-food drink to you. We hope that, with a little help from your Vitamix and the recipes and tips in this book, we contribute in some small way to your own vitality.

To your health!

—Jodi Berg

The Vitamix Cookbook

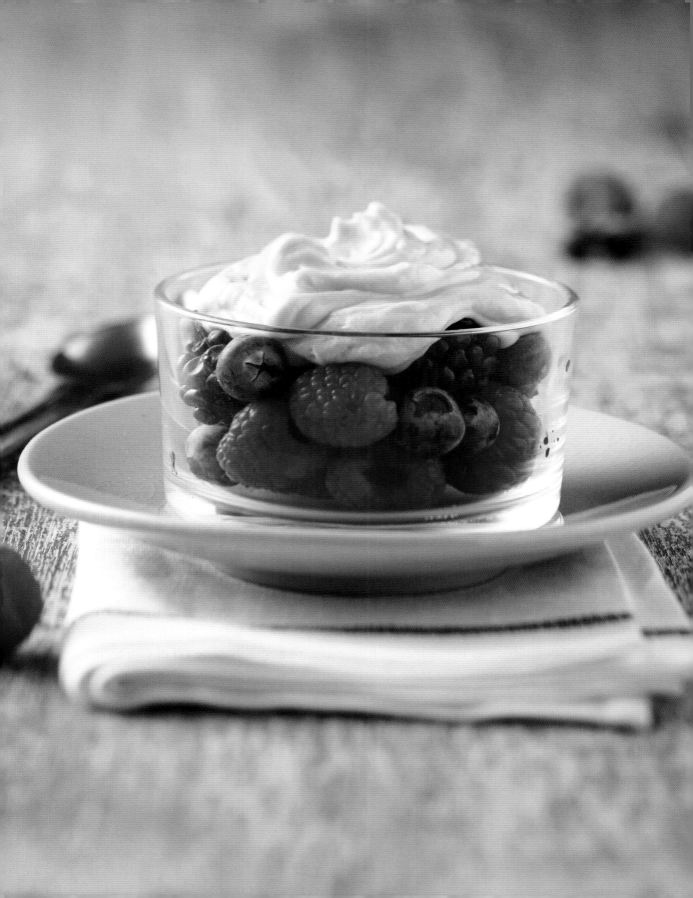

Chapter 1

Why Whole Foods?

With health, we have wealth!' declared Papa Barnard in the first infomercial in 1949. 'With our health, we're the richest person on Earth!' He went on to show us how, by using the Vitamix to blend the amazing flavours and nutrients of whole foods, we can consume more of already healthy foods: peels, seeds and all. He showed us how we can improve our diets and our health without sacrificing flavour or convenience. Papa may have been more of a salesperson than a scientist, but over the years, the research in favour of whole food has stacked up. And however one defines wealth, there is no question that there is tremendous value to good health.

And yes, people may choose to define wealth differently, but there is no doubt that a lot of money is being spent on health care annually. The NHS currently spends about £60 billion on long-term conditions, of which 80 per cent could be prevented by healthier lifestyles.

But how do we get people eating a better diet? Here at Vitamix, we strongly believe that whole foods are key.

Whole Food Health Benefits

There is a lot of talk about whole foods and for good reasons. In 2014 in the Annual Review of Public Health, Dr David Katz and Dr Stephanie Meller from Yale University published a study comparing different popular diets. As *The Atlantic*, reporting on their work, concluded:

> A diet of minimally processed food close to nature, predominantly plants, is decisively associated with health promotion and disease prevention.
>
> [N]utritionally-complete, plant-based diets are supported by a wide array of favorable health outcomes, including fewer cancers and less heart disease. These diets ideally include not just fruits and vegetables, but whole grains, nuts, and seeds as well.

We can, it appears, make a positive impact on our health by eating more whole foods. Papa would not be surprised.

Before we talk about why we should eat more whole foods and how, let me clarify what we here at Vitamix believe they are. To us, whole foods are foods in, or very close to, their natural state, complete with most or all of their nutrients, fibre, phytochemicals, minerals and the like. Fresh or frozen fruits, vegetables, nuts and seeds are all whole foods. Whole grains – unprocessed whole grains such as whole oat, whole wheat kernels and brown rice – are also whole foods. You get the idea.

Besides just plain tasting good, whole foods usually offer more nutrition. As a group, whole foods generally have higher nutrient density. What is nutrient density? It simply means that the foods have a large per cent of nutrients relative to the total number of calories. Blueberries and kale, for example, considered to be superfoods by some, have a very large number of nutrients relative to their calories. Not all whole foods are low in calories, of course, but even foods like avocados and nuts are much more nutrient-dense than a serving of a more processed snack – even if you eat the same number of calories. Great taste and good nutrition together? Absolutely!

Whole foods are clearly very good for us, but do we eat enough of them? Sadly the answer is no, and we can't really say it is for lack of awareness about the health benefits of fruits and vegetables. This information was fairly common knowledge even back in Grandpa and Grandma's day.

The National Diet and Nutrition Survey in 2014 showed that adults between 19 and 64 consumed an average 4.1 portions of fruit and vegetables every day, which children between the ages of 11 and 18 ate 3.0–2.7 portions per day. Only 10% of boys and 7% of girls ate their 5-a-day. Think about this. We need to do better – our health depends upon it! We logically know we should eat more produce, yet we don't. How can this be?

Processed Foods

Let's talk about processed food. If American adults are eating too few fruits and vegetables, we are arguably eating too many processed foods. A whopping 70 per cent of the food purchased in America is processed. What counts as processed food? The Academy of Nutrition and Dietetics identifies a range. First there are minimally processed foods like bagged greens. Next they identify foods processed at their peak to preserve nutrition, such as frozen vegetables. Then foods with ingredients – such as sweeteners, fats or preservatives – added for flavour and texture. Finally the last category of processed foods includes items like packaged baking mixes or bottled sauces and ready-to-eat foods like crackers and frozen meals.

Just as all whole foods are not created equal, not all processed foods are created equal either – nutritionally speaking. Cut and bagged vegetables or greens can make vegetables a more accessible, although slightly more expensive, option. Just be sure to check the labels. Some cut and bagged vegetables have added sugar, salt or fat to enhance the flavour or texture, so steer clear of those if your desire is for the least-processed whole foods.

The 2010 Dietary Guidelines for Americans, a report produced by the departments of Agriculture and Health and Human Services, explains the problem bluntly:

> Americans currently consume too much sodium and too many calories from solid fats, added sugars, and refined grains. These replace nutrient-dense foods and beverages and make it difficult for people to achieve recommended nutrient intake while controlling calorie and sodium intake.

The more a food is processed and refined, the more likely it is to lose its naturally occurring fibre, minerals, vitamins and so forth.

Health Benefits of Whole Foods

The health benefits of whole foods are vast. Because whole foods tend to have higher nutrient density, you can often eat more of them while taking in fewer calories overall, which in turn support maintaining a healthy ideal weight. Fresh fruits and vegetables usually contain fibre, so you are likely to feel fuller for longer, an added advantage.

Cooking and eating whole foods can also be important if you are on a restricted diet. When you prepare whole foods at home, you know exactly what is going into your food. If you put spinach, grapes, banana, berries and ice in your blender for a smoothie, you will simply get a delicious drink, no hidden ingredients, preservatives or other such surprises.

By preparing foods at home, you can also control the amounts of salt and sugar added to your food. There may very well be a health benefit to the peace of mind of knowing exactly what you are putting into your body, but the scientists have not discovered this yet!

We know that whole foods are important to good health, so the question becomes not why should we eat a more whole-foods-focused diet, but how? If flavour and convenience are important, we here at Vitamix have great news. With this cookbook in hand, you will quickly discover that healthy cooking can be both simple and delicious.

JOHN BARNARD

My dad, John Barnard, grew up as a vegetarian and in a family that emphasised the importance of eating whole foods at a time when neither practice was common.

After Dad left home for college, he says he turned his back on his childhood diet. In college and after he got married, he ate a pretty typical American diet. My family ate more fruits and vegetables than most when I was growing up, but we were not vegetarians like my dad's parents. Dad returned to Ohio and the family business in 1981. In 2004, after reading T. Colin Campbell and Thomas Campbell III's *The China Study*, which advocates a diet based primarily on plant foods, Dad decided to return to his healthier-eating roots.

Never much of a cook, my dad now loves to use his Vitamix to make green smoothies for himself and my mum. Dad's favourite smoothie often contains grapes, part of a whole lime, broccoli and pineapple, chia or flax seeds, a little water and at least three different kinds of greens – filling up at least half of the container. Dad makes a big batch a few times a week and puts it in the fridge, so they can enjoy a delicious green smoothie every day.

My parents, now in their seventies, have more energy than people a fraction their age. Dad even completed a forty-mile hike the day before his seventy-fourth birthday! Our goal at Vitamix is to increase our customers' vitality so they can live a long, full life. My dad and mum are walking, talking examples of this goal in action!

—Jodi Berg

THE DIRTY DOZEN
AND
THE CLEAN FIFTEEN

Often when we reflect on what we are consuming, the subject of eating organic comes up. Many of us have to strike a compromise between what we might like to eat and what is financially and logistically possible. If you want to buy some organic produce, but are unable or unwilling to buy all organic, there is a great resource to guide your choices.

Every year, the Environmental Working Group (EWG) publishes 'The Dirty Dozen' list and 'The Clean Fifteen', ranking common produce on the amounts of pesticide residue found on conventionally grown produce even after it had been washed. The EWG website (www.ewg.org/foodnews/index.php) publishes this list, and it is worth taking a few minutes to read the full report. For example, leafy greens and hot peppers were on the 'Dirty Dozen' list recently even though the number of pesticides found after washing was low, because they contained residues from particularly toxic insecticides that can damage the nervous system. The EWG recommended that customers who frequently eat these vegetables buy organic if possible. The two lists from 2015 are presented on the opposite page.

DIRTY DOZEN PLUS

1. Apples
2. Peaches
3. Nectarines
4. Strawberries
5. Grapes
6. Celery
7. Spinach
8. Sweet peppers
9. Cucumbers
10. Cherry tomatoes
11. Imported sugar snap peas
12. Potatoes
13. Hot peppers
14. Kale / collard greens

CLEAN FIFTEEN

1. Avocado
2. Sweetcorn
3. Pineapple
4. Cabbage
5. Peas (frozen)
6. Onions
7. Asparagus
8. Mangoes
9. Papaya
10. Kiwi fruit
11. Aubergine
12. Grapefruit
13. Cantaloupe
14. Cauliflower
15. Sweet potatoes

The EWG encourages us to try to limit our exposure to pesticides but states, 'The health benefits of a diet rich in fruits and vegetables outweigh the risks of pesticide exposure. Use EWG's Shopper's Guide to reduce your exposures as much as possible, but eating conventionally grown produce is better than not eating fruits and vegetables at all'. Papa Barnard would doubtlessly agree.

Better Nutrition Made Simple

As we learned in the introduction, Papa was thrilled after he first encountered the blender. This was the way to bring more whole foods into their diets! He was clearly on to something. Similarly, just as my grandma realised back in 1937, a sustainable whole foods diet needs to taste good and have variety. To meet the demands of our busy lives, at Vitamix we strongly believe it's important that food be simple and quick to prepare. You may not want to sit down to a big bowl of leafy greens first thing in the morning, but drop those greens in a Vitamix with fresh fruit, whip up a delicious smoothie, and suddenly you have a nutritious and delicious breakfast on the go. Especially the kids; try giving toddlers a smoothie in their sippy cups and they may not let you take it away.

As our Vitamix nutritionist Anne Thacker notes, you can hide a lot of greens in a smoothie, get all of the good nutrition that comes with them and not alter the flavour of the other ingredients. Combining leafy greens with fruit brings out the sweetness in the greens, allowing the flavours to blend right in. That's a lot of nutrient-dense foods first thing in the morning that make for a powerful way to prepare your body for anything that fills your day! Smoothies are a great place to start, but they aren't the only easy way to add more whole foods to your diet. Tomato Vinaigrette (page 234) contains raw tomatoes. Imagine, getting a healthy dose of vegetables in both the dressing and the salad!

Want more whole foods in your diet but worry that you don't have the culinary skills or the time? With the Vitamix vegetables for soups and salads can be chopped in seconds. Fruit and vegetables can be whipped into tasty, silky drinks in under a minute. (You can even make a large batch of your favourite smoothie every few days and store it in the fridge like my dad does. Just stir or shake it to re-emulsify, and enjoy.) Whole-grain cereals, quick breads, savoury soups and hearty tomato sauces come together in a snap. Each recipe contains lots of nutrient-dense whole foods and most come together in less than 30 minutes, including prep and cleanup.

Why Blended Recipes?

There are lots of ways that you can incorporate whole foods into your diet, but it is quite a challenge to eat the volume of whole food and get the nutrition your body needs without a Vitamix. A Vitamix allows you to use the whole food so you retain all the nutrients within the food. The sweet pineapple core is too fibrous to chew, but can be blended up into a juice, smoothie or sauce. You can purée a whole tomato – skin, seeds and all – and make a soup or hearty tomato sauce. You can't chew up an orange seed or a flax seed very easily, but a Vitamix can pulverise it almost instantly, where other blenders may struggle with these tougher ingredients. Using the whole food lets you consume all of the available nutrients. And preparing it quickly allows you to squeeze healthy eating into even the busiest day. We don't just talk the talk here at Vitamix. It is not uncommon to see one of our employees bring a bag of vegetables into the office and whip up a hot, steaming soup for lunch in a matter of minutes. Of course it helps to work for a company that has a Vitamix station in every break room.

When We Say Delicious

It is easier to eat healthier foods when they taste delicious, and all of the nearly 250 recipes in this book will not disappoint! Our culinary team, registered dietician nutritionist Anne Thacker and chef and manager of recipe development, Bev Shaffer, worked together to create recipes that were tasty and met our own rigorous nutritional standards. They created delicious and nutritious recipes with little to no refined sugar, little added salt and no more than 15 grams of total fat. In this book you will find a huge variety of tempting treats, savoury soups and hearty entrees for every meal. Our goal is to help you eat more whole foods. Our sincere hope is these recipes will allow you to eat healthier in an efficient and delicious way.

How to Use This Book

All the recipes in this book are intended to be made in the Vitamix. Although some recipes may also work in another blender, the Vitamix engineering allows us to do a lot of things other blenders may not be able to do as well, if at all. The instructions for blending speeds and times have been created with optimal taste and texture in mind. The Vitamix is powerful and built to be reliable and durable. Don't worry about using it on its highest speeds or using the tamper, the machine is made for it! The end product will be worth it.

Our culinary team created these recipes to demonstrate how easy it is to get healthy whole food into the foods you already love to eat, as well as suggesting some foods you may not have tried before. The focus of this book is whole foods, so some recipes do include dairy or meat products, but feel free to experiment on your own with substitutions if you choose not to use these ingredients.

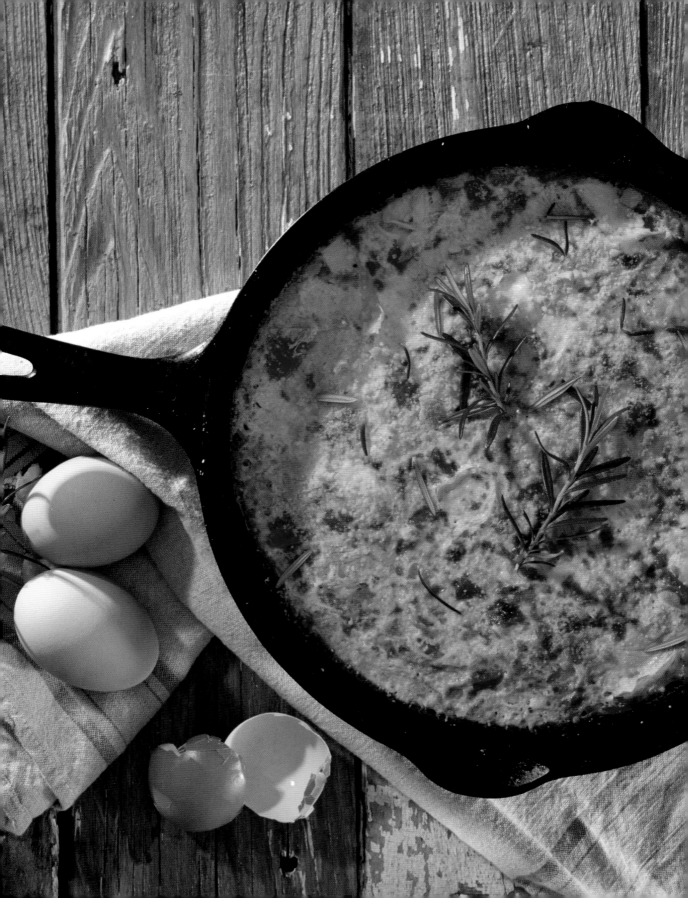

Chapter 2

Breakfast and Brunch

The alarm clock sounds. The children wake up hungry for breakfast. Pets want food and attention. There are showers to take, teeth to brush, shoes and socks to find. There are workouts to squeeze in, lunches to pack and jobs to get to. Sound familiar? Most of us are busy from the moment our feet hit the ground. My family is no exception. Even the weekends, which can be a respite from the usual hustle and bustle, are usually hectic. Saturday and Sunday quickly fill up with softball and volleyball practice, gardening, errands galore and time with family and friends. It is hard to imagine that we have time for any sort of breakfast, much less a healthy one.

Many of us are told from a tender age that breakfast is the most important meal of the day. The link between children who eat breakfast, particularly a healthy one with nutrients and fibre, and academic success, is well established. Research aside, starting the day with a healthy meal, complete with whole foods, may just feel good to you, as it does to me, as right and proper as a hot shower and a cup of coffee. Enter the Vitamix! In this chapter, we explore all of the healthy, delicious and fast ways that you can start your day.

Drink Your Breakfast

When you think about making breakfast in your Vitamix, many of you will think first of making a smoothie or whole-fruit or vegetable juice. This sort of drink can be quickly assembled and can use whatever produce you have in your fruit bowl, fridge or freezer. The potential combinations are nearly endless. We've included a handful of delicious smoothies here, but Chapter 8, Drinks, offers many other recipes you many want to consider for your morning meal.

More Than Just Smoothies

Smoothies aren't the only healthy breakfast choice, of course. In this chapter, you will also find delicious recipes for quick breads, muffins and breakfast cakes. How do you use a Vitamix to make foods like these? The Vitamix has always been more than a blender. Dry ingredients can be chopped and ground and wet ingredients are whipped, blended or mixed together in the Vitamix. Wet ingredients get stirred into dry, the batter gets poured into a loaf tin, a cake tin, or muffin tins and into the oven it goes. (You will also learn how to make your own flours for some of these recipes.) In almost no time at all, your kitchen will smell amazing, and your stomach will be rumbling!

After they have cooled, the quick breads and muffins in this chapter freeze beautifully. Consider making an extra batch of your favourite recipe, so you have a healthy breakfast or snack on hand even on your busiest days. To freeze quick breads, cool the bread completely. Wrap the slices individually in foil and store in a freezer-safe bag or a container with a tight--fitting lid to prevent freezer burn. Slices can be thawed at room temperature. Leave a wrapped slice or two on the counter before you go to sleep, and they will be thawed and ready to eat by morning.

Home-made Granola and Hot Cereals

The cereal aisle in your local supermarket has an endless bounty of options, from the marshmallow-sprinkled to the flax-seed-full. Our home-made granola is a delicious alternative to these processed options, and you can adjust the recipe to include the nuts, seeds and dried fruits that you like best. Egg whites, honey, brown sugar, a little canola oil, cinnamon and a pinch of sea salt can be blended together in the Vitamix and poured over a bowl of oats, nuts and seeds. Toasty, crunchy clusters emerge from the oven, ready to be mixed with your favourite dried fruits. This granola is delicious on yoghurt, with milk or straight out of the jar for a healthy snack.

On the mornings you crave a hot, hearty, whole-grain cereal, try Apple Raisin Cracked Wheat Cereal (page 38), Oat Porridge (page 42) or Creamy Rice Cereal (page 40). Extras will keep in the fridge for 4 days, so once again, consider making enough for leftovers.

Pancakes, Waffles and More

Some mornings we crave something heartier for breakfast. The many pancake, waffle and crepe recipes in this book will be sure to please. Try Curried Sweet Potato Pancakes (page 50), Breakfast Crepes (page 63) or Buttermilk Cornmeal Waffles (page 57) to name just a few. Oatmeal Pancakes (page 52) will fill you up, and we pair them with a Dried Cranberry Topping so delicious that you will find yourself making extra, just to have it on hand for oatmeal, yoghurt, maybe even a smoothie. Vegan French Toast (page 62) will tempt breakfast lovers everywhere, even those who are not avoiding animal products. These delicious dishes come together quickly enough to be a weekday morning staple and yet are tempting enough to be welcome at a leisurely brunch.

Pancakes and waffles also freeze well, and extras can be put aside for busier mornings. Cool the cooked items and store them in a freezer-safe bag. Frozen pancakes and waffles can be easily warmed up in a toaster or microwave.

Toast and Toppings

Grandpa and Grandma loved to make their famous Vitamix whole wheat bread for their children and grandchildren during our family reunions in Ohio. I remember how my grandfather used to make dozens of loaves of bread at a time. He would put his yeast into warm water, and while that developed, he would grind his wheat berries into fresh flour. Adding the yeast mixture and any other ingredients, possibly raisins for sweetness, he would knead the bread dough in the Vitamix and have a loaf tin of dough ready to rise in 3 minutes flat. We used to time him. He would do it over and over again. The only time it took longer than 3 minutes was when we would distract him and cause him to break out in a belly laugh or remind him of a joke.

Few scents can match the heavenly aroma of baking bread, and if you like to start your mornings with a slice of toast, consider using your Vitamix to make the dough for your own hearty, healthy whole wheat bread, just as my grandpa loved to do. This bread is delicious toasted or for sandwiches. Top it with home-made nut butter or Raisin Almond Breakfast Spread in Chapter 6 for a tasty and protein-packed treat.

Grind Your Own Flours for a Reliably Gluten-Free Morning

Our scrumptious Gluten-Free Buttermilk Pancake Mix (page 53) – along with two delicious variations – will delight those who avoid gluten as well as those that don't. You can purchase the appropriate flours, or you can quickly grind your own in a Vitamix dry grains container, which was designed with specially angled and spaced blades and a container design that efficiently grinds dry ingredients with excellent results time after time. In this chapter, you will also learn how to make your own cornmeal (page 60) and whole-grain flour (page 64). It begins to lose its nutritional value once it is ground, so use it immediately if possible. If not, store in the freezer for up to one month.

Let's eat!

Cracked Wheat Cereal

With a whopping 9 grams of fibre, 8 grams of protein and a delicious nutty flavour, you will find yourself making this cracked wheat cereal again and again. Delicious on its own or topped with fresh or dried fruit, toasted nuts, maple syrup or your favourite milk.

Preparation: **10 minutes**   Processing: **15 seconds**   Cook time: **15–20 minutes**
Yield: **720 g cooked cereal**

180 g whole wheat kernels

720 ml water

½ teaspoon salt

1. Place the wheat into the Vitamix Dry Grains container and secure the lid. Select Variable 1. Turn the machine on and slowly increase the speed to Variable 7 or 8. Grind to desired degree of fineness, or for about 15 seconds.

2. Combine the water and salt in a pan and bring to a boil. Slowly add the cracked wheat to the boiling water, whisking constantly. Reduce the heat to low, cover and simmer until cooked, 15–20 minutes.

AMOUNT PER 240 ML SERVING: calories 210, total fat 1.5 g, saturated fat 0 g, cholesterol 0 mg, sodium 400 mg, total carbohydrate 45 g, dietary fibre 9g, sugars 0 g, protein 8 g

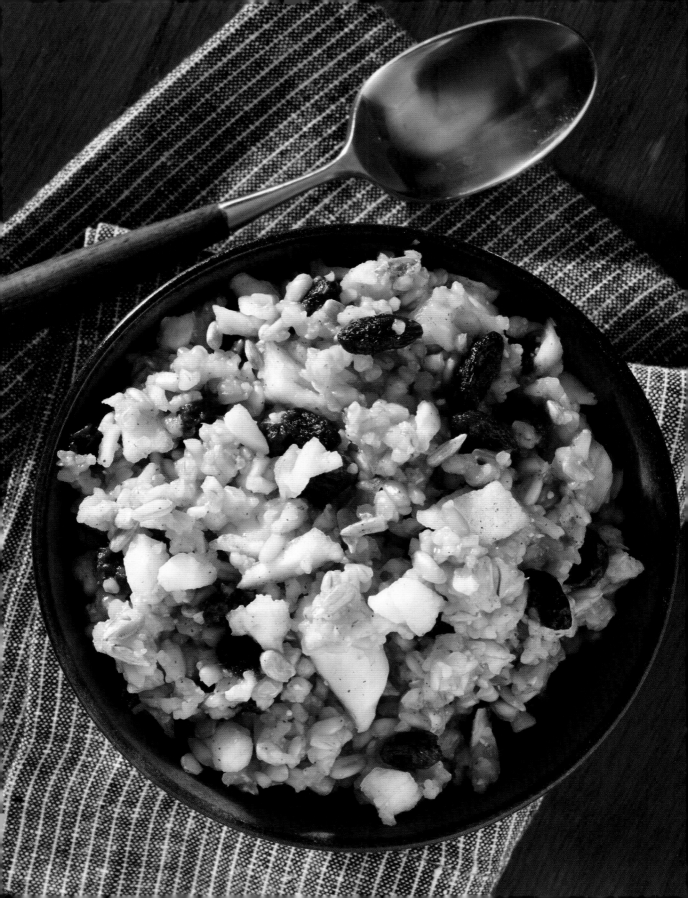

Apple Raisin Cracked Wheat Cereal

In the late 1930s, my grandma Ruth and my papa participated in one of Bernarr Macfadden's 265-mile hikes from Cleveland, Ohio, to Danville, New York. These walks were sometimes called 'cracked wheat derbies' because of the limited and healthy diet that the participants were fed. You don't need to go on a long walk to appreciate this hearty, cracked wheat cereal in the morning, but we suspect that this delicious dish would have been popular on Macfadden's hikes!

Preparation: **15 minutes** Processing: **25 seconds** Cook time: **15–20 minutes**
Yield: **720 g cooked cereal**

180 g whole wheat kernels

360 ml water

¼ teaspoon salt

1 tart apple (170 g), peeled, cored and quartered

⅛ teaspoon ground cinnamon

75 g raisins

2 tablespoons sunflower seeds

1. Place the whole wheat kernels into the Vitamix Dry Grains container and secure the lid. Select Variable 1. Turn the machine on and slowly increase the speed to Variable 7. Grind to the desired degree of fineness (ideally a coarse texture), about 15 seconds.

2. Combine the water and salt in a pan and bring to a boil. Slowly add the cracked wheat to the boiling water, whisking constantly. Reduce the heat to low, cover, and simmer, stirring frequently, until cooked but still al dente, 15–20 minutes.

3. Meanwhile, switch the container to the standard Vitamix container. Secure the lid and remove the lid plug. Select Variable 1. Turn the machine on and slowly increase the speed to Variable 4. With the machine running, drop the apple quarters through the lid plug opening (using the tamper as needed) to chop the apples.

4. Remove the pan from the heat and add the chopped apple, cinnamon, raisins and sunflower seeds and stir to combine.

5. Cover and let the mixture stand for 5 minutes before serving.

AMOUNT PER 240 ML SERVING: calories 360, total fat 3.5 g, saturated fat 0 g, cholesterol 0 mg, sodium 210 mg, total carbohydrate 75 g, dietary fibre 13 g, sugars 25 g, protein 10 g

Creamy Rice Cereal

This creamy, soothing cereal is the perfect use for that last ½ cup of rice. You can make the cereal with pretty much any variety of rice that you have on hand, and you won't lose a bit of the nutritional goodness because you are grinding it yourself. Brown rice will take slightly longer to cook, but the nutty, hearty flavour will be worth the wait!

Preparation: **10 minutes**   Processing: **10 seconds**   Cook time: **8 to 10 minutes**
Yield: **420 ml cooked cereal**

90 g uncooked rice

480 ml water

¼ teaspoon salt (optional)

1. Place the rice into the Vitamix Dry Grains container and secure the lid. Select Variable 1. Turn the machine on and slowly increase the speed to Variable 7 or 8. Grind to the desired degree of fineness, about 10 seconds. If a finer cereal is desired, grind longer.

2. Combine the water and salt (if using) in a pan and bring to a boil. Slowly add the cracked rice to the boiling water, whisking constantly. Reduce the heat to low, cover and simmer, stirring frequently, until cooked, 8–10 minutes (slightly longer for brown rice).

AMOUNT PER 240 ML SERVING: calories 170, total fat 0 g, saturated fat 0 g, cholesterol 0 mg, sodium 340 mg, total carbohydrate 40 g, dietary fibre 0 g, sugars 0 g, protein 3 g

Apricot Brown Rice Cereal

Why limit delicious and undeniably nutritious brown rice to lunch or dinner? This hearty cereal, complete with dried apricots and sunflower seeds, will encourage you to see this healthy grain's good-morning potential.

Preparation: **10 minutes**   Processing: **10 seconds**   Cook time: **20 minutes**
Yield: **840 ml cooked cereal**

185 g uncooked brown rice

840 ml water

½ teaspoon salt

8 unsweetened dried apricots

2 tablespoons sunflower seeds

¼ teaspoon almond extract (optional)

1. Place the brown rice into the Vitamix Dry Grains container and secure the lid. Select Variable 1. Turn the machine on and slowly increase the speed to Variable 7 or 8. Grind to the desired degree of fineness, about 10 seconds. If a finer cereal is desired, grind longer.

2. Combine the water and salt in a pan and bring to a boil. Slowly add the cracked rice to the boiling water, whisking constantly. Reduce the heat to low, cover and simmer, stirring frequently, until cooked, about 20 minutes.

3. Meanwhile, switch to the standard Vitamix container. Select Variable 1. Secure the lid and remove the lid plug. Turn the machine on and slowly increase the speed to Variable 5. With the machine running, drop the apricots through the lid plug opening. If necessary, adjust the Variable speed for a finer chop.

4. Remove the pan from the heat and add the chopped apricots, sunflower seeds and almond extract (if using) and stir to combine.

5. Cover and let the mixture stand for 5 minutes before serving.

AMOUNT PER 240 ML SERVING: calories 260, total fat 3 g, saturated fat 0.5 g, cholesterol 0 mg, sodium 350 mg, total carbohydrate 52 g, dietary fibre 4 g, sugars 8 g, protein 5 g

Oat Porridge

Whole oats – with just the outermost inedible hull removed – are the least processed form of oat that you can buy at the grocery store. (Steel-cut oats are whole oats that have been cut just enough to reduce the cooking time.) This porridge will sustain you on even the most blustery of winter days!

Preparation: **10 minutes**   Processing: **10 seconds**   Cook time: **35 minutes**   Yield: **840 ml cooked cereal**

160 g whole oats (NOT oatmeal)

960 ml water

½ teaspoon salt (optional, to taste)

1. Place whole oats into the Vitamix Dry Grains container and secure the lid. Select Variable 1. Turn the machine on and slowly increase the speed to Variable 7. Grind to the desired degree of fineness, about 10 seconds. If a finer cereal is desired, grind longer.

2. Combine the water and salt (if using) in a pan and bring to a boil. Slowly add the cracked oats to the boiling water, whisking constantly. Reduce the heat to low, cover and simmer, stirring frequently, until cooked, about 30 minutes.

AMOUNT PER 240 ML SERVING: calories 130, total fat 3 g, saturated fat 0 g, cholesterol 0 mg, sodium 340 mg, total carbohydrate 31 g, dietary fibre 5 g, sugars 1 g, protein 8 g

Crunchy Customised Granola

Once you start making this wonderful, crunchy granola you may wonder why you ever bought it! Feel free to get creative and use whatever nuts and seeds you have to hand.

Preparation: **15 minutes**   Processing: **20 seconds**   Bake time: **40–55 minutes**   Yield: **1.7 litres**

2 large egg whites

80 ml honey

60 ml vegetable oil

2 tablespoons light brown sugar

½ teaspoon sea salt

1 teaspoon ground cinnamon

240 g rolled oats

75 g unsalted raw almonds

60 g unsalted pecan pieces

60 g unsalted walnut pieces

80 g unsweetened desiccated coconut

80 g pumpkin seeds

40 g golden flax seeds

130 g assorted unsweetened dried fruit (such as apricots, tart cherries, cranberries), cut into pieces

1. Pre-heat the oven to 150°C. Line 1 or 2 rimmed baking sheets (the mixture needs to be in a single layer) with baking paper or silicone baking mats.

2. Place the egg whites, honey, vegetable oil, brown sugar, salt and cinnamon into the Vitamix container in the order listed and secure the lid. Select Variable 1. Turn the machine on and slowly increase the speed to Variable 10, then to High. Blend for 20 seconds or until well blended.

3. Combine the oats, nuts, coconut, pumpkin seeds and flax seeds in a large bowl. Pour in the egg white mixture and stir well to combine.

4. Spread the mixture on the baking sheet(s) and bake for 40–55 minutes, stirring every 10 or 15 minutes, until light golden brown.

5. Cool on the baking sheet(s) on a wire rack for 10 minutes, then transfer to a large bowl and stir in the dried fruit pieces. (The granola will crisp as it cools.)

6. Store airtight at room temperature.

AMOUNT PER 60 ML SERVING: calories 170, total fat 11 g, saturated fat 2.5 g, cholesterol 0 mg, sodium 50 mg, total carbohydrate 16 g, dietary fibre 3 g, sugars 7 g, protein 4 g

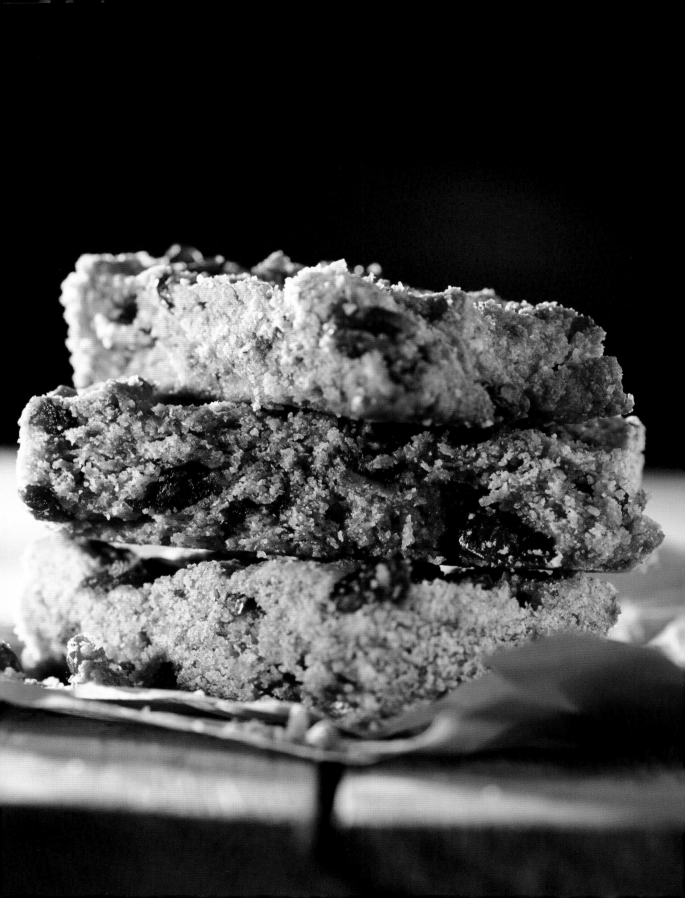

Vitamix Granola Bars

These granola bars are full of grains, nuts and fruit (both fresh and dried), and they are destined to become a staple in your household! They have terrific flavour with much less fat and sugar than many other granola bars.

Preparation: **10 minutes**   Processing: **1 minute 10 seconds**   Bake time: **25 minutes**   Yield: **12 bars**

50 g wheat berries or ½ 60 g whole grain flour, preferably home-made (page 64)

28 g wheatgerm

70 g raw almonds

155 g rolled oats

1 medium to large apple, cubed, or 210 g unsweetened apple sauce

¼ teaspoon salt

1 teaspoon ground cinnamon

1 teaspoon vanilla extract

3 tablespoons honey or agave nectar

60 g dried unsweetened cranberries

1. Pre-heat the oven to 180°C. Grease a 20-cm square baking tin.

2. Place the wheat berries, wheatgerm, almonds and oats into the Vitamix container and secure the lid. Select Variable 1. Turn the machine on and slowly increase to speed to Variable 10, then to High. Blend for 30 seconds.

3. Turn the machine off and pour the mixture out into a bowl.

4. If using an apple, place it into the Vitamix container and secure the lid. Select Variable 1. Turn the machine on and slowly increase the speed to Variable 10, then to High. Blend for 35–40 seconds, until the consistency of apple sauce, using the tamper to press the apple into the blades.

5. Add the applesauce to the bowl with the dry ingredients. Add the salt, cinnamon, vanilla, honey and cranberries to mixture. Mix gently by hand to combine.

6. Spread the mixture into the baking tin. Bake for 25 minutes. Cool completely on wire rack, then cut bars in pan.

AMOUNT PER SERVING: calories 120, total fat 4 g, saturated fat 0 g, cholesterol 0 mg, sodium 50 mg, total carbohydrate 21 g, dietary fibre 3 g, sugars 10 g, protein 3 g

Artichoke, Red Pepper and Parmesan Frittata

You may already be adding vegetables to your morning smoothie, but don't forget to add a few servings to your frittata. Here, the marinated artichokes and roasted red peppers are puréed in the Vitamix along with eggs, garlic, milk and spices to produce a breakfast bursting with flavour. With only 10–15 minutes of cooking time, it is fast enough for a quick breakfast or supper.

Preparation: **10 minutes**   Processing: **20 seconds**   Cook time: **10–15 minutes**   Yield: **5 servings**

2 tablespoons olive oil

60 ml skimmed milk

3 large eggs

3 large egg whites

1 garlic clove, roasted and peeled

¼ teaspoon red pepper flakes

¼ teaspoon freshly cracked black pepper

1 x 213-g jar grilled marinated artichoke hearts, drained

100 g marinated roasted red pepper, drained

35 g freshly grated Parmesan

Sea salt (optional)

1. Heat a 20-cm heavy-based frying pan (which can go under the grill) over a medium heat. Add the olive oil.

2. Meanwhile, place the milk, whole eggs, egg whites, garlic, red pepper flakes and black pepper into the Vitamix container in the order listed and secure the lid. Select Variable 1. Turn the machine on and slowly increase the speed to Variable 4. Blend for 10 seconds or until smooth.

3. Stop the machine and remove the lid. Add the artichoke hearts and roasted red peppers and secure the lid. Select Variable 1. Turn the machine on and slowly increase the speed to Variable 3. Blend for 10 seconds.

4. Pour the egg mixture into the frying pan. Cook over a medium heat until the edges are lightly browned, 8–10 minutes. Sprinkle with the Parmesan.

5. Place the frying pan under the grill pre-heated to high. Grill for 1–2 minutes, until the top is lightly browned and no longer wet. Season to taste with sea salt, if desired.

AMOUNT PER SERVING: calories 190, total fat 14 g, saturated fat 3 g, cholesterol 115 mg, sodium 410 mg, total carbohydrate 5 g, dietary fibre 2 g, sugars 1 g, protein 9 g

Corned Beef Hash

Chopping the ingredients for this tasty hash in your Vitamix makes the dish come together in a flash. Adding water with your vegetables – wet-chopping – helps the ingredients float above the blades, resulting in more evenly sized pieces. A few quick pulses and everything is ready! Drain the chopped food and proceed with the recipe as directed.

Preparation: **15 minutes**   Processing: **pulsing**   Cook time: **20 minutes**   Yield: **5 servings**

560 g small red potatoes, halved

½ small onion, halved

1 small green pepper, cut into eighths

110 g deli corned beef (sliced 1 cm thick), cut into 4 cm pieces

1 tablespoon (30 ml) olive oil

¼ teaspoon ground black pepper

5 large eggs (optional)

1. Place the potatoes, onion and pepper into the Vitamix container. Add water to just cover the vegetables and secure the lid. Select Variable 4. Use the On/Off switch to quickly pulse 5 times.

2. Pour the contents into a colander and drain well.

3. Add the corned beef to the Vitamix container and secure the lid. Select Variable 5. Use the On/Off switch to quickly pulse 4 times.

4. Heat the oil in a heavy-based, 30-cm non-stick frying pan over a medium heat. Add the potato mixture and the corned beef. Stir in the black pepper. Cook, turning the mixture over 2 or 3 times, until browned and crisp, 8–10 minutes.

5. If desired, make 5 depressions in the surface of the hash and crack an egg into each depression. Cover, reduce the heat to low and cook until the potatoes are tender (and the eggs are cooked to desired doneness), 8–10 minutes.

AMOUNT PER SERVING (WITHOUT EGGS): calories 130, total fat 4 g, saturated fat 1 g, sodium 280 mg, total carbohydrate 20 g, dietary fibre 3 g, sugars 3 g, protein 6 g

Apple Pancakes

An apple a day may or may not keep the doctor away, but apples do add wonderful flavour, moisture and sweetness to these delicious pancakes. Try them topped with home-made apple sauce (page 247).

Preparation: **15 minutes**   Processing: **15 seconds**   Yield: **enough batter for 10 pancakes**

120 g whole grain flour, preferably home-made (page 64)

1 tablespoon baking powder

½ teaspoon bicarbonate of soda

½ teaspoon salt

3 tablespoons (38 g) granulated sugar

¼ teaspoon ground nutmeg

240 ml skimmed milk

1 large egg

1½ teaspoons unsalted butter

1½ teaspoons vanilla extract

½ medium apple (85 g), cut into chunks

1. Combine the flour, baking powder, bicarbonate of soda, salt, sugar and nutmeg in a medium bowl and stir lightly. Set aside.

2. Place the milk, egg, butter, vanilla and apple into the Vitamix container in the order listed and secure the lid. Select Variable 1. Turn the machine on and slowly increase the speed to Variable 8. Blend for 15 seconds.

3. Pour the milk mixture into the flour mixture and mix by hand just until combined.

4. For the best texture and flavour, let the batter sit for 5–10 minutes before using.

AMOUNT PER PANCAKE: calories 80, total fat 1.5 g, saturated fat 0.5 g, cholesterol 20 mg, sodium 340 mg, total carbohydrate 15 g, dietary fibre 2 g, sugars 6 g, protein 3 g

Oatmeal Cranberry Pancakes

After you whip up this tasty pancake batter, be sure to let it rest for 5–10 minutes at room temperature. The resting time allows the oats and flax meal to soften a bit, resulting in a more delicious and tender pancake.

Preparation: **15 minutes**   Processing: **35 seconds**   Yield: **10 pancakes**

360 ml skimmed milk

90 g whole grain flour, preferably home-made (page 64)

2 teaspoons baking powder

½ teaspoon bicarbonate of soda

½ teaspoon salt (optional)

40 g flax meal

60 g rolled oats

30 g cranberries

2 tablespoons (20 g) unsalted sunflower seeds

1. Place the milk, flour, baking powder, bicarbonate of soda and salt (if using) into the Vitamix container in the order listed and secure the lid. Select Variable 1. Turn the machine on and slowly increase the speed to Variable 10, then to High. Blend for 20 seconds.

2. Stop the machine and remove the lid. Add the flax meal, oats, cranberries and sunflower seeds and secure the lid. Select Variable 2. Turn the machine on and blend for 15 seconds, using the tamper if necessary to press the ingredients into the blades.

3. For the best texture, let the batter sit for 5–10 minutes before using.

AMOUNT PER PANCAKE: calories 110, total fat 2.5 g, saturated fat 0 g, cholesterol 0 mg, sodium 180 mg, total carbohydrate 18 g, dietary fibre 3 g, sugars 4 g, protein 4 g

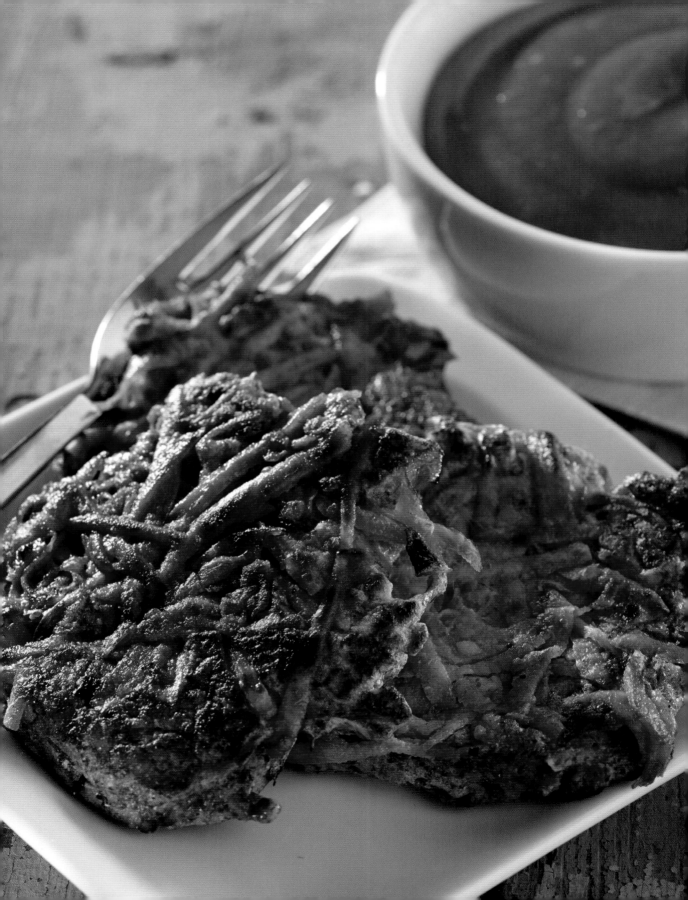

Curried Sweet Potato Pancakes

These pancakes are perfect for the mornings when you want something warm but aren't hungry for something sweet. Not only will you be able to skip the maple syrup here, but you will get a serving of vegetables too.

Preparation: **15 minutes**   Processing: **35 seconds**   Cook time: **45 minutes**   Yield: **12 pancakes**

2 large eggs

60 ml low-fat (1%) milk

2 tablespoons (30 ml) light olive oil or vegetable oil

25 g flax meal

2 tablespoons fresh thyme leaves

480 ml grated peeled sweet potato (about 1 medium to large sweet potato)

2 tablespoons grated onion

40 g whole grain flour, preferably home-made (page 64)

1 teaspoon baking powder

½ teaspoon salt

½ teaspoon curry powder

1. Place the eggs, milk, olive oil and flax meal into the Vitamix container in the order listed and secure the lid. Select Variable 1. Turn the machine on and slowly increase the speed to Variable 10. Blend for 20 seconds.

2. Stop the machine and remove the lid. Add the thyme to the container and secure the lid. Select Variable 1. Turn the machine on and slowly increase the speed to Variable 4. Blend for 15 seconds.

3. Combine the sweet potato, onion, flour, baking powder, salt and curry powder in a medium bowl.

4. Pour the egg mixture into the sweet potato mixture and stir by hand just until combined.

5. Drop 2 tablespoons of batter for each pancake on to a hot non-stick griddle. Cook until golden on the bottom, about 5 minutes, Flip, then press lightly and continue to cook until golden and cooked through, about 8 minutes longer.

AMOUNT PER PANCAKE: calories 80, total fat 4 g, saturated fat 0.5 g, cholesterol 30 mg, sodium 160 mg, total carbohydrate 8 g, dietary fibre 2 g, sugars 1 g, protein 3 g

Oatmeal Pancakes with Dried Cranberry Topping

These hearty pancakes give you another great way to add oats to your morning meal. The dried cranberry topping comes together in a snap and is so delicious you will find yourself spooning it on everything – a turkey sandwich, a dish of yoghurt, maybe even into an autumn-inspired smoothie!

Preparation: **15 minutes**   Processing: **15 seconds**   Yield: **18 pancakes (2 per serving)**

TOPPING:

2 tablespoons (30 ml) pure maple syrup

95 g unsweetened dried cranberries

PANCAKES:

2 large eggs

480 ml skimmed milk

2 tablespoons vegetable oil

1½ tablespoons light brown sugar

125 g unbleached plain flour

90 g whole grain flour, preferably home-made (page 64)

2 teaspoons baking powder

½ teaspoon ground cinnamon

¼ teaspoon salt

85 g rolled oats

1. For the topping: Combine 160 ml water, the maple syrup and cranberries in a small pan and bring to a boil. Remove from the heat and set aside, covered, until ready to serve.

2. For the pancakes: Place the eggs, milk, oil and brown sugar into the Vitamix container in the order listed and secure the lid. Select Variable 1. Turn the machine on and slowly increase the speed to Variable 8. Blend for 15 seconds until mixture is creamy.

3. Combine the flours, baking powder, cinnamon, salt and oats in a medium bowl.

4. Pour the milk mixture into the flour mixture and fold by hand just until blended.

5. Portion and cook, turning after 3 minutes or once the bottom side is golden brown. Cook until both sides are golden brown and firm to touch (page 51). Serve hot with the topping.

AMOUNT PER SERVING: calories 210, total fat 5 g, saturated fat 1 g, cholesterol 40 mg, sodium 210 mg, total carbohydrate 35 g, dietary fibre 3 g, sugars 9 g, protein 7 g

Gluten-Free Buttermilk Pancake Mix

Whip up this delicious gluten-free pancake mix in your Vitamix and you can have pancakes for breakfast or dinner at a moment's notice. Consider grinding your own brown rice and white rice flours too. (See page 56 for instructions.)

Preparation: **15 minutes**   Processing: **15 seconds**   Yield: **1.2 litres, enough to make 20 pancakes**

370 g brown rice flour*

160 g potato starch flour

60 g amaranth flour

42 g white rice flour*

120 g low-fat buttermilk powder

50 g granulated sugar

4 teaspoons gluten-free baking powder

1 tablespoon bicarbonate of soda

½ teaspoon salt

1½ teaspoons xanthum gum

***Make brown rice flour and white rice flour in Vitamix Dry Grains Container**

1. Place all the ingredients into the Vitamix container and secure the lid. Select Variable 1. Turn the machine on and slowly increase the speed to Variable 2 or 3. Blend for 15 seconds or until combined, using the tamper as needed.

2. Store the mix, tightly covered in an airtight container in the fridge, for up to 3 months. Whisk thoroughly to recombine before each use.

AMOUNT PER 60 ML SERVING: calories 150, total fat 1 g, saturated fat 0 g, cholesterol 5 mg, sodium 280 mg, total carbohydrate 31 g, dietary fibre 2 g, sugars 3 g, protein 4 g

Gluten-Free Pancakes

Once you have home-made gluten-free buttermilk pancake mix on hand, you can whip up these delicious pancakes any time using basic store-cupboard staples. Serve them up with fresh fruit or maple syrup for a dish that will delight everyone at the table.

Preparation: **10 minutes**   Processing: **20 seconds**   Yield: **12 pancakes (about 3 pancakes per serving)**

2 large eggs

360 ml water

2 tablespoons vegetable oil

195 g Gluten-Free Buttermilk Pancake Mix (page 53)

1. Place the eggs, water and oil into the Vitamix container in the order listed and secure the lid. Select Variable 1. Turn the machine on and slowly increase the speed to Variable 5. Blend for 20 seconds.

2. Place the pancake mix in a medium bowl. Pour the egg mixture into the pancake mix and combine by hand until blended.

3. Let the batter rest for 5 minutes while you heat a non-stick heavy-based frying pan or griddle.

4. Cook the pancakes in batches. Pour about 4 tablespoons (60 ml) of batter for each pancake into the pan and cook until golden on each side.

AMOUNT PER SERVING: calories 360, total fat 14 g, saturated fat 2.5 g, cholesterol 130 mg, sodium 490 mg, total carbohydrate 49 g, dietary fibre 2 g, sugars 4 g, protein 11 g

Gluten-Free Ricotta Pancakes

The most delicious, aromatic, light and fluffy pancakes you have ever tasted! And gluten-free too. Wonderful with the blueberries or without.

Preparation: **15 minutes**   Processing: **20 seconds**   Yield **12 pancakes**

120 ml skimmed milk

2 tablespoons vegetable oil

4 large egg whites, lightly beaten

120 ml half-fat ricotta

120 ml 0% natural Greek yoghurt, stirred

75 g light brown sugar

Grated zest of 1 lemon

90 g Gluten-Free Flour Mix (page 56)

¼ teaspoon xanthum gum

1 teaspoon gluten-free baking powder

75 g blueberries, washed and patted completely dry

1. Place the milk, oil, egg whites, ricotta, yoghurt, brown sugar and lemon zest into the Vitamix container in the order listed and secure the lid. Select Variable 1. Turn the machine on and slowly increase the speed to Variable 10, then to High. Blend for 20 seconds.

2. Combine the gluten-free flour mix, xanthum gum and baking powder in a medium bowl and whisk by hand.

3. Pour the ricotta mixture into the flour mixture and whisk together until mixture is well blended. Fold in the blueberries.

4. Let the batter rest for 5 minutes. Lightly coat a non-stick frying pan or griddle with cooking spray and place over a low-medium heat.

5. Cook the pancakes in batches: drop about 4 tablespoons of batter for each pancake and cook until cooked through and golden brown on both sides.

AMOUNT PER PANCAKE: calories 100, total fat 3.5 g, saturated fat 1 g, cholesterol 5 mg, sodium 80 mg, total carbohydrate 14 g, dietary fibre 1 g, sugars 8 g, protein 4 g

Gluten-Free Flour Mix

You can buy gluten-free flours, of course, but if you have the Dry Grains container for your Vitamix, you should consider grinding your own. This mix comes together quickly and will keep well in an airtight container in the fridge (several months) or in the freezer (6–8 months).

Preparation: **10 minutes**   Processing: **30 seconds**   Yield: **700 g**

555 g brown rice

320 g cornflour

180 g tapioca flour

1. Place the brown rice into the Vitamix Dry Grains container and secure the lid. Select Variable 1. Turn the machine on and slowly increase the speed to Variable 10, then to High. Blend for 30 seconds, or until the desired flour consistency is reached.

2. Pour into a large bowl and whisk in the cornflour and tapioca flour until completely blended.

3. Store in an airtight container and whisk together before each use.

AMOUNT PER 25 G SERVING: calories 110, total fat 0 g, saturated fat 0 g, cholesterol 0 mg, sodium 0 mg, total carbohydrate 24 g, dietary fibre 1 g, sugars 0 g, protein 1 g

Buttermilk Cornmeal Waffles

Tempted by this recipe but out of buttermilk? Pour 450 ml of 1% or 2% milk into a bowl. Add 2 tablespoons of lemon juice or vinegar to the milk and allow it to thicken at room temperature, 10–15 minutes. Proceed with the recipe as directed!

Preparation: **10 minutes**   Processing: **15 seconds**   Yield: **10 waffles**

2 large eggs

480 ml low-fat buttermilk

60 ml vegetable oil

1 tablespoon light brown sugar

95 g unbleached plain flour

150 g whole grain flour, preferably home-made (page 64)

118 g cornmeal, preferably home-made (page 60)

2 teaspoons baking powder

1 teaspoon bicarbonate of soda

¼ teaspoon salt

¼ teaspoon ground cinnamon

⅓ teaspoon ground ginger

1. Place the eggs, buttermilk, vegetable oil and brown sugar into the Vitamix container in the order listed and secure the lid. Select Variable 1. Turn the machine on and slowly increase the speed to Variable 10, then to High. Blend for 15 seconds.

2. Combine the flours, cornmeal, baking powder, bicarbonate of soda, salt, cinnamon and ginger in a medium bowl.

3. Pour the buttermilk mixture into the flour mixture and fold by hand just until combined.

AMOUNT PER WAFFLE: calories 220, total fat 8 g, saturated fat 1 g, cholesterol 40 mg, sodium 350 mg, total carbohydrate 32 g, dietary fibre 2 g, sugars 4 g, protein 7 g

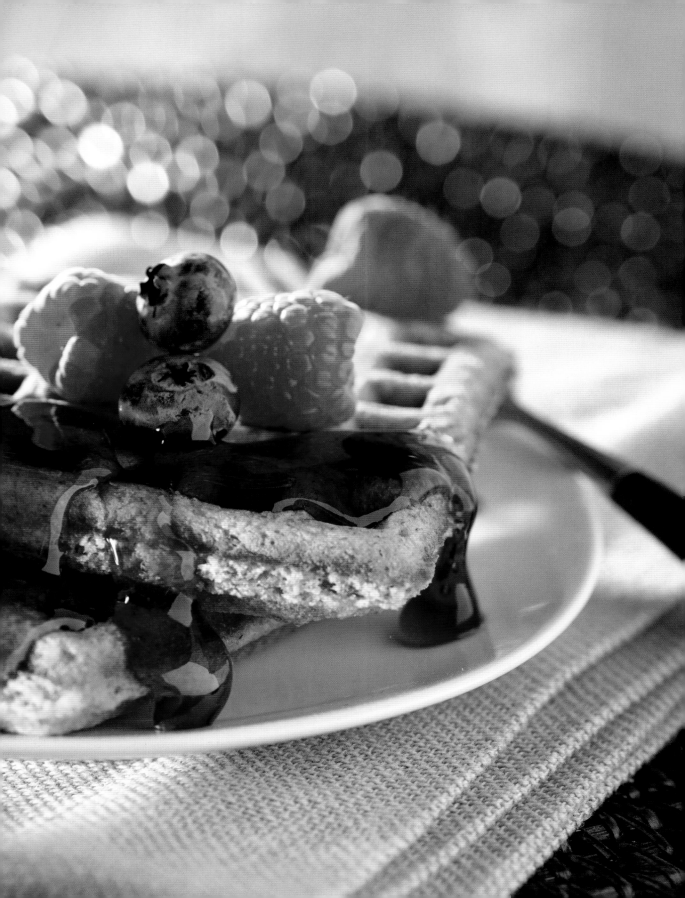

Banana Waffles

Like banana bread in your waffle maker! These sweet waffles, loaded with potassium, are lovely plain, as the bread for a peanut butter sandwich, or simply topped with maple syrup or fresh fruit.

Preparation: **10 minutes**   Processing: **40 seconds**   Yield: **10 waffles**

240 g whole grain, preferably home-made (page 64)

1 tablespoon baking powder

1 teaspoon salt

3 large eggs

360 ml skimmed milk

2 ripe bananas, peeled

3 tablespoons (40 g) unsalted butter

1. Combine the flour, baking powder and salt in a medium bowl and stir lightly. Set aside.

2. Place the eggs, milk, bananas and butter into the Vitamix container in the order listed and secure the lid. Select Variable 1. Turn the machine on and slowly increase the speed to Variable 6. Blend for 20 seconds.

3. Stop the machine and remove the lid. Add the flour mixture and secure the lid. Select Variable 1. Turn the machine on and slowly increase the speed to Variable 6. Blend for 20 seconds, using the tamper to press the ingredients into the blades.

4. For best texture and flavour, let the batter sit 5–10 minutes before using.

AMOUNT PER WAFFLE: calories 170, total fat 6 g, saturated fat 3 g, cholesterol 65 mg, sodium 420 mg, total carbohydrate 25 g, dietary fibre 3 g, sugars 5 g, protein 7 g

Cornmeal

Making home-made flours, like this fresh cornmeal, is a snap in your Vitamix. Whip up a batch to use in the Cornmeal Pumpkin Spice Loaf (page 79) and save the leftover in a tightly sealed container for another use.

Preparation: **5 minutes**   Processing: **1 minute**   Yield: **460 g**

390 g unpopped popcorn kernels

Place the popcorn kernels into the Vitamix container and secure the lid. Select Variable 1. Start the machine and slowly increase the speed to Variable 10, then to High. Grind to the desired degree of fineness. The longer the machine runs, the finer the consistency of the cornmeal, up to 1 minute.

AMOUNT PER 60 ML SERVING: calories 130, total fat 1.5 g, saturated fat 0 g, cholesterol 0 mg, sodium 0 mg, total carbohydrate 26 g, dietary fibre 4 g, sugars 0 g, protein 4 g

Baked Whole Wheat French Toast

Fragrant with vanilla, cinnamon and nutmeg, this whole wheat French toast will quickly become a regular at your breakfast table! Baking the French toast gives you a golden brown, crispy result without any added oil.

Preparation: **10 minutes**   Processing: **15 seconds**   Bake time: **8 minutes**   Yield: **6 servings**

1 large egg

2 large egg whites

180 ml skimmed milk

1 tablespoon honey

1 teaspoon vanilla extract

¼ teaspoon ground cinnamon

⅓ teaspoon ground nutmeg

½ teaspoon baking powder

6 slices whole wheat bread

Fresh seasonal fruit (optional)

1. Place the whole egg, egg whites, milk, honey, vanilla, cinnamon, nutmeg and baking powder into the Vitamix container in the order listed and secure the lid. Select Variable 1. Turn the machine on and slowly increase the speed to Variable 6. Blend for 15 seconds.

2. Place the bread slices in a large, deep baking dish in a single layer. Pour the egg mixture over the bread, cover and chill for 30 minutes.

3. Pre-heat the oven to 220°C. Line a large baking sheet with non-stick baking paper or a silicone baking mat.

4. Remove the bread from the egg mixture and arrange them on a lined baking sheet. Bake for 8 minutes, flip and bake 8 minutes longer, or until crisp and golden.

5. Serve hot, topped with fresh fruit, if desired.

AMOUNT PER SERVING: calories 140, total fat 2 g, saturated fat 0 g, cholesterol 30 mg, sodium 200 mg, total carbohydrate 24 g, dietary fibre 3 g, sugars 7 g, protein 8 g

Vegan French Toast

This delicious vegan French toast is fast to make and full of flavour! Baking the French toast helps you make a tasty breakfast without adding any oil.

Preparation: **10 minutes**　Processing: **30 seconds**　Bake time: **25 minutes**　Yield: **4 servings**

225 g silken tofu

180 ml water

1 teaspoon maple syrup

½ teaspoon ground cinnamon

1 tablespoon flax meal

1 medium banana

8 slices whole wheat bread

Fresh seasonal berries and maple syrup, for serving (optional)

1. Pre-heat the oven to 190°C. Line a baking sheet with non-stick baking paper or a silicone baking mat.

2. Place the tofu, water, maple syrup, cinnamon, flax meal and banana into the Vitamix container in the order listed and secure the lid. Select Variable 1. Turn the machine on and slowly increase the speed to Variable 10, then to High. Blend for 30 seconds.

3. Pour the mixture into a 23 x 33 cm baking dish. Place the bread in the batter and turn to coat both sides. Arrange the bread on the baking sheet.

4. Bake for 25 minutes, or until golden. Serve with fresh berries and maple syrup, if desired.

AMOUNT PER SERVING: calories 250, total fat 4 g, saturated fat 0 g, cholesterol 0 mg, sodium 270 mg, total carbohydrate 42 g, dietary fibre 5 g, sugars 9 g, protein 11 g

Breakfast Crepes

These nutty breakfast crepes are wonderfully adaptable. Fill the cooked crepes with your favourite sweet or savoury filling, depending on your mood and contents of your store cupboard. Cooked crepes keep, covered, in the fridge for 2 days.

Preparation: **10 minutes plus resting time**   Processing time: **25 seconds**   Yield: **8 large crepes**

3 large eggs

120 ml low-fat (1%) milk

2 teaspoons vegetable oil

90 g whole grain flour, preferably home-made (page 64)

30 g unbleached plain flour

¼ teaspoon sea salt

120 ml seltzer water

1. Place the eggs, milk, vegetable oil, flours and salt into the Vitamix container in the order listed and secure the lid. Select Variable 1. Turn the machine on and slowly increase the speed to Variable 10, then to High. Blend for 25 seconds until smooth. Stop the machine, remove the lid, and scrape the sides of the container as needed.

2. Transfer the batter to a bowl. Cover and chill for at least 1 hour and up to overnight.

3. When ready to cook, whisk the seltzer water into the batter.

4. Coat a medium frying pan with cooking spray. Heat over a medium-high heat.

5. Ladle 60–80 ml of batter into the centre of the pan and immediately tilt and rotate the pan to spread the batter evenly over the bottom. Cook until the underside is lightly browned, 30 seconds to 1 minute. Flip crepe and cook until lightly browned on second side, about 20 seconds.

AMOUNT PER SERVING: calories 100, total fat 3.5 g, saturated fat 1 g, cholesterol 70 mg, sodium 105 mg, total carbohydrate 12 g, dietary fibre 1 g, sugars 1 g, protein 5 g

Whole-Grain Flour

Talking about the benefits of whole-grain flours, Adam Wilson, our Senior Culinary Manager at Vitamix, says, 'A grain kernel consists of three parts: the innermost germ, the endosperm that surrounds the germ and the bran that envelops both. Most of the kernel's nutrients are locked into the germ and bran. Whole-grain products, therefore, provide us with the full nutrient content of the grain kernel.'

By grinding your own flour, you keep all of the nutrition of the whole grain, even after the grain is processed. But if we can buy whole-grain flours, why should we grind our own? There are a number of reasons. The flavour and aroma of ground flours are something special, and these qualities come through when you use the flour. If you are using a lot of speciality flours – teff, millet and oat, for example – grinding your own flours from whole grains can be cheaper. Home-made flours can also be safer if you are avoiding gluten, because you can reduce the risk of cross-contamination. Please do note that, because the fresh flour will contain some oil, plan on either using the flour within a day or two or storing it in the fridge, so the flour does not become rancid.

Read the Whole Foods Success Stories about Shauna Ahern (page 80) and Janice Summers (page 257) for more about grinding your own flours.

Preparation: **5 minutes**   Processing: **1 minute**   Yield: **50-400 g**

50–400 g whole-kernel grains

1. Place up to 400 g whole-kernel grain into the Vitamix Dry Grains container and secure the lid. Select Variable 1.

2. Turn machine on and slowly increase the speed to Variable 10, then to High. Grind to the desired degree of fineness, up to 1 minute. The longer the machine runs, the finer the consistency of the flour.

Whole Wheat Muffins

These delicious, homey muffins can be enjoyed plain or split, toasted and spread with your favourite topping. If you want to add a little extra flavour, fold in a cup of chopped dried fruit or chocolate chips once the wet and dry ingredients have been combined for an extra tasty treat!

Preparation: **10 minutes**   Processing: **30 seconds**   Bake time: **18–25 minutes**   Yield: **12 muffins**

180 g whole grain flour, preferably home-made (page 64)

2 teaspoons baking powder

½ teaspoon salt

1 large egg

120 ml low-fat (1%) milk

120 ml unsweetened apple sauce

55 g light brown sugar

60 ml light olive oil

1 tablespoon pure maple syrup

1 tablespoon water

200 g pitted dates

1. Pre-heat the oven to 190°C. Line 12 cups of a muffin tin with paper cases.

2. Combine the flour, baking powder and salt in a medium bowl.

3. Place the egg, milk, apple sauce, brown sugar, olive oil, maple syrup, water and dates into the Vitamix container in the order listed and secure the lid. Select Variable 1. Turn the machine on and slowly increase the speed to Variable 10, then to High. Blend for 30 seconds or until well blended and creamy.

4. Pour the wet mixture into the flour mixture and fold by hand just until blended. Fill the muffin cases three-quarters full.

5. Bake for 18–25 minutes, until a toothpick inserted in the centre comes out clean. Immediately transfer to a wire rack.

AMOUNT PER MUFFIN: calories 180, total fat 6 g, saturated fat 1 g, cholesterol 15 mg, sodium 190 mg, total carbohydrate 32 g, dietary fibre 3 g, sugars 19 g, protein 3 g

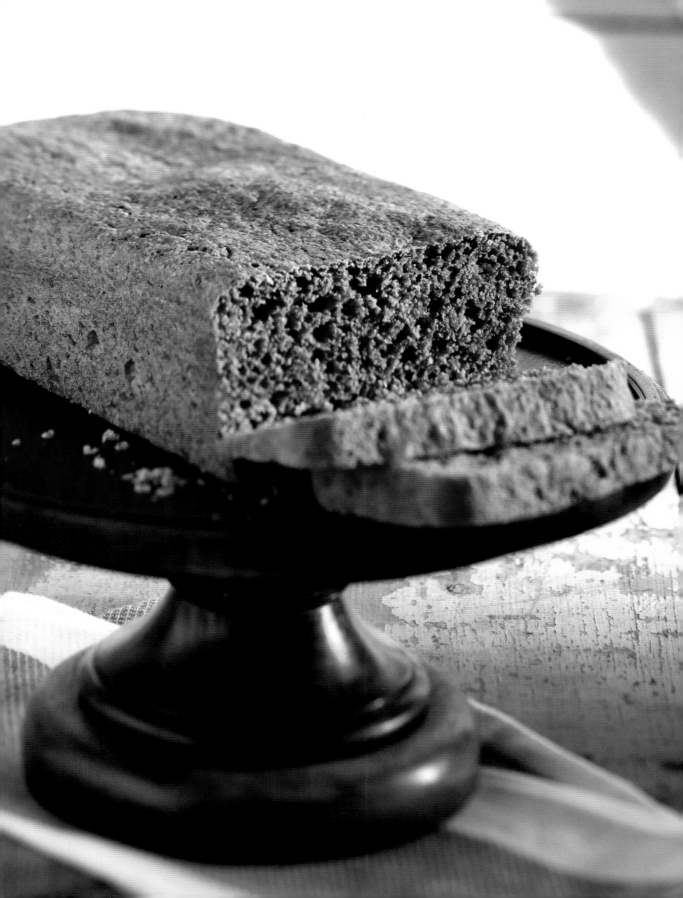

Whole Wheat Bread

In the introduction, you heard a story about my grandpa Bill taking time away from a family reunion to explain to a customer, step-by-step, how to make Vitamix bread. Grandpa Bill taught us the basics but Vitamix chef and recipe developer Bev Shaffer has added some advice of her own.

Pay careful attention to the instructions for this delicious bread. Not significantly more difficult than making a smoothie, but definitely more precise! Shaffer says that the most common mistake is overworking the dough once the liquid is added. Mixing the dough too long will overdevelop the gluten, and the resulting bread will be tough. Making bread in the Vitamix, just as without, takes practice. If at first you don't succeed, try and try again! The results are worth it.

Preparation: **10 minutes**   Processing: **35 seconds**   Bake time: **35 minutes**   Yield: **1 loaf (10 slices)**

1 tablespoon honey

300 ml warm water (40–46°C)

1 tablespoon active dry yeast

270 g whole kernel wheat or 270 g whole grain flour, preferably home-made (page 64)

1 teaspoon salt (optional)

1 tablespoon light olive or grapeseed oil

1 teaspoon fresh lemon juice

1 egg white mixed with 1 tablespoon water (optional), for brushing dough

1. Combine the warm water, honey and yeast in a bowl and stir quickly to combine. Set aside for 5 minutes to proof.

2. When starting with whole kernel wheat: Place the wheat and salt (if using) into the Vitamix Dry Grains container and secure the lid. Select Variable 1. Turn the machine on and slowly increase the speed to Variable 10, then to High. Grind the wheat for 1 minute. (Do not overprocess.) Stop the machine to allow the flour to cool for a few minutes.

3. When starting with whole wheat flour: Place the flour and salt into the Vitamix Dry Grains container and secure the lid. Select Variable 1. Turn the machine on and slowly increase the speed to Variable 6. Blend until a hole forms in the centre of the mixture, about 5 seconds.

4. Select Variable 3. Turn the machine on and remove the lid plug. Pour the oil, lemon juice and the yeast mixture through the lid plug opening. Stop the machine.

5. Replace the lid plug. Select High speed. Use the On/Off switch to quickly pulse 2 times. Stop the machine and remove the lid. Let the dough rest while greasing the pan.

6. Lightly coat a 22 x 11 cm loaf tin with cooking spray.

7. Use a spatula to scrape the sides of the Vitamix container. Pull the dough away from the container sides and into the centre of the mixture. Replace the lid. Select High speed. Use the On/Off switch to quickly pulse 5 times. (Add additional water, 1 tablespoon at a time, only if the dough seems exceptionally dry.) Repeat the process 5 times, scraping the sides of the container each time, until the dough binds together into a soft, elastic mixture.

8. To remove the dough from the container, use the On/Off switch to quickly pulse 5 times (to assist in lifting the dough up and away from the blades). Invert the container over the loaf tin and let the dough fall into the tin. Use a wet spatula to remove any remaining dough.

9. Use a wet or oiled spatula (or lightly floured fingers) to shape the loaf. Allow the dough to rise, covered with a clean, dry tea towel, until the top of it is as high as the top of the loaf tin, 20–25 minutes.

10. Meanwhile, pre-heat the oven to 180°C.

11. If desired, brush the loaf quickly and gently with the egg white wash. Using a sharp serrated knife, make 3 or 4 diagonal slits about 5 mm deep on the top of the loaf.

12. Bake for 35 minutes, or until the bread is well browned and reaches an internal temperature of 88°C when tested with an instant-read thermometer.

13. Cool in the tin on a wire rack 10 minutes, then carefully turn out of the tin on to the rack to cool completely before slicing.

AMOUNT PER SLICE: calories 140, total fat 2 g, saturated fat 0 g, cholesterol 0 mg, sodium 240 mg, total carbohydrate 26 g, dietary fibre 4 g, sugars 2 g, protein 5 g

Wholesome Hearty Grain Breakfast 'Cake'

What could be more exciting than cake for breakfast? True, this cake is not dripping with chocolate icing or sprinkles, but it's full of hearty, nutty flavour that will keep you coming back for more.

Preparation: **20 minutes**   Processing: **15 seconds**   Bake time: **35–45 minutes**   Yield: **10 servings**

125 g unbleached plain flour

240 g whole grain flour, preferably home-made (page 64)

42 g quick-cook oats, plus 1–2 tablespoons for garnish

1 tablespoon baking powder

½ teaspoon sea salt

360 ml low-fat (1%) milk

3 tablespoons vegetable oil

55 g light brown sugar

1 large egg

1. Pre-heat the oven to 180°C. Lightly coat the bottom only of a 20-cm round cake tin with cooking spray.

2. Combine the flours, oats, baking powder and salt in a medium bowl.

3. Place the milk, oil, brown sugar and egg into the Vitamix container in the order listed and secure the lid. Select Variable 1. Turn the machine on and slowly increase the speed to Variable 8. Blend for 15 seconds, until the mixture is a smooth, creamy consistency.

4. Pour the milk mixture into the flour mixture and fold by hand just until moistened. Spread the batter in the tin and sprinkle with additional oats for garnish.

5. Bake for 35–45 minutes, until golden brown and a toothpick inserted into the centre comes out clean. Cool for 15 minutes in the tin, then turn out of the tin on to a wire rack to cool. Cut into 10 wedges before serving.

AMOUNT PER SERVING: calories 230, total fat 6 g, saturated fat 1 g, cholesterol 20 mg, sodium 290 mg, total carbohydrate 38 g, dietary fibre 3 g, sugars 8 g, protein 7 g

Yoghurt Bread with Fruit and Nuts

This moist, flavourful bread is full of grains, dried fruit and crunchy chopped nuts. Just sweet enough to taste like a treat, but with enough nutritional oomph to feel like a treat that you could have every day.

Preparation: **15 minutes**   Processing: **15 seconds**   Bake time: **45 minutes**
Yield: **2 loaves (16 slices per loaf)**

240 ml low-fat buttermilk

165 g light brown sugar

120 ml natural 0% Greek yoghurt, stirred

2 tablespoons unsalted butter, melted

1 large egg

150 g whole grain flour, preferably home-made (page 64)

125 g unbleached plain flour

75 g bran flake cereal

2 teaspoons baking powder

2 teaspoons ground cinnamon

1 teaspoon bicarbonate of soda

¼ teaspoon sea salt

140 g chopped almonds

160 g unsweetened dried fruit (such as raisins or chopped apricots, pineapple or apples)

1. Pre-heat the oven to 180°C. Lightly coat two 22 x 11 cm loaf tins with cooking spray.

2. Place the buttermilk, brown sugar, yoghurt, melted butter and egg into the Vitamix container in the order listed and secure the lid. Select Variable 1. Turn the machine on and slowly increase the speed to Variable 10. Blend for 10 to 15 seconds, until a creamy consistency is reached.

3. Combine the flours, cereal, baking powder, cinnamon, bicarbonate of soda and salt in a large bowl.

4. Pour the buttermilk mixture into the flour mixture and stir by hand just until combined. Stir in the almonds and dried fruit.

5. Bake for 45 minutes, or until a toothpick inserted in the centre comes out clean. Cool for 10 minutes in the tins, then turn out on to a wire rack to cool completely.

AMOUNT PER SLICE: calories 110, total fat 3.5 g, saturated fat 1 g, cholesterol 10 mg, sodium 120 mg, total carbohydrate 19 g, dietary fibre 2 g, sugars 10 g, protein 3 g

Bran Cherry Muffins

With crunchy toasted almonds, chewy dried cherries and cosy spices, these bran muffins are great for a quick breakfast or an afterschool snack. Enjoy these along with the knowledge that you are getting a good dose of calcium, protein and fibre along with an unbeatable taste!

Preparation: **10 minutes**   Processing: **15 seconds**   Bake time: **20–25 minutes**   Yield: **12 muffins**

90 g wheat bran

300 ml skimmed milk

2 large eggs

80 ml molasses

4–5 tablespoons natural 0% Greek yoghurt, stirred

1 tablespoon light brown sugar

180 g whole grain flour, preferably home-made (page 64)

1 tablespoon baking powder

½ teaspoon bicarbonate of soda

1 teaspoon ground cinnamon

¾ teaspoon ground ginger

¼ teaspoon sea salt

100 g coarsely chopped almonds, toasted

80 g unsweetened dried cherries

1. Pre-heat the oven to 180°C. Lightly coat 12 cups of a muffin tin with cooking spray or line with paper cases.

2. Combine the wheat bran and milk in a medium bowl. Let stand for 10 minutes, or until most of the milk is absorbed.

3. Transfer the milk and bran to the Vitamix container. Add the eggs, molasses, 4 tablespoons of the yoghurt and brown sugar in the order listed and secure the lid. Select Variable 1. Turn the machine on and slowly increase the speed to Variable 10, then to High. Blend for 15 seconds. If batter is too dry, add another tablespoon of yoghurt.

4. Combine the flour, baking powder, bicarbonate of soda, cinnamon, ginger and salt in a medium bowl.

5. Pour the egg mixture into the flour mixture and fold by hand just until combined. Stir in the almonds and cherries.

6. Scrape the batter into the muffin cases and bake 20–25 minutes, or until a toothpick inserted in the centre comes out with a few moist crumbs. Serve warm.

AMOUNT PER MUFFIN: calories 200, total fat 6 g, saturated fat 0.5 g, cholesterol 30 mg, sodium 260 mg, total carbohydrate 33 g, dietary fibre 6 g, sugars 14 g, protein 7 g

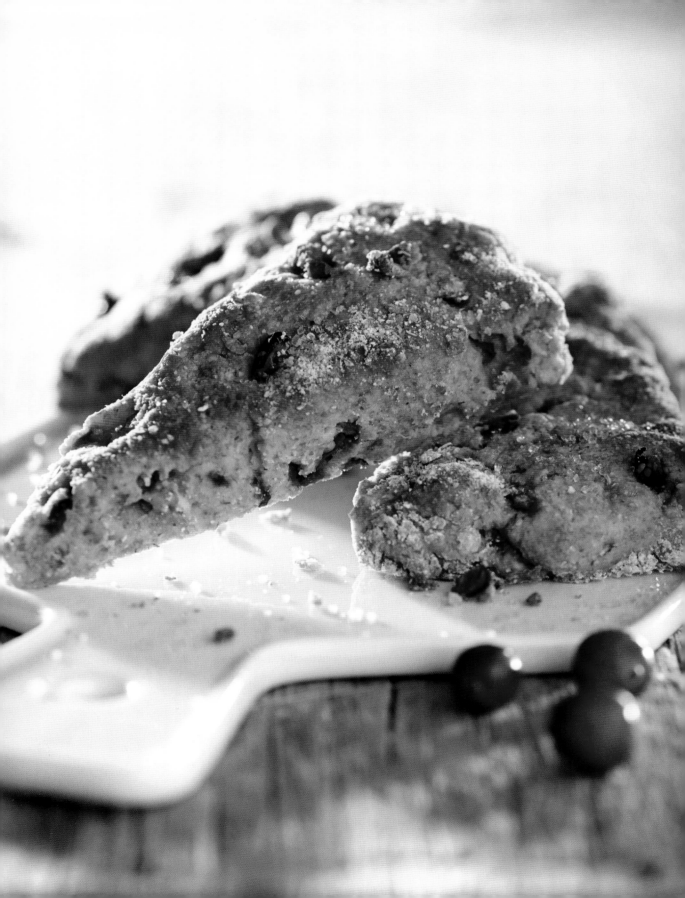

Individual Orange Cranberry Scones

Perfect for an autumn brunch or a breakfast treat, these tender scones are bursting with tart cranberries, orange zest and the gentle perfume of vanilla.

Preparation: **15 minutes**   Processing: **20 seconds**   Bake time: **30–35 minutes**   Yield: **12 biscuits**

150 g whole grain flour, preferably home-made (page 64)

125 g unbleached plain flour

2¼ teaspoons baking powder

½ teaspoon bicarbonate of soda

¼ teaspoon sea salt

285 g natural 0% Greek yoghurt, stirred

60 ml fresh orange juice (page 303)

75 g light brown sugar

1 tablespoon grated orange zest

1 teaspoon vanilla extract

100 g frozen cranberries, coarsely chopped

60 ml semi-skimmed milk

1. Pre-heat the oven to 200°C. Line a baking sheet with non-stick baking paper or a silicone baking mat.

2. Combine the flours, baking powder, bicarbonate of soda and salt in a medium bowl.

3. Place the yoghurt, orange juice, brown sugar, orange zest and vanilla into the Vitamix container in the order listed and secure the lid. Select Variable 1. Turn the machine on and slowly increase the speed to Variable 10, then to High. Blend for 20 seconds.

4. Pour the yoghurt mixture into the flour mixture and fold in the cranberries.

5. On a floured surface, pat the dough into a 23-cm round about 1 cm thick. Cut into 12 wedges.

6. Place the wedges on the baking sheet and brush the tops with the milk. Bake for 30–35 minutes, until lightly browned. Remove from the baking sheet and cool on a wire rack.

AMOUNT PER BISCUIT: calories 130, total fat 0.5 g, saturated fat 0 g, cholesterol 0 mg, sodium 210 mg, total carbohydrate 26 g, dietary fibre 2 g, sugars 8 g, protein 5 g

Oatmeal Breakfast Muffins with Raisins

All of the wonderful and cosy flavours we love in a bowl of oatmeal – the raisins, cinnamon and brown sugar – in a convenient, handheld package. Perfect with a cup of tea or tucked in a lunchbox for a not-too-sweet dessert.

Preparation: **15 minutes**   Processing: **20 seconds**   Bake time: **18–20 minutes**   Yield: **12 muffins**

80 g rolled oats

240 ml low-fat buttermilk

90 g whole grain flour, preferably home-made (page 64)

¾ teaspoon bicarbonate of soda

½ teaspoon baking powder

¼ teaspoon salt

½ teaspoon ground cinnamon

2 large eggs

75 g light brown sugar

3 tablespoons natural 0% Greek yoghurt, stirred

3 tablespoons olive oil

50 g raisins

1. Combine the oats and buttermilk in a bowl and set aside to soften for 15 minutes.

2. Pre-heat the oven to 190°C. Coat 12 cups of a muffin tin with cooking spray or line with paper cases.

3. Combine the flour, bicarbonate of soda, baking powder, salt and cinnamon in a medium bowl.

4. Place the eggs, brown sugar, yoghurt and olive oil into the Vitamix container in the order listed and secure the lid. Select Variable 1. Turn the machine on and slowly increase the speed to Variable 10, then to High. Blend for 20 seconds or until a creamy consistency is reached.

5. Stir the soaked oats and any remaining liquid into the flour mixture. Pour in the egg mixture and stir just until combined. Fold in the raisins.

6. Spoon the batter into the muffin cases, filling them about two-thirds full. Bake for 18–20 minutes, or until a toothpick inserted in the centre comes out with a few moist crumbs.

7. Let the muffins cool in the tin 10 minutes, then transfer to a wire rack to cool.

AMOUNT PER MUFFIN: calories 140, total fat 5 g, saturated fat 1 g, cholesterol 30 mg, sodium 190 mg, total carbohydrate 21 g, dietary fibre 2 g, sugars 11 g, protein 4 g

Pumpkin Purée

This home-made pumpkin purée is a snap to make and perfect for quick breads like Pumpkin Bread (page 77) or Cornmeal Pumpkin Spice Loaf (page 79)! We like to make a double or even triple batch of this purée and freeze the leftovers. Simply thaw the purée as you need it for soups, quick breads or muffins.

Preparation: **5 minutes**   Processing: **30 seconds**   Yield: **600 ml**

440 g cubed, roasted fresh pumpkin

120 ml low-sodium vegetable stock

¼ teaspoon ground ginger

¼ teaspoon ground cinnamon

1. Place all the ingredients into the Vitamix container in the order listed and secure the lid. Select Variable 1. Turn the machine on and slowly increase the speed to Variable 10, then to High. Blend for 30 seconds, using the tamper to push the ingredients into the blade.

Use this simple recipe in place of canned pumpkin.

AMOUNT PER 120 ML SERVING: calories 20, total fat 0 g, saturated fat 0 g, cholesterol 0 mg, sodium 25 mg, total carbohydrate 5 g, dietary fibre 1 g, sugars 2 g, protein 1 g

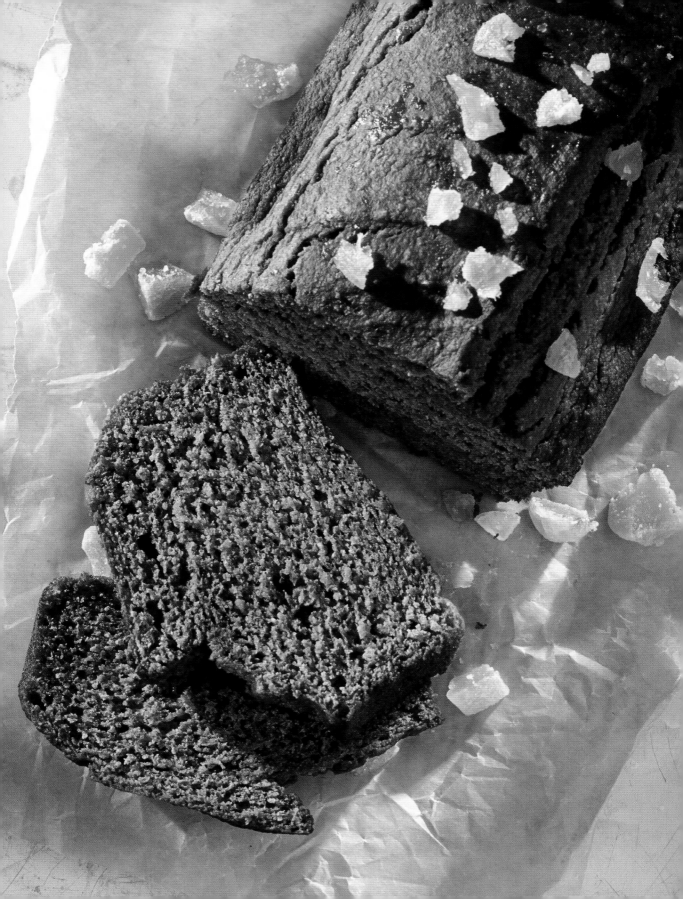

Pumpkin Bread

The recipe for this delicious, tender, lightly spiced pumpkin bread makes two loaves: one to enjoy now, the other to share or freeze. Be sure to try toasting the thickly sliced bread and serving it with your favourite spread.

Preparation: **15 minutes**   Processing: **30 seconds**   Yield: **2 loaves (16 slices per loaf)**

120 ml low-fat (1%) milk

160 ml unsweetened apple sauce

1 x 425 g can unsweetened pumpkin purée, or use home-made (page 75)

2 teaspoons vanilla extract

2 large eggs

4 large egg whites

60 ml honey

110 g dark brown sugar

240 g whole grain flour, preferably home-made (page 64)

125 g unbleached plain flour

2 teaspoons bicarbonate of soda

½ teaspoon baking powder

1 teaspoon salt

1 teaspoon ground cinnamon

½ teaspoon ground cloves

1. Pre-heat the oven to 180°C. Lightly coat the bottoms only of two 22 x 11 cm loaf tins with cooking spray.

2. Place the milk, apple sauce, pumpkin purée, vanilla, whole eggs, egg whites, honey and brown sugar into the Vitamix container in the order listed and secure the lid. Select Variable 1. Turn the machine on and slowly increase the speed to Variable 10, then to High. Blend for 30 seconds until mixture is creamy and smooth.

3. Combine the flours, bicarbonate of soda, baking powder, salt, cinnamon and cloves in a large bowl.

4. Pour the pumpkin mixture into the flour mixture and fold by hand just until blended.

5. Scrape the batter into the pans and bake 45–55 minutes, until a toothpick inserted into the centre comes out clean.

6. Cool in the tins for 20 minutes, then turn out of the tins on to a wire rack.

AMOUNT PER HALF SLICE: calories 80, total fat 0.5 g, saturated fat 0 g, cholesterol 10 mg, sodium 170 mg, total carbohydrate 16 g, dietary fibre 2 g, sugars 7 g, protein 3 g

Flecks of Courgette Cornbread

A perfect recipe for the days when gardens, supermarkets, and farmer's markets are overflowing with courgettes. This tasty bread gets a gentle sweetness from brown sugar and dates and a whole-grain boost from whole wheat flour and cornmeal.

Preparation: **15 minutes**   Processing: **15 seconds**   Bake time: **45–55 minutes**   Yield: **1 loaf (16 slices)**

120 ml natural 0% Greek yoghurt, stirred

2 large eggs

120 ml low-fat buttermilk

75 g light brown sugar

2 pitted dates

125 g unbleached plain flour

60 g whole grain flour, preferably home-made (page 64)

90 g whole-grain cornmeal, preferably home-made (page 60)

1 teaspoon baking powder

½ teaspoon bicarbonate of soda

½ teaspoon sea salt

1 large courgette (284 g), coarsely grated and well drained

1. Pre-heat the oven to 180°C. Lightly coat a 33 x 13 cm loaf tin with cooking spray.

2. Place the yoghurt, eggs, buttermilk, brown sugar and dates into the Vitamix container in the order listed and secure the lid. Select Variable 1. Turn the machine on and slowly increase the speed to Variable 10. Blend for 15 seconds or until well blended and creamy.

3. Combine the flours, cornmeal, baking powder, bicarbonate of soda and salt in a medium bowl.

4. Stir the courgette into the flour mixture. Pour the yoghurt mixture into the bowl and fold by hand; mix just until blended.

5. Scrape the batter into the tin and gently smooth the top. Bake until golden and a toothpick inserted in the centre comes out clean, 45–55 minutes. Cool in the tin for 15 minutes, then turn out of the tin on to a wire rack to cool completely.

AMOUNT PER SLICE: calories 110, total fat 1 g, saturated fat 0 g, cholesterol 25 mg, sodium 70 mg, total carbohydrate 21 g, dietary fibre 1 g, sugars 8 g, protein 4 g

Cornmeal Pumpkin Spice Loaf

Pumpkin, spices, whole-grain flours and chocolate chips too? This tasty loaf is equally at home at breakfast, tucked in a briefcase for an on-the-go snack, or alongside a cup of tea in the afternoon.

Preparation: **15 minutes**   Processing: **20 seconds**   Bake time: **35–40 minutes**   Yield: **1 loaf (16 slices)**

60 g whole-grain cornmeal, preferably home-made (page 60)

150 g whole grain flour, preferably home-made (page 64)

2½ teaspoons baking powder

½ teaspoon bicarbonate of soda

¼ teaspoon salt

½ teaspoon ground cinnamon

½ teaspoon ground nutmeg

½ teaspoon ground ginger

⅓ teaspoon ground allspice

⅓ teaspoon ground black pepper

180 ml low-fat buttermilk

80 ml light olive oil

2 large eggs

1 large egg white

75 g light brown sugar

240 ml unsweetened pumpkin purée (page 75)

60 g plain chocolate chips

1. Pre-heat the oven to 180°C. Lightly coat a 22 x 11 cm loaf tin with cooking spray.

2. Combine the cornmeal, flour, baking powder, bicarbonate of soda, salt, cinnamon, nutmeg, ginger, allspice and pepper in a medium bowl. Set aside.

3. Place the buttermilk, oil, whole eggs, egg white, brown sugar and pumpkin purée into the Vitamix container in the order listed and secure the lid. Select Variable 1. Turn the machine on and slowly increase the speed to Variable 10, then to High. Blend for 20 seconds or until mixture is a creamy consistency.

4. Pour the pumpkin mixture into the flour mixture. Add the chocolate chips and fold by hand just until blended.

5. Scrape the batter into the loaf tin and bake for 35–40 minutes, until a toothpick inserted in the centre comes out clean. Cool for 15 minutes on a wire rack, then remove from the pan to cool completely before cutting.

AMOUNT PER SLICE: calories 140, total fat 7 g, saturated fat 2 g, cholesterol 25 mg, sodium 140 mg, total carbohydrate 18 g, dietary fibre 2 g, sugars 7 g, protein 3 g

SHAUNA AHERN

When expecting a first baby, many people expect to get baby clothes or perhaps a car seat. But a Vitamix? That's just what Shauna and Danny Ahern received when they were expecting their daughter back in 2008. Shauna, a writer, and Danny, a chef, collaborate on the award-winning blog, Gluten-Free Girl and the Chef (www.glutenfreegirl.com). After the couple announced their news on their site, a generous reader sent the couple a Vitamix to celebrate all of the changes that a new baby would bring.

Shauna and Danny began using it immediately, and like many Vitamix users, they use their machine almost daily. Their daughter, Lucy, is six now, and both she and the machine are going strong. The Aherns appreciate their Vitamix's ability to produce delightfully smooth soups and perfectly emulsified smoothies. Shauna also loves to make whole-grain crepe batter. Says Shauna, 'If I want to make buckwheat crepes in the morning, I mix whole buckwheat groats with a bit of yoghurt and water and let it sit all night. In the morning I add a bit of baking powder, a touch of sugar and some salt, and whirl it up with eggs. Perfect crepe batter, every time.'

Shauna has coeliac disease – hence the gluten-free focus of their blog – so the Aherns also like being able to grind their own flours. Shauna says that there are many good sources of reliably gluten-free whole grains and that, in her experience, grinding her own flours is generally cheaper than buying them. The Aherns grind teff, millet, oat, sorghum and buckwheat flours, usually just grinding enough for the particular recipe. (As 100 grams of teff is the equivalent of 100 grams of teff flour, it is simple to just grind what you need. As with much of baking, and particularly gluten-free baking, using a digital scale and measuring ingredients by weight will give you the best, most consistent product.) 'Fresh flours taste the best in baked goods', Shauna tells us.

To make flour, Shauna says 'I put a bit of grain in the blender, grind it on low speed. Turn off the blender and scrape down the sides with a rubber spatula. And then I turn the Vitamix on high. Afterwards, I sift the flour through a fine-mesh sieve, to catch any parts of the bran or hull that wasn't fully ground. The whole thing takes about 10 minutes.' By using gluten-free grains and grinding them herself, Shauna can fully enjoy her baked goods without any fear of cross-contamination. And the bread she is able to make? 'The sandwich bread we make with our ground flours tastes like warm, home-made bread.' And thanks to their home-made flours, it's delicious and reliably gluten-free too.

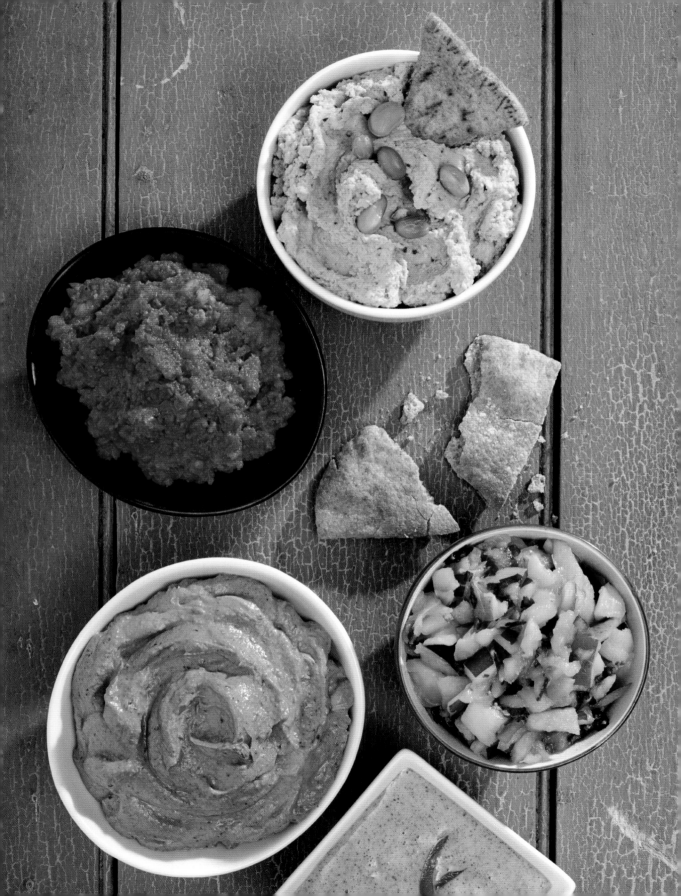

Chapter 3

Appetisers

My grandma embraced healthy eating as passionately as Grandpa and Papa did. After all, it was her father's health that inspired our family to explore health through whole foods in the first place! She, like many of us, loved to entertain and she struggled with having enough nutritious recipes that tasted fantastic in order to keep her guests coming back. She was on a mission. Over the years, Grandma worked tirelessly to develop ever more delicious and diverse recipes and techniques for the Vitamix, so she and others would have lots of tasty options to choose from.

Flash forward to 2015. My grandma would certainly not have to wonder what to offer her guests now. The delicious recipes in this chapter would have given her lots of good choices. These recipes are quick to assemble, delicious and of course – nutritious. Many of the recipes use staples you may already have in your store cupboard or fridge, such as canned beans, lemons and herbs. By making your own appetizers instead of buying prepared items from a store, you can control the amount of added salt and fat in your offerings – not to mention eliminating preservatives and other hidden additives. You can easily accommodate a vegan, vegetarian or gluten-free guest as well.

You can serve these delicious dips and spreads with accompaniments as diverse as the recipes themselves. Baked tortilla chips or pepper strips are delicious with the bean dip, the bean and cheese dip, the guacamole or any of the salsas. Scoop up Avocado Tahini Dip (page 86), Cannellini Bean Houmous (page 90) or Two-Cheese Spread with Spinach (page 110) with whole-grain crackers or steamed asparagus and green beans. Goats' Cheese Crostini with Roasted Red Pepper Spread (page 107) and Edamame Pâté (page 93) spread on home-made crostini are both elegant appetizers.

Buy at the Store or DIY

Many of the dips and snacks in this chapter include foods such as salsa and tahini. To control the amount of added salt or fat in these foods, we recommend making them at home.

Home-made roasted red peppers: Use the recipe included in Roasted Red Pepper Houmous (page 91).

Home-made salsa: Our California Salsa (page 100) is so fresh, fast, simple and delicious, you'll think twice before buying another jar at the store. The cheese and bean dip in this chapter calls for ½ cup salsa, so simply whip up the full recipe of salsa, use what you need for the cheese dip, and serve the remainder alongside the bean dip.

Home-made tahini: Tahini, a sesame seed paste, is a common ingredient in houmous, and we use it in several of the bean dips in this chapter. To make your own, use the recipe on page 244.

Home-made pitta chips or crostini: You can buy pitta chips and crackers, of course, but you can easily make your own. Both DIY pitta chips and crostini are a great way to use up slightly stale bread. Plus you can add your favourite spices and herbs while also controlling the amount of salt and fat that is added. Win-win!

TO MAKE PITTA CHIPS OR CROSTINI: Pre-heat the oven to 190°C. Slice 6 pittas into eighths or cut one whole-grain baguette crosswise into 5-mm-thick slices. Toss with 2 tablespoons olive oil or coat with olive oil cooking spray. Sprinkle with

¼ teaspoon sea salt. (You can also add a pinch of chilli powder or a teaspoon of your favourite finely chopped herb.) Spread the pitta wedges or bread slices in an even layer on a foil-lined baking sheet. Bake until golden brown and crisp, turning occasionally, 8–10 minutes. Store the cooled crisps in a container with a tight-fitting lid.

Great at a Party, Delicious in a Packed Lunch

These dips, spreads and nibbles will all be so delicious that you will hope for leftovers. Bringing your own lunch to school or work can be healthier and cheaper than buying it, and many of these tasty dips are delicious additions to your lunchbox. My dad, John, may have felt a bit self-conscious about the healthy lunch his mother packed, but times have changed. You will feel glad to have your own nutritious meal on hand. Spread leftover Black Bean Houmous (page 89) or Edamame Chickpea Dip (page 94) on whole-grain bread and top with fresh veggies for a delicious sandwich. The bean spread would also be delicious in a quesadilla with a little grated Cheddar, spinach and a spoonful of salsa. Pack a small container of leftover Avocado Tahini Dip (page 87) or houmous with cut veggies, pretzels or pitta bread for a tasty lunch or snack. If you have access to a microwave, treat yourself to a little warm Crab and Artichoke Heart Dip (page 105) with crostini for dipping and perhaps a small salad on the side.

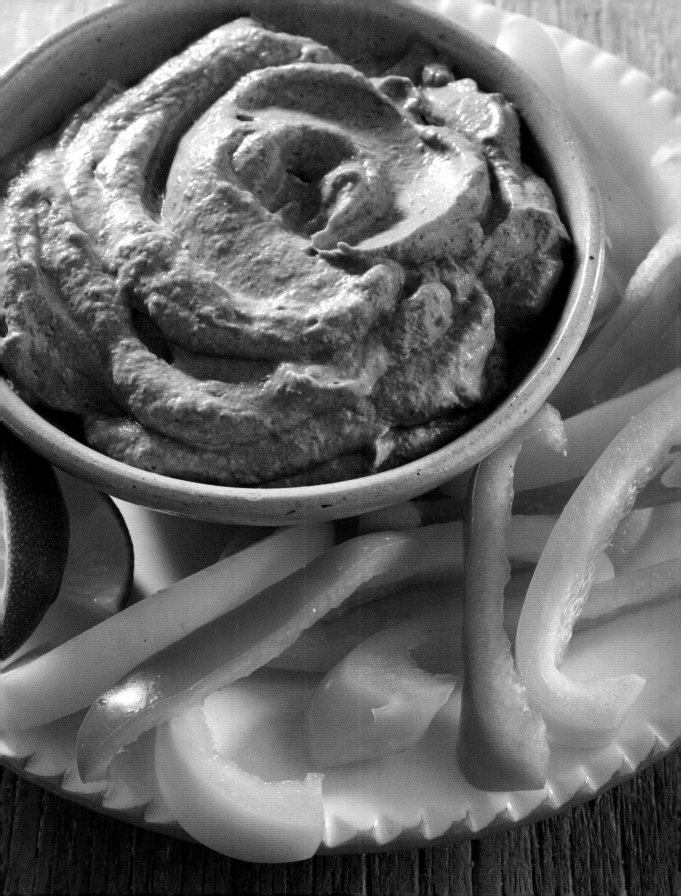

Avocado Tahini Dip

This vibrantly green dip will be the star of your next party! It is creamy with avocado, a little nutty from the tahini, bursting with herby flavour and beautifully green, thanks to the herbs and a little steamed spinach or rocket. Great as a sandwich spread too.

Preparation: **10 minutes**   Processing: **35–40 seconds**   Yield: **540 ml**

80 ml tahini (page 244)

Juice of 1 lemon (about 3 tablespoons)

1 large avocado, halved, pitted and peeled

½ teaspoon ground cumin

1 tablespoon fresh parsley leaves

1 tablespoon fresh dill leaves

¼ teaspoon ground black pepper

115 g baby spinach or rocket, steamed for 20 minutes then cooled

60 ml water

Place all the ingredients into the Vitamix container in the order listed and secure the lid. Select Variable 1. Turn the machine on and slowly increase the speed to Variable 10, then to High. Blend for 35–40 seconds, using the tamper to press the ingredients into the blades if necessary.

AMOUNT PER 30 ML SERVING: calories 50, total fat 4 g, saturated fat 0.5 g, cholesterol 0 mg, sodium 10 mg, total carbohydrate 3 g, dietary fibre 1 g, sugars 0 g, protein 1 g

Houmous

Many houmous recipes call for tahini (including several in this book), but we also like the fresh, nutty flavour that comes from using raw sesame seeds. Thanks to the Vitamix's unparalleled blending power, the texture of this classic houmous is still silky smooth.

Preparation: **10 minutes**   Processing: **1 minute**   Yield: **840 ml**

2 x 425 g cans chickpeas

35 g raw sesame seeds

1 tablespoon olive oil

60 ml fresh lemon juice

1 garlic clove, peeled

1 teaspoon ground cumin

1 teaspoon kosher salt

1. Rinse and drain one can of chickpeas. Leave the other undrained.

2. Place all the chickpeas (and the liquid from the second can) into the Vitamix container along with the other ingredients in the order listed and secure the lid. Select Variable 1. Turn the machine on and slowly increase the speed to Variable 10, then to High. Blend for 1 minute, using the tamper to press the ingredients into the blades.

AMOUNT PER 30 ML SERVING: calories 35, total fat 1.5 g, saturated fat 0 g, cholesterol 0 mg, sodium 125 mg, total carbohydrate 5 g, dietary fibre 1 g, sugars 0 g, protein 1 g

Black Bean Houmous

Out of chickpeas? Whip up this tasty black bean houmous instead. You can use it as a spread in a sandwich or as a dip with crunchy vegetables for dipping.

Preparation: **10 minutes**   Processing: **30 seconds**   Yield: **720 ml**

2 x 425 g cans no-salt-added black beans

¼ teaspoon sea salt

¼ teaspoon ground black pepper

2 garlic cloves, peeled

60 ml tahini (page 244)

½ teaspoon grated lemon zest

2 tablespoons fresh lemon juice

1 tablespoon olive oil

1. Drain and rinse one of the cans of beans. Leave the second can undrained.

2. Place all the beans (including liquid from undrained can) and all the remaining ingredients into the Vitamix container in the order listed and secure the lid. Select Variable 1. Turn the machine on and slowly increase the speed to Variable 10, then to High. Blend for 30 seconds, using the tamper to press the ingredients into the blades.

Change the flavour profile by using roasted or sautéed garlic instead of raw or add cumin or chilli powder.

AMOUNT PER 30 ML SERVING: calories 40, total fat 2 g, saturated fat 0 g, cholesterol 0 mg, sodium 30 mg, total carbohydrate 4 g, dietary fibre 1 g, sugars 0 g, protein 2 g

Cannellini Bean Houmous

Canned beans should be a store cupboard staple, and this delicious cannellini bean houmous may very well convince you to always keep them in stock. This dip is packed with flavour from ingredients you may already have on hand. It has the brightness of lemon and a little hot sauce, the herbiness of thyme, a gentle heat from the garlic and the creamy goodness of cannellini beans all in a single dip! Spread it on crudités for a snack or in a pitta for a quick sandwich.

Preparation: **10 minutes**   Processing: **45 seconds**   Yield: **840 ml**

2 x 425 g cans no-salt-added
cannellini beans

1 teaspoon grated lemon zest

½ lemon, peeled

60 ml tahini (page 244)

3 garlic cloves, roasted and peeled

½ teaspoon chilli powder

1 tablespoon fresh thyme leaves

½ teaspoon sea salt

2 dashes of hot sauce

1. Drain and rinse one of the cans of beans. Leave the second can undrained.

2. Place all the beans (including liquid from undrained can) and all the remaining ingredients into the Vitamix container in the order listed and secure the lid. Select Variable 1. Turn the machine on and slowly increase the speed to Variable 5. Blend for 15 seconds.

3. Slowly increase the speed to Variable 10, then to High. Blend for 30 seconds, using the tamper to push the ingredients into the blades.

AMOUNT PER 30 ML SERVING: calories 30, total fat 1.5 g, saturated fat 0 g, cholesterol 0 mg, sodium 50 mg, total carbohydrate 4 g, dietary fibre 1 g, sugars 0 g, protein 1 g

Roasted Red Pepper Houmous

Red peppers, botanically a fruit, are bursting with vitamins A, C and B6 as well as a number of phytochemicals. You can buy roasted red peppers or roast your own. If you want to make them yourself, here's how: Place whole peppers on a foil-lined baking sheet. Roast them at 190°C, turning them carefully with tongs every 20 minutes or so for 1 hour, or until they are soft and have begun to brown. Cool for 20–30 minutes. Peel and seed the peppers over a bowl or the sink (cooked peppers will contain a few tablespoons of liquid, and peeling them can be a messy job). Cut into strips or slices if desired.

Preparation: **10 minutes**   Processing: **1 minute**   Yield: **720 ml**

2 x 425 g cans chickpeas, rinsed and drained

170 g roasted red peppers, in water

60 ml fresh lemon juice

1 garlic clove, peeled

1 teaspoon salt (or to taste)

Place all the ingredients into the Vitamix container in the order listed and secure the lid. Select Variable 1. Turn the machine on and slowly increase the speed to Variable 10, then to High. Blend for 1 minute, using the tamper to press the ingredients into the blades.

AMOUNT PER 30 ML SERVING: calories 50, total fat 0.5 g, saturated fat 0 g, cholesterol 0 mg, sodium 330 mg, total carbohydrate 8 g, dietary fibre 1 g, protein 2 g

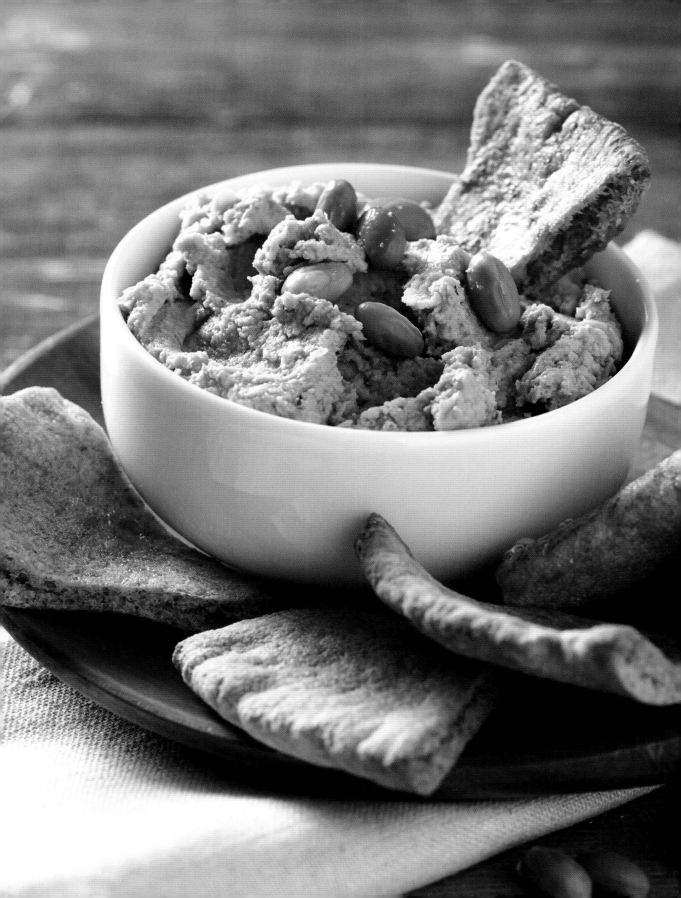

Edamame Dip or Pâté

Sometimes a bowl of bean dip and pitta chips is the perfect snack at a party, but sometimes you want something a bit more elegant. At those times, this simple, flavourful edamame pâté is the perfect appetizer. Spread the pâté on thin slices of toasted whole wheat baguette and garnish with a little extra mint or a drizzle of Garlic-Parsley Crème Sauce (page 244).

Preparation: **10 minutes**   Processing: **30 seconds**   Yield: **300 ml**

3 tablespoons low-sodium vegetable stock

3 tablespoons fresh lemon juice

190 g frozen shelled edamame, thawed

2 tablespoons chopped spring onions

½ teaspoon sea salt

60 g walnut pieces

8 g fresh mint leaves

Place all the ingredients into the Vitamix container in the order listed and secure the lid. Select Variable 1. Turn the machine on and slowly increase the speed to Variable 8. Blend for 30 seconds, using the tamper to press the ingredients into the blades, until desired consistency is reached. (For a thinner consistency, add more vegetable stock.)

AMOUNT PER 30 ML SERVING: calories 70, total fat 4.5 g, saturated fat 0 g, cholesterol 0 mg, sodium 130 mg, total carbohydrate 4 g, dietary fibre 1 g, sugars 1 g, protein 3 g

Edamame Chickpea Dip

Edamame (green soybeans) are flavourful as a snack, simply boiled and sprinkled with sea salt. But if you are looking for a different way to serve them, whip up this delightful dip. A tasty spin on houmous, creamy with Greek yoghurt and tahini; bright with lemon, garlic and a little cayenne; gently green from the parsley and the edamame. Serve it as a dip with pitta chips or celery sticks.

Preparation: **15 minutes**   Processing: **35–40 seconds**   Yield: **480 ml**

90 ml natural 0% Greek yoghurt, stirred

2 tablespoons tahini (page 244)

3 tablespoons fresh lemon juice

150 g fresh or frozen shelled edamame, steamed until tender and cooled

2 garlic cloves, peeled

¼ teaspoon sea salt

12 g fresh flatleaf parsley leaves

114 g drained canned chickpeas

Pinch of cayenne pepper

1 teaspoon ground cumin

Place all the ingredients into the Vitamix container in the order listed and secure the lid. Select Variable 1. Turn the machine on and slowly increase the speed to Variable 10, then to High. Blend for 35–40 seconds, using the tamper to press the ingredients into the blades, adding 60–20 ml water if needed, until the desired consistency is reached.

AMOUNT PER 30 ML SERVING: calories 40, total fat 1.5 g, saturated fat 0 g, cholesterol 0 mg, sodium 60 mg, total carbohydrate 4 g, dietary fibre 1 g, sugars 0 g, protein 2 g

Bean Spread

Beans may be small in size but they pack an outsized nutritional punch. An excellent source of protein and fibre, beans also have iron, zinc, folate and potassium. They are tasty and usually inexpensive to boot. Make this delicious bean spread for your next burrito or quesadilla, or enjoy it at your next party, with crunchy vegetables or baked tortilla chips for dipping.

Preparation: **15 minutes**   Processing: **1 minute**   Yield: **840 ml**

2 tablespoons olive oil

320 g chopped onion

2 garlic cloves, peeled

1 jalapeño pepper, halved and seeded

1 teaspoon ground cumin

½ teaspoon chilli powder

½ teaspoon sea salt

¼ teaspoon ground black pepper

120 ml medium salsa

2 x 425 g cans red kidney beans, rinsed and drained

1. Heat the oil in a large frying pan over a medium-high heat. Add the onion, garlic and jalapeño and cook until the onions are translucent. Stir in the cumin, chilli powder, salt and black pepper and cook for 1 minute. Remove from the heat and cool slightly.

2. Place the onion mixture, salsa and beans into the Vitamix container in the order listed and secure the lid. Select Variable 1. Turn the machine on and slowly increase the speed to Variable 10, then to High. Blend for 1 minute, using the tamper to press the ingredients into the blades.

AMOUNT PER 60 ML SERVING: calories 80, total fat 2.5 g, saturated fat 0 g, cholesterol 0 mg, sodium 220 mg, total carbohydrate 11 g, dietary fibre 3 g, sugars 2 g, protein 4 g

Cheese and Bean Dip

Warm and hearty, this cheese and bean dip served with unsalted blue corn tortilla chips will be the hit of your next football party. Spread any leftover dip in a tortilla for a quick, delicious snack.

Preparation: **10 minutes**   Processing: **30 seconds**   Yield: **480 ml**

120 ml California Salsa (page 100)

1 x 114 g can chopped green chillies, undrained

1 x 440 g can red kidney beans, rinsed and drained

¼ teaspoon chilli powder

⅛ teaspoon ground cumin

30 g grated reduced-fat Cheddar

1 tablespoon fresh coriander leaves (optional), for garnish

1. Place the salsa, chillies (and their liquid), beans, chilli powder and cumin into the Vitamix container in the order listed and secure the lid. Select Variable 1. Turn the machine on and slowly increase the speed to Variable 10, then to High. Blend for 30 seconds using the tamper to press the ingredients into the blades.

2. Transfer to a pan and heat, stirring frequently, until hot, about 4 minutes.

3. Place in a serving bowl and stir in the Cheddar. If desired, garnish with coriander. Serve with tortilla chips.

AMOUNT PER 30 ML SERVING: calories 45, total fat 1 g, saturated fat 0 g, cholesterol 0 mg, sodium 125 mg, total carbohydrate 7 g, dietary fibre 2 g, sugars 0 g, protein 3 g

Guacamole

Nutrient-dense avocados contain fibre, potassium, vitamin K, folate, vitamin B6 and more. They do have more fat than most vegetables, but 75 per cent of the fat in avocados is unsaturated, still making it a sensible choice in place of foods higher in saturated fat. Whip all of this nutritional goodness and mellow, creamy flavour into this satisfying guacamole. Try it with tortilla chips or strips of red, yellow and green peppers for dipping.

Preparation: **20 minutes**   Processing: **40–50 seconds**   Yield: **900 ml**

1 Roma (plum) tomato, quartered

4 ripe avocados, halved, pitted and peeled

10 g fresh coriander leaves

40 g chopped red onion

2 tablespoons fresh lemon juice

1 teaspoon salt

1. Place 1 tomato quarter, 1 avocado half, the coriander, onion, lemon juice and salt into the Vitamix container in that order and secure the lid. Select Variable 3. Turn the machine on and blend for 15–20 seconds, until the ingredients are mixed, using the tamper to press the ingredients into the blades.

2. Stop the machine and remove the lid. Add the remaining tomato quarters and avocado halves into the Vitamix container and secure the lid. Select Variable 5. Turn the machine on and blend for 20–30 seconds, using the tamper to press the ingredients into the blades. Leave chunky. Do not overmix.

AMOUNT PER 30 ML SERVING: calories 30, total fat 3 g, saturated fat 0 g, cholesterol 0 mg, sodium 0 mg, total carbohydrate 2 g, dietary fibre 1 g, sugars 0 g, protein 0 g

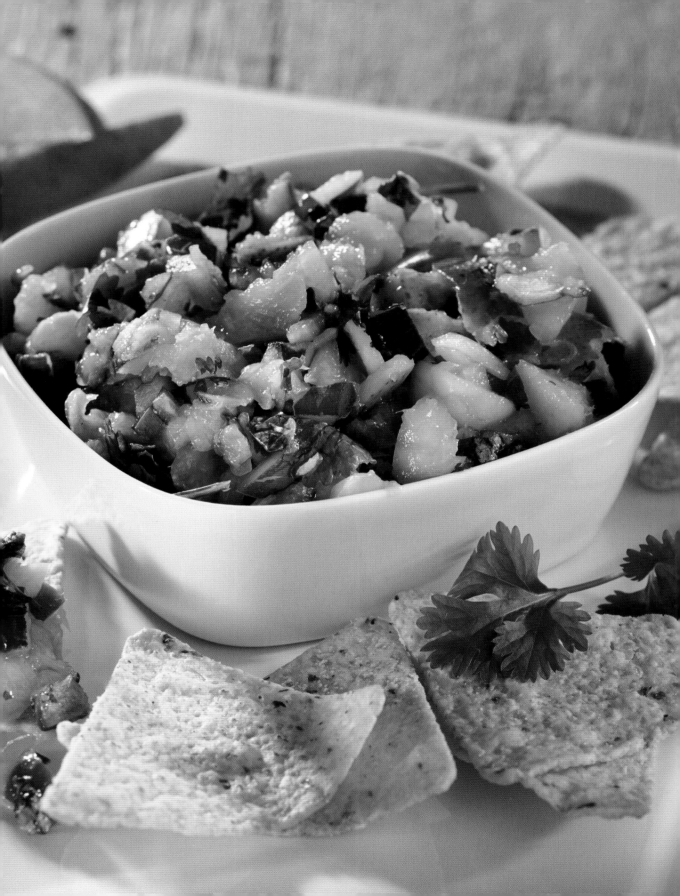

Mango Salsa

A fruity twist on the classic salsa, this recipe uses the whole mango (minus the pit), so no peeling or chopping required. Delicious with chips or spooned over baked fish or chicken.

Preparation: **10 minutes**   Processing: **15 seconds**   Yield: **720 ml**

2 semi-ripe mangoes, pitted but unpeeled, chunked

16 g fresh coriander

½ medium red onion, peeled and chopped (about 120 g)

1 jalapeño pepper, halved and seeded

1 tablespoon fresh lime or lemon juice

1. Place all the ingredients into the Vitamix container in the order listed and secure the lid. Select Variable 1. Turn the machine on and slowly increase the speed to Variable 4. Blend for 15 seconds, or until the desired consistency is reached, using the tamper to press the ingredients into the blades.

AMOUNT PER 30 ML SERVING: calories 20, total fat 0 g, saturated fat 0 g, cholesterol 0 mg, sodium 0 mg, total carbohydrate 5 g, dietary fibre 1 g, sugars 4 g, protein 0 g

California Salsa

Once you have made this fresh, bright salsa, you may hesitate to buy a jar at the shop again. This salsa is simple and bursting with flavour. Delicious with tortilla chips or spooned over a burrito.

Preparation: **15 minutes**   Processing: **30 seconds**   Yield: **720 ml**

½ **medium onion (55 g), peeled**

1 **jalapeño pepper, halved and seeded**

5 g **fresh coriander leaves**

1 **teaspoon fresh lemon juice**

½ **teaspoon salt**

6 **Roma (plum) tomatoes, quartered**

1. Place the onion, jalapeño, coriander, lemon juice, salt and 6 of the tomato quarters into the Vitamix container in the order listed and secure the lid. Select Variable 1. Turn the machine on and blend for 10 to 15 seconds, using the tamper to press the ingredients into the blades.

2. Stop the machine. Add the remaining tomato quarters. Select Variable 1. Blend until a chunky consistency is reached, using the tamper to press the ingredients into the blades. Increase the speed as necessary to attain that consistency. Do not overmix.

AMOUNT PER 30 ML SERVING: calories 5, total fat 0 g, saturated fat 0 g, cholesterol 0 mg, sodium 50 mg, total carbohydrate 1 g, dietary fibre 0 g, sugars 1 g, protein 0 g

Pineapple Salsa

Pineapple, while available to most of us all year, is at its best in season, from December to March. Luckily for salsa lovers, you can enjoy this vibrant pineapple salsa when you need a different dip for your tortilla chips, especially when good tomatoes are not in season.

Preparation: **20 minutes**   Processing: **10 seconds plus pulsing**   Yield: **540 ml**

2 tablespoons olive oil

½ lime, peeled

500 g large pieces peeled pineapple

½ teaspoon kosher salt

40 g chopped onion

75 g red pepper pieces
(2.5 cm square)

2 tablespoons chopped fresh
coriander leaves

¼ jalapeño pepper

1. Place the oil, lime, half the pineapple and salt into the Vitamix container in the order listed and secure the lid. Select Variable 1. Turn the machine on and slowly increase the speed to Variable 4. Blend for 10 seconds, using the tamper to press the ingredients into the blades.

2. Stop the machine and remove the lid. Add the remaining pineapple, the onion, pepper, coriander and jalapeño to the Vitamix container in the order listed and secure the lid. Select Variable 7. Use the On/Off switch to quickly pulse 7 to 10 times, until desired consistency is reached.

Don't worry about getting all the pineapple peel off. The Vitamix will break it down so you'll never know it's there, yet you'll benefit from the extra nutrition.

AMOUNT PER 30 ML SERVING: calories 30, total fat 1.5 g, saturated fat 0 g, cholesterol 0 mg, sodium 55 mg, total carbohydrate 4 g, dietary fibre 0 g, sugars 3 g, protein 0 g

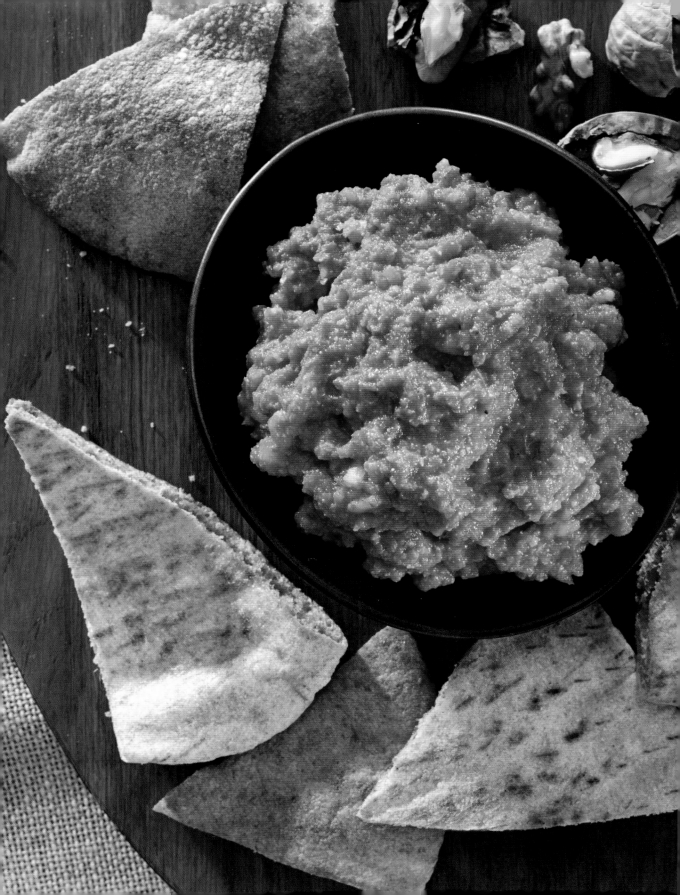

Muhammara
(Red Pepper and Walnut Dip)

This bright, tangy Middle-Eastern dip hails from Syria. Pomegranate molasses, which is simply pomegranate juice that has been reduced to a thick syrup, has a deep, tart flavour. It can be found at Middle-Eastern markets and now, more frequently, at your local grocery or health food store.

Preparation: **15 minutes**   Processing: **20 seconds**   Yield: **480 ml**

2 tablespoons olive oil

1 slice whole wheat bread

315 g roasted red peppers (page 91)

½ lemon, peeled and pips removed

2 teaspoons sweet paprika

¼ teaspoon cayenne pepper

2 teaspoons pomegranate molasses

1 garlic clove, peeled

½ teaspoon sea salt

¼ teaspoon ground black pepper

1. Heat the oil in a non-stick frying pan over a medium heat. Add the bread and fry both sides. Remove from the heat.

2. Place the toasted bread and oil from the frying pan into the Vitamix container, then add all the remaining ingredients in the order listed and secure the lid. Select Variable 1. Turn the machine on and slowly increase the speed to Variable 8. Blend for 20 seconds, using the tamper to press the ingredients into the blades.

AMOUNT PER 30 ML SERVING: calories 50, total fat 2 g, saturated fat 0 g, cholesterol 0 mg, sodium 280 mg, total carbohydrate 6 g, dietary fibre 0 g, sugars 1 g, protein 1 g

Aubergine Onion Dip

Garam masala is a spice blend that is used in Indian cooking. The ingredients vary regionally and by personal taste, but garam masala usually includes turmeric, black and white peppercorns, cumin seeds, cloves and cardamom seeds. The spice blend's gentle warmth is the perfect complement to the mellowness of roasted aubergine. Serve this delicious dip with toasted pitta chips.

Preparation: **10 minutes**   Processing: **40 seconds**   Bake time: 30 minutes   Yield: **480 ml**

1 medium aubergine (about 560 g), quartered lengthwise

3 tablespoons olive oil

270 g chopped onion

2 garlic cloves, peeled

2 tablespoons fresh mint leaves

2 tablespoons fresh coriander leaves

½ teaspoon garam masala

1. Pre-heat the oven to 240°C. Line a baking sheet with foil or a silicone baking mat.

2. Place the aubergine, skin side down, on the baking sheet and brush with 2 tablespoons of the olive oil.

3. Toss the onions and garlic with the remaining olive oil and place on the baking sheet.

4. Roast for 15 minutes. Rotate the baking sheet front to back and continue roasting until browned and tender, about 15 minutes longer.

5. When cool enough to handle, carefully peel the skin off of the aubergine.

6. Transfer all the roasted vegetables to the Vitamix container and secure the lid. Select Variable 1. Turn the machine on and slowly increase the speed to Variable 8. Blend for 30 seconds, using the tamper to press the ingredients into the blades.

7. Stop the machine and remove the lid plug. Add the mint, coriander and garam masala to the Vitamix container and secure the lid. Select Variable 1. Turn the machine on and slowly increase the speed to Variable 8. Blend for 10 seconds, using the tamper to press the ingredients into the blades.

AMOUNT PER 30 ML SERVING: calories 40, total fat 2.5 g, saturated fat 0 g, cholesterol 0 mg, sodium 0 mg, total carbohydrate 4 g, dietary fibre 2 g, sugars 2 g, protein 1 g

Hot Crab and Artichoke Dip

Hot, creamy and just plain delicious, this dip is sure to become a tradition at your winter festive parties. Serve with pitta chips or toast triangles for dipping.

Preparation: **15 minutes**   Processing: **30 seconds**   Bake time: **25–30 minutes**   Yield: **360 ml**

80 ml natural 0% Greek yoghurt, stirred

3 tablespoons fat-free mayonnaise

32 g grated Parmesan

2 garlic cloves, cut into pieces

170 g crabmeat, chopped

1 x 400 g can artichoke hearts, drained and coarsely chopped

⅓ teaspoon sweet paprika

1 x 115 g can chopped green chillies, drained

1. Pre-heat the oven to 180°C. Coat a 2-litre capacity baking dish with cooking spray.

2. Place the yoghurt, mayo, Parmesan and garlic into the Vitamix container in the order listed and secure the lid. Select Variable 1. Turn the machine on and slowly increase the speed to Variable 4. Blend for 20 seconds.

3. Stop the machine, remove the lid and scrape the sides of the container. Secure the lid. Select Variable 1. Turn the machine on and slowly increase the speed to Variable 3. Blend for 10 seconds until smooth.

4. Combine the crabmeat, artichoke hearts, paprika and chillies in the baking dish. Scrape the yoghurt mixture on top and stir gently to combine. Bake uncovered for 25–30 minutes, until a light golden brown and bubbling.

AMOUNT PER 30 ML SERVING: calories 40, total fat 1 g, saturated fat 0.5 g, cholesterol 5 mg, sodium 320 mg, total carbohydrate 5 g, dietary fibre 1 g, sugars 2 g, protein 3 g

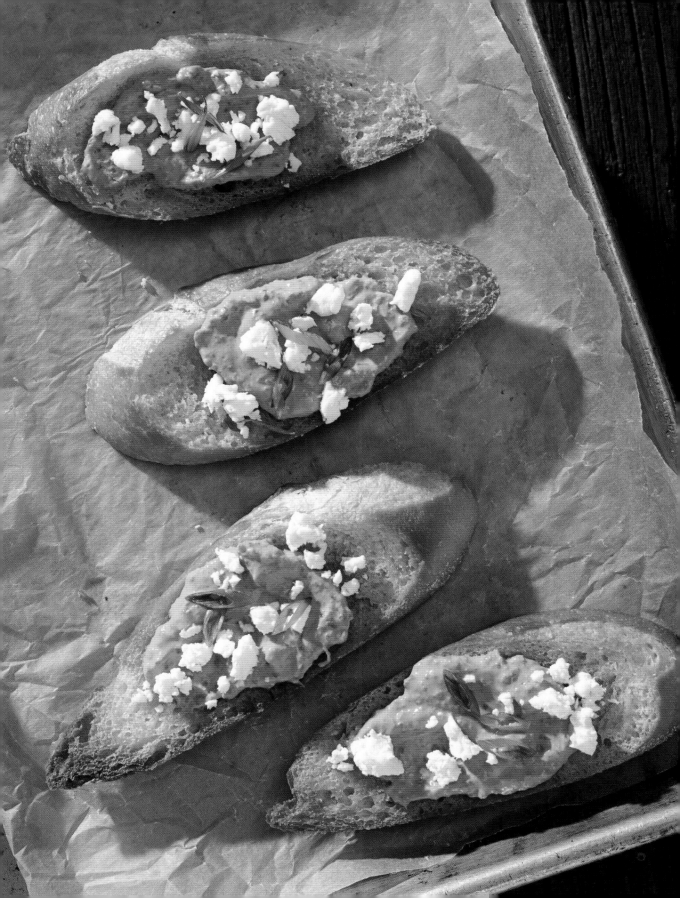

Goats' Cheese Crostini with Roasted Red Pepper Spread

An elegant appetizer for your next gathering. Both the toasts and the red pepper spread can be made a day in advance so these tasty snacks will come together in a snap! This spread is also wonderful on a sandwich with whole-grain bread, sharp Cheddar and spinach.

Preparation: **15 minutes**   Processing: **30 seconds**   Yield: **10 servings (2 crostini each); 360 ml spread**

1 baguette

2 tablespoons olive oil

115 g roasted red peppers (page 91)

1 spring onion, halved

1 roasted garlic clove, peeled

¼ teaspoon grated lemon zest

¼ teaspoon ground black pepper

¼ teaspoon sea salt

115 g Neufchâtel (⅓-less-fat cream cheese)

115 g goats' cheese, crumbled

1. Slice the baguette crossways into at least 20 slices and brush lightly with olive oil. Set aside.

2. Place the roasted peppers, spring onion, garlic, lemon zest, black pepper, salt and Neufchâtel into the Vitamix container in the order listed and secure the lid. Select Variable 1. Turn the machine on and slowly increase the speed to Variable 6. Blend for 30 seconds, using the tamper to press the ingredients into the blades.

3. Brush both sides of the sliced bread with olive oil. Toast in the oven at 170 degrees, turning until golden brown.

4. Spread the roasted pepper spread evenly on the baguette toasts. Top with goats' cheese and serve immediately.

AMOUNT PER SERVING: calories 280, total fat 8 g, saturated fat 3.5 g, cholesterol 15 mg, sodium 670 mg, total carbohydrate 41 g, dietary fibre 2 g, sugars 1 g, protein 12 g

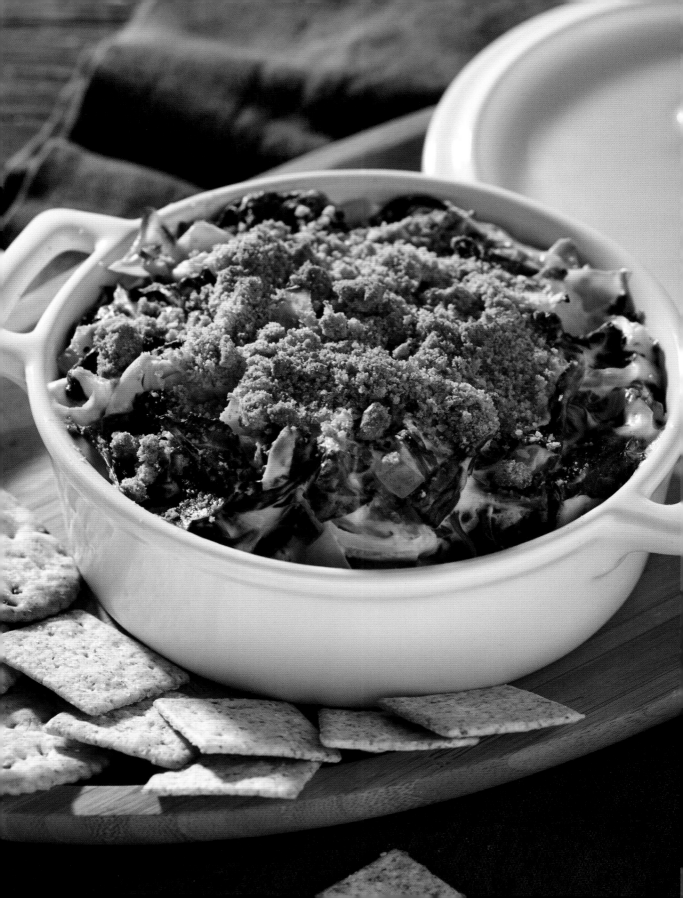

Yoghurt, Spinach and Artichoke Dip

Warm and hearty, this savoury spinach and artichoke dip will be a welcome addition to your next winter gathering. Serve it with pitta chips or home-made toasts.

Preparation: **20 minutes**   Processing: **20 seconds**   Bake time: **15 minutes**   Yield: **1.4 litres**

28 g whole-grain crackers, crushed

¼ teaspoon garlic powder

¼ teaspoon onion powder

2 tablespoons grated Parmesan

170 g natural 0% Greek yoghurt, stirred

115 g Neufchâtel (⅓-less-fat cream cheese)

1 teaspoon grated lemon zest

2 teaspoons chopped fresh oregano

2 teaspoons chopped fresh mint leaves

½ teaspoon sea salt

½ teaspoon ground black pepper

1 tablespoon olive oil

1 large onion (170 g), cut into pieces

1 garlic clove, peeled and finely chopped

140 g fresh spinach

1 x 400 g can water-packed artichoke hearts, rinsed, drained and cut into pieces

1. Pre-heat the oven to 200°C.

2. Combine the cracker crumbs, garlic powder, onion powder and Parmesan in a small bowl. Set aside.

3. Place the yoghurt, Neufchâtel, lemon zest, oregano, mint, salt and pepper into the Vitamix container in the order listed and secure the lid. Select Variable 1. Turn the machine on and slowly increase the speed to Variable 4. Blend for 20 seconds, using the tamper to press the ingredients into the blades.

4. Heat the oil in a frying pan over a medium heat. Add the onion and garlic and cook until soft, 4–6 minutes. Add the spinach and cook until soft and the liquid has evaporated, 4–6 minutes.

5. Remove from the heat and scrape in the artichokes and yoghurt mixture, stirring to combine. Spoon into a 20-cm square baking dish.

6. Sprinkle with the cracker crumb mixture and bake for 15 minutes, or until hot and bubbling. Serve hot.

AMOUNT PER 30 ML SERVING: calories 20, total fat 1 g, saturated fat 0 g, cholesterol 0 mg, sodium 100 mg, total carbohydrate 2 g, dietary fibre 1 g, sugars 0 g, protein 1 g

Two-Cheese Spread with Spinach

Bright and creamy and full of fresh spinach, this isn't your standard spinach dip. Feta, goats' cheese and 0% Greek yoghurt give this spread a decadent, smooth texture. Serve with crackers or pitta chips for an appetizer, or along with cut veggies and pitta wedges for a healthy lunch.

Preparation: **15 minutes**   Processing: **1 minute**   Yield: **480 ml**

55 g feta, at room temperature, crumbled

115 g goats' cheese, at room temperature, crumbled

180 ml natural 0% Greek yoghurt, stirred

75 g fresh spinach

1 garlic clove, peeled

2 teaspoons fresh mint leaves

1 teaspoon grated lemon zest

1 teaspoon fresh lemon juice

⅛ teaspoon sea salt

⅛ teaspoon ground black pepper

1. Place all the ingredients into the Vitamix container in the order listed and secure the lid. Select Variable 1. Turn the machine on and slowly increase the speed to Variable 10, then to High. Blend for 45 seconds.

2. Stop the machine, remove the lid, and scrape the mixture into the blades. Secure the lid. Select Variable 1. Turn the machine on and slowly increase the speed to Variable 10, then to High. Blend for 15 seconds.

AMOUNT PER 30 ML SERVING: calories 35, total fat 2.5 g, saturated fat 1.5 g, cholesterol 5 mg, sodium 95 mg, total carbohydrate 1 g, dietary fibre 0 g, sugars 1 g, protein 3 g

MARY LOU BUKAR

....

SALESPERSON AND PRODUCT REP FOR NATIONAL KITCHENWARE RETAILER, CHICAGO, ILLINOIS

As you read the nearly 250 recipes in this book, you will learn about all of the different jobs a Vitamix can do. Sure, smoothies, but did you know your machine could make hot soup, no stove required? That it can chop? That it can grind both fresh flours and meat? Or that it can make frozen treats that taste better than ice cream? The possibilities are endless, and once you know the ins and outs of your Vitamix, you can get creative. Make up your own family recipe for a smoothie or a whole-fruit margarita. Make a crisper-cleansing soup or juice. With your Vitamix and your imagination, you can make any number of delicious meals and snacks.

Mary Lou Bukar, an Illinois-based salesperson and product rep for a national kitchenware retailer, purchased her first Vitamix in 2009. Like many a fan, Mary Lou uses her machine a lot, taking advantage of multiple Vitamix techniques. Mary Lou loves using her Vitamix to 'think outside the box' when she tackles meal preparation. Some days she uses her machine to grate cheese, whip up a quick dressing or chop veggies. Other times, Mary Lou will make a fresh pesto or nut butter. All very fast to make, each finished dish is delicious. And she really appreciates being able to make different dishes at home using whole foods instead of having to buy processed products at the shop. 'It's not surprising to me how easy it is to substitute whole, raw foods for processed food products when you use a Vitamix in meal preparation', remarks Mary Lou.

Using the machine's diverse capacities has allowed Mary Lou to bring more whole foods into her daily diet in a number of different forms. Her favourite thing to make is whole-food juices, using a variety of vegetables, fruits and spices to whip up drinks 'brightly coloured by nature, not by chemicals'. Later she might make fresh salsa or peanut butter for a healthy snack. When it comes to dinner, Mary Lou uses her Vitamix to whip up a fresh, nutritious sauce or dressing. A delicious dessert often rounds out the day; whipping up cream, mixing a cake batter or making a quick frozen yoghurt. In a day, she might very well make a recipe from every category in this book! And in the process, she is eating lots of scrumptious, nutritious food, too. A whole food success story for sure!

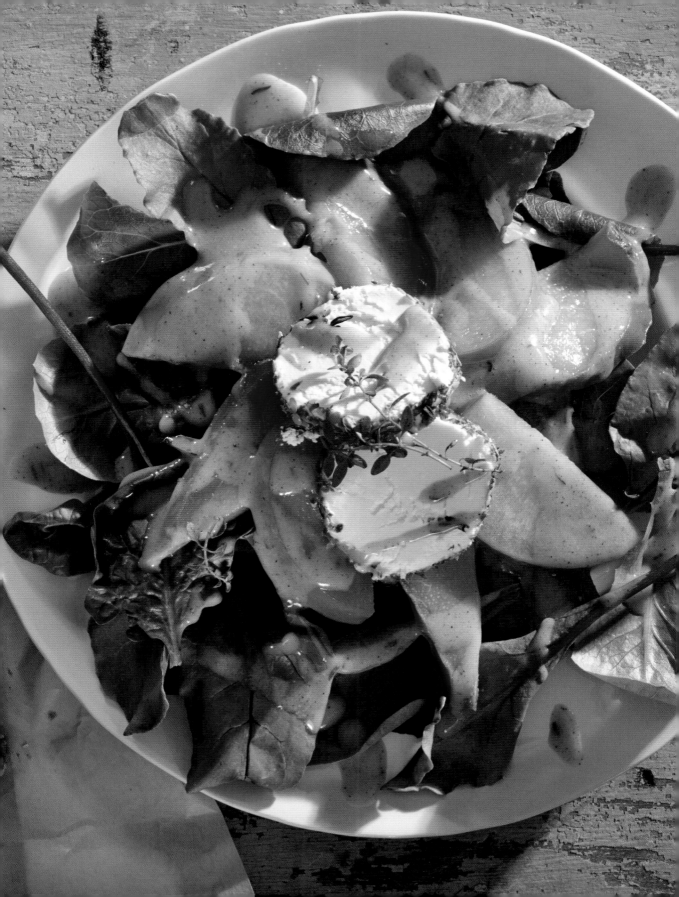

Chapter 4

Soups, Salads and Sides

Soups, side dishes and salads are a wonderful way to get more fruits, vegetables and whole grains into your diet. In this chapter, you will find recipes for fresh and crunchy vegetable salads, hearty grain salads, gluten-free rolls, and cooked vegetable dishes. And the soups! Hearty, chunky soups perfect for the coldest winter days, soothing puréed soups bursting with flavour and refreshing cold soups for the most sweltering summer days. There are even soups that are made completely in the Vitamix, without using the stove.

Any of these soups and sides would be a wonderful addition to a meal or a great light lunch or supper in and of themselves.

Soups

Restaurants value our products because they can create silky smooth sauces, soups and vinaigrettes, among other things. In this chapter, you'll find recipes that allow you to achieve similarly sumptuous results at home. Recipes such as Beetroot Soup with Goats' Cheese and Almonds (page 121), Carrot with Fennel Soup (page 129), Garden-Fresh Tomato Soup (page 150) allow you to enjoy lusciously smooth and just plain delightful soup.

Here are a few tips to keep in mind when you are puréeing hot soups.

- Be careful! The very act of transferring hot soup to a blender can be tricky for some, and there is no harm in letting the soup cool for a few minutes before beginning to purée it!

- Position lid on container with lid flaps midway between the spout and the handle. Push the lid on to the container until it locks in place. The lid must always be secured when processing, especially hot liquids that may scald.

- Don't overfill the container. Hot liquids expand. It is usually safer to fill the canister a little over half-full, so that the hot liquid doesn't overflow while you are blending it.

- When blending hot ingredients, start your Vitamix on a low speed.

My husband, Frank, learned about checking the lid and the speed the hard way. We were hosting our first Thanksgiving dinner. The table was set, the turkey was cooked and all the side dishes were prepared and ready to go. We called everyone to dinner as Frank started to make his famous gravy by putting the pan drippings and vegetables in the Vitamix with his secret ingredient – fresh apple. So as we are all gathering around the table, which was right next to the counter, which was right next to the gas hob – it was a very tiny kitchen – he turned the Vitamix on without the lid. And on top of the fact that there was no lid, the speed was on high. Hot grease went straight up in the air, coated the ceiling and splashed down on the hob, bursting into flames. No one was hurt and everyone jumped in to put out the fire and clean up the walls, ceiling and counter. It managed to completely miss the table and all the guests. Thirty minutes later we sat down with one more thing to be thankful for. And of course, he has never forgotten to put the lid on again!

Silky smooth soups are wonderful, but sometimes we crave something more substantial. No problem. After blending your soup until it is steamy and hot, simply add additional ingredients and pulse the blades several times to give it a chunkier, heartier texture. This is the technique used in some soups, like Tuscan Bean Soup with Whole Grains (page 157). In others, such as Garden-Fresh Minestrone (page 156), stock, tomatoes and beans are puréed to make a lovely, nutrient-rich stock, and this stock is used, in turn, to simmer the vegetables. Puréeing a portion of a cooked soup, as you do in Barley and Vegetable Soup (page 149), makes a slightly heartier, less brothy soup without making it entirely smooth.

One of the most amazing features of the Vitamix is its ability to make a soup ready to serve directly from the blender – no hob required. The fact that you can make a cold soup in the Vitamix will be less of a revelation, although you will appreciate Chilled Cucumber and Avocado Soup (page 148) and Avocado Soup with Chipotle Yoghurt (page 117) on a hot day just the same. Still, on that crazy-busy day when you come through the door and just want to eat right now – yes, this very minute, the fact that you can put raw vegetables in the Vitamix and make hot soup so quickly is something pretty special. You can toss the ingredients for Easy 'Cheesey' Vegan Broccoli Soup (page 134), Black Bean Tortilla Soup (page 132) or Chicken Potato Soup (page 144) – my family's favourite; we serve it in a bread bowl – into the Vitamix and make hot soup in the time it takes to unload the dishwasher . . . maybe even a little faster. Not only will you be able to get a meal on the table quickly, but your food will contain whole foods and less sodium than many other convenience dishes. Fast, healthy and delicious food! A truly winning combination.

Salads and Sides

Fresh, crunchy salads, gluten-free rolls (and a recipe for flour), hearty grain salads and cooked vegetable sides abound in this chapter too. Any of these would be a perfect accompaniment to a main dish, or you could build a whole meal out of one or two of these recipes.

You may enjoy a nice bowl of simply dressed leafy greens, but it may be easier to eat more veggies if you expand your salad repertoire with the recipes found in this chapter. There are lots of kale salads on restaurant menus these days, but we would challenge any of them to hold a candle to our nutrient-packed Kale Salad with Avocado-Tahini Dressing (page 167). This salad is full of veggies and has a dressing that contains the healthy fats found in avocado and sesame seeds, plus a handful of kale. Both Fiesta Salad (page 170) and Lime-Dressed Ginger Carrot Slaw (page 169) use whole fruits to bring flavour and nutrients to salads with lots of different crunchy vegetables. Pear and Apple Salad (page 171) pairs greens and lightly poached fruit with a maple and flax seed oil vinaigrette and goats' cheese encrusted with flax seeds and fresh thyme. This composed salad would make an elegant first course for your next dinner party or a lovely light lunch.

Salads can be made from more than just vegetables of course; this chapter contains a number of grain- and seed-based salads. These hearty sides are perfect as part of a meal or as a substantial lunch or entree. Chewy barley is featured in two delightful salads. The first, our Barley and Sweetcorn Salad (page 162), dresses barley, sweetcorn, cucumbers and tomatoes with a yoghurt and chive dressing. The second, our Festive Barley Salad (page 165), has both raw and steamed vegetables tossed with a red wine vinaigrette with fresh herbs. In our Southwestern Quinoa Salad (page 172), quinoa, technically a seed, shines in a hearty salad with a slightly spicy dressing, black beans, sweetcorn, peppers, chillies and red onion. This salad travels well and would be an excellent addition to a potluck or packed lunch. Try bulghar, a quick-cooking whole wheat similar to couscous, in the herb-packed Lebanese Tabbouleh (page 173).

There are just a handful of cooked vegetable sides in this chapter, but all are worthy of a place on your table. In our Bulghar-Stuffed Baby Potatoes (page 176), cooked and cooled red potatoes are stuffed with a delicious mixture of bulghar, leeks, sweetcorn and parsley-pistachio pesto. These flavour-packed potatoes are the perfect appetizer or side dish. They can also be made ahead of time and served at room temperature. A wild-rice stuffing dish pairs cooked seeds (that's the wild rice) with a few veggies, lots of dried fruit and crunchy pumpkin seeds. The perfect, naturally gluten-free stuffing for your holiday meal.

With so many ways to bring variety, nutrition and amazing flavour, getting more whole foods into your diet will be a snap!

Avocado Soup with Chipotle Yoghurt

Cold soups are the perfect meal for a steamy summer day. This mellow, creamy-without-cream avocado soup with the gently smoky chipotle yoghurt will fill you up without making you feel too hot or too full. This soup would be delicious with Southwestern Quinoa Salad (page 172) on the side.

Preparation: **15 minutes**   Processing: **2 minutes 30 seconds**   Cook time: **5 minutes**   Yield: **2 litres**

CHIPOTLE YOGHURT:

240 ml natural 0% Greek yoghurt, stirred

1 teaspoon chipotle peppers in adobo sauce, coarsely chopped

SOUP:

2 tablespoons olive oil

160 g chopped onion

1 garlic clove, peeled

1.4 litres fat-free low-sodium chicken stock

1 teaspoon grated lime zest

2 tablespoons fresh lime juice

2 tablespoons fresh coriander leaves

1 teaspoon sea salt

4 avocados, halved, pitted and peeled

1. For the chipotle yoghurt: Place the yoghurt and chipotle peppers with their sauce into the Vitamix container and secure the lid. Select Variable 1. Turn the machine on and slowly increase to Variable 4. Blend for 10 seconds. Stop the machine, scrape the sides and repeat 2 times. Spoon into a bowl and chill until serving time.

2. For the soup: Heat the olive oil in a frying pan over a medium-high heat. Add the onion and garlic and cook until translucent, about 5 minutes. Do not brown. Let cool.

3. Place half the chicken stock, half of the onion and garlic mixture, ½ teaspoon of the lime zest, 1 tablespoon of the lime juice, 1 tablespoon of the coriander, ½ teaspoon of the sea salt and 4 avocado halves in the Vitamix container in the order listed and secure the lid. Select Variable 1. Turn the machine on and slowly increase the speed to Variable 10, then to High. Blend for 1 minute.

4. Pour the puréed soup into a large bowl. Repeat with the remaining ingredients. Stir together both batches to combine. Chill slightly before serving. Store leftovers in a covered container for up to 2 days. Use leftover yoghurt as a salad dressing or a dip for fresh vegetables.

**AMOUNT PER 240 ML SOUP (WITH 1 TABLESPOON CHIPOTLE YOGHURT):
calories 160, total fat 13 g, saturated fat 2 g, cholesterol 0 mg, sodium 340 mg, total carbohydrate 9 g, dietary fibre 5 g, sugars 2 g, protein 5 g**

Potato and Cauliflower Bisque

This thick richly flavoured soup with fresh herbs has a pop of freshness from the bright essential oils of the lemon zest. The Bisque is delicious on a cold Autumn or Winter afternoon, or for a light dinner with fresh baked bread and a green salad.

Preparation: **15 minutes**   Processing: **6 minutes 40 seconds**   Cook time: **4–6 minutes**   Yield: **1.5 litres**

1 tablespoon olive oil

60 g chopped onion

50 g diced celery

2 small garlic cloves, peeled

½ teaspoon fresh thyme leaves

½ teaspoon fresh rosemary leaves

240 ml low-fat (1%) milk

600 ml low-sodium chicken stock

365 g quartered Yukon Gold potatoes, parboiled (see note)

105 g cauliflower florets, blanched

1 teaspoon sea salt

¼ teaspoon ground black pepper

¼ teaspoon grated lemon zest

OPTIONAL GARNISHES:

Finely chopped chives (or other herbs)

Cracked black pepper

Chilli oil

1. Heat the olive oil in a frying pan over a medium heat. Add the onion, celery and garlic and cook until translucent, 4–6 minutes. Do not brown. Add the thyme and rosemary and stir to coat.

2. Place the milk, stock, potatoes, cauliflower, sautéed vegetable mixture, salt and pepper into the Vitamix container in that order and secure the lid. Select Variable 1. Turn the machine on and slowly increase the speed to Variable 10, then to High. Blend for 6 minutes 30 seconds, or until heavy steam escapes from the vented lid.

3. Reduce the speed to Variable 2 and remove the lid plug. Through the lid plug opening, add the lemon zest and blend for an additional 10 seconds.

4. Serve hot. If desired, garnish with chopped chives (or other herbs), cracked pepper or chilli oil.

Note: To parboil the potatoes and blanch the cauliflower for this recipe, place the potatoes in a medium pan and cover them with cold water by about 5 cm. Add a pinch of sea salt, cover and bring to the boil over a high heat. Meanwhile, cut the cauliflower into florets. When the potatoes come to a boil, add the cauliflower and continue cooking until both are just tender, about 4 minutes longer. Drain the potatoes and cauliflower and proceed with the recipe as directed.

AMOUNT PER 240 ML SERVING (WITHOUT GARNISHES): calories 100, total fat 2.5 g, saturated fat 0.5 g, cholesterol 0 mg, sodium 450 mg, total carbohydrate 14 g, dietary fibre 1 g, sugars 3 g, protein 5 g

Bean and Squash Soup

This soup is the perfect last-minute supper, composed almost entirely of store cupboard staples. The ginger, Tabasco sauce and lemon juice balance out the natural sweetness of the squash. The chickpeas add fibre and protein, making the soup more filling. Vegetarian and vegan as is. Make extra to freeze!

Preparation: **15 minutes**   Processing: **30 seconds**   Cook time: **30–35 minutes**   Yield: **1.7 litres**

2 tablespoons olive oil

170 g onion, peeled and cut into small pieces

2 garlic cloves, peeled

½ teaspoon ground cinnamon

½ teaspoon ground cumin

½ teaspoon ground ginger

¼ teaspoon ground cloves

1 tablespoon light brown sugar

900 g butternut squash, peeled, seeded and cut into small pieces

720 ml low-sodium vegetable stock

1 x 440 g can chickpeas, rinsed and drained

Dash of Tabasco sauce

1 teaspoon fresh lemon juice

1. Heat the olive oil in a large pan over a medium heat. Add the onion and garlic and cook until the onions are translucent. Stir in the cinnamon, cumin, ginger, cloves, brown sugar and squash. Cook, stirring frequently, until the squash is fragrant and just beginning to soften, about 5 minutes.

2. Add the stock and bring to a boil. Reduce to a simmer, cover, and cook until the squash is tender, 20–25 minutes. Add the chickpeas, Tabasco and lemon juice.

3. Ladle the hot soup into the Vitamix container and secure the lid. Select Variable 1. Turn the machine on and slowly increase the speed to Variable 10, then to High. Blend for 30 seconds.

4. Serve hot.

AMOUNT PER 240 ML SERVING: calories 160, total fat 5 g, saturated fat 0.5 g, cholesterol 0 mg, sodium 140 mg, total carbohydrate 27 g, dietary fibre 3 g, sugars 7 g, protein 4 g

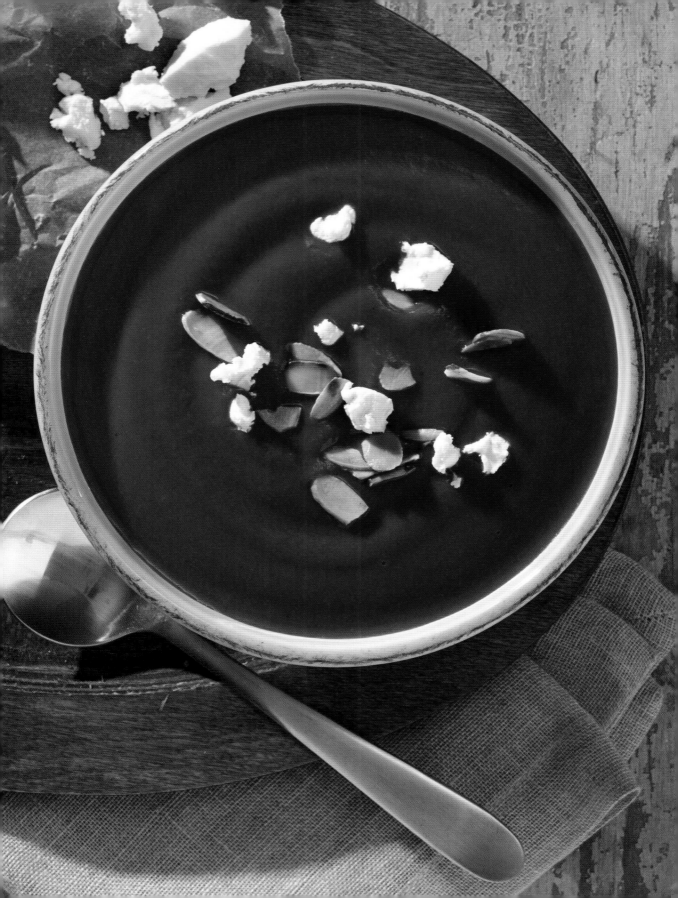

Beetroot Soup with Goats' Cheese and Almonds

In season through the autumn, beetroots add a wonderful splash of colour when the colours on our plates begin to lose the brilliant cornucopia of summer. You won't be able to taste the roasted Roma tomatoes in the final product, but their acidity will keep the beetroot flavour from being too sweet.

Preparation: **45 minutes**   Processing: **1 minute**   Cook time: **30 minutes**   Yield: **1.7 litres**

2 tablespoons olive oil

225 g chopped onion

1 garlic clove, peeled and halved

4 medium beetroots (570 g total), roasted, cooled, peeled and diced

4 Roma (plum) tomatoes, halved, roasted and cooled

½ teaspoon sea salt

¼ teaspoon ground black pepper

720 ml low-sodium chicken stock

GARNISHES:

115 g goats' cheese, crumbled

100 g flaked almonds, lightly toasted

1. Heat the olive oil in a large pan over a medium heat. Add the onion and garlic and cook until the onion is translucent, 6–8 minutes.

2. Add the beetroots, tomatoes, salt and pepper and cook for 4 minutes until the tomatoes have released most of their liquid.

3. Add the stock and bring to a boil. Reduce to a simmer, cover and cook for 15 minutes.

4. Ladle the hot soup into the Vitamix container and secure the lid. Select Variable 1. Turn the machine on and slowly increase the speed to Variable 10, then to High. Blend for 1 minute.

5. Serve the soup hot. Garnish with goats' cheese and almonds.

AMOUNT PER 240 ML SERVING: calories 220, total fat 14 g, saturated fat 3.5 g, cholesterol 5 mg, sodium 360 mg, total carbohydrate 17 g, dietary fibre 5 g, sugars 9 g, protein 10 g

Broccoli Cheese Soup

One of the wonders of the Vitamix is the machine's ability to take raw ingredients and transform them into steaming hot soup. Imagine taking the store cupboard staples for this soup, putting them in your Vitamix, and having dinner in the time it takes to set the table! The rest of our busy lives should be so easy. And because you are making the soup yourself, you can avoid the extra fat and sodium that would likely be in a canned soup.

Preparation: **10 minutes**   Processing: **5–6 minutes**   Yield: **600 ml**

240 ml skimmed milk

60 g grated Cheddar

150 g fresh or frozen broccoli or cauliflower florets, steamed

1 teaspoon diced onion

80 ml low-sodium vegetable stock

Place all the ingredients into the Vitamix container in the order listed and secure the lid. Select Variable 1. Turn the machine on and slowly increase the speed to Variable 10, then to High. Blend for 5–6 minutes, or until heavy steam escapes from the vented lid.

AMOUNT PER 240 ML SERVING: calories 110, total fat 2 g, saturated fat 1 g, cholesterol 5 mg, sodium 250 mg, total carbohydrate 13 g, dietary fibre 3 g, sugars 7 g, protein 11 g

Sassy Sweet Potato Soup

Because sweet potatoes are bursting with beta-carotene, vitamin B6 and potassium and because this soup is simple and quick to assemble, you may reach for this recipe instead of chicken soup the next time you are feeling under the weather. And it is so delicious, you will enjoy this in times of sickness and health!

Preparation: **15 minutes**   Processing: **45 seconds**   Cook time: **25 minutes**   Yield: **840 ml**

1 tablespoon olive oil

1 teaspoon toasted sesame oil

17 g chopped fresh ginger

420 g cubed peeled sweet potato

1 tablespoon honey

½ teaspoon sea salt

1. Heat both oils in a medium frying pan over a medium-high heat. Add the ginger and cook until fragrant and lightly golden. Remove the frying pan from the heat.

2. Bring 730 ml water to a boil in a medium pan. Add the sweet potato, honey and salt. Reduce to a simmer and cook until sweet potatoes are very tender, 15–20 minutes.

3. Scrape the sautéed ginger into the Vitamix container. Pour in the hot sweet potato mixture and secure the lid. Select Variable 1. Turn the machine on and slowly increase the speed to Variable 10, then to High. Blend for 45 seconds.

4. Serve hot.

AMOUNT PER 240 ML SERVING: calories 170, total fat 5 g, saturated fat 1 g, cholesterol 0 mg, sodium 400 mg, total carbohydrate 30 g, dietary fibre 4 g, sugars 10 g, protein 2 g

Autumn Flavours Bisque

This mellow bisque is like autumn in a bowl. Pumpkin purée, a little apple juice and maple syrup, cinnamon, thyme and cloves. And vanilla? And white balsamic vinegar? Yes and yes! The vanilla adds a wonderful aroma while the vinegar brightens up the otherwise mellow soup.

Preparation: **20 minutes**   Processing: **40 seconds**   Yield: **1.2 litres**

1 tablespoon olive oil

35 g coarsely chopped onion

35 g chopped shallots

5-mm-thick slice of peeled fresh ginger

2 tablespoons unbleached plain flour

720 ml fat-free low-sodium chicken stock

4 tablespoons 100% apple juice

284 g pumpkin purée, preferably home-made (page 75)

1 tablespoon pure maple syrup

¼ teaspoon ground cinnamon

¼ teaspoon ground thyme

¼ teaspoon sea salt

⅛ teaspoon ground black pepper

Pinch of ground cloves

120 ml unsweetened almond milk

¼ teaspoon vanilla extract

1 teaspoon white balsamic vinegar

1. Heat the olive oil in a stock pot over a medium-high heat. Add the onion, shallots and ginger. Cook, stirring, until the shallots and onion are tender, about 2 minutes. Do not brown.

2. Add the flour, stir to coat all the vegetables, then add the stock and apple juice. Bring to a boil, then reduce to a simmer and cook until slightly thickened.

3. Whisk in the pumpkin, maple syrup, cinnamon, thyme, salt, pepper and cloves. Bring to a boil, then reduce to a low heat and simmer for 15 minutes until flavours are blended.

4. Ladle the hot mixture into the Vitamix container. Add the almond milk, vanilla and vinegar and secure the lid. Select Variable 1. Turn the machine on and slowly increase the speed to Variable 10, then to High. Blend for 40 seconds.

5. Serve hot.

AMOUNT PER 240 ML SERVING: calories 90, total fat 3.5 g, saturated fat 0 g, cholesterol 0 mg, sodium 410 mg, total carbohydrate 14 g, dietary fibre 3 g, sugars 7 g, protein 2 g

Coconut Green Curry Soup

The green curry paste that makes up the base for this soup is traditionally made with green chillies, lemon grass, kaffir lime peel, shallots, garlic, galangal, coriander seeds, cumin seeds, shrimp paste, red turmeric, white peppercorns, coriander root and salt. This wonderful array of ingredients adds up to a deep, nuanced flavour for this delicious soup.

Preparation: **20 minutes**   Processing: **1 minute**   Cook time: **25 minutes**   Yield: **1.5 litres**

2 tablespoons sesame oil

2 garlic cloves, chopped

55 g chopped spring onions (white parts only), green tops reserved

20 g thinly sliced lemon grass (cut on an angle)

1 tablespoon chopped fresh ginger

215 g julienned shiitake mushroom caps

960 ml white miso broth

420 ml canned light coconut milk

2 tablespoons green curry paste

35 g diced red pepper

28 g thinly sliced spring onion greens (cut on an angle)

38 g sweetcorn kernels

OPTIONAL GARNISHES:

Thinly sliced chillies

Fresh coriander leaves

Beansprouts

Lime wedges

1. Heat 1 tablespoon of the sesame oil in a large pan. Add the garlic, spring onion whites, lemon grass and ginger and cook until aromatic, 2–3 minutes. Add half the shiitakes and cook until soft and wilted, 4–6 minutes.

2. Add the broth, coconut milk and green curry paste and bring to a boil. Reduce to a simmer, cover and cook for 15 minutes until the flavours are blended.

3. Ladle the hot soup into the Vitamix container and secure the lid. Select Variable 1. Turn the machine on and slowly increase the speed to Variable 10, then to High. Blend for 1 minute.

4. Wipe out the pan and return to a medium-high heat. Add the remaining oil, pepper, spring onion greens, sweetcorn and remaining shiitakes. Cook just until soft, 2–3 minutes.

5. Add the puréed broth and bring to a simmer. Cover and cook for 15 minutes until heated through.

6. Serve hot. If desired, garnish with sliced chillies, coriander or beansprouts, and serve with a lime wedge to squeeze over.

AMOUNT PER 240 ML SERVING (WITHOUT GARNISHES): calories 100, total fat 7 g, saturated fat 2.5 g, cholesterol 0 mg, sodium 300 mg, total carbohydrate 7 g, dietary fibre 2 g, sugars 2 g, protein 2 g

Roasted Sweetcorn, Pepper and Tomato Chowder

Roasting the sweetcorn, tomatoes and red peppers concentrates their flavours and gives them a slight smokiness. This smokiness, complemented by a little chipotle powder, gives this soup wonderful depth.

Preparation: **20 minutes plus roasting times**   Processing: **3 minutes**
Cook time: **35 minutes**   Yield: **1.9 litres**

680 g tomatoes, halved

3 tablespoons extra virgin olive oil

295 g sweetcorn kernels

3 red peppers (625 g), halved and roasted

200 g chopped onion

2 garlic cloves, finely chopped

¼ teaspoon chipotle powder

¼ teaspoon sea salt

¼ teaspoon ground black pepper

720 ml fat-free low-sodium chicken stock

280 g cooked brown rice

35 g diced avocado, for garnish

2 tablespoons finely chopped fresh herbs or spring onions, for garnish

1. Pre-heat the grill to high.

2. Place the tomato halves in a large bowl with 1 tablespoon of the olive oil and toss to coat. Place cut side down on a foil-lined baking sheet. Grill for 12 minutes, or until charred. Set aside to cool.

3. Add the sweetcorn kernels to a large bowl and toss with 1 tablespoon of the olive oil. Spread on a baking sheet and grill for 8 minutes, or until charred.

4. Once cooled, peel the tomatoes. Cut the peppers and tomatoes into large pieces and combine in a large bowl with the roasted sweetcorn kernels.

5. Heat the remaining olive oil in a large pan over a medium-high heat. Add the onion and garlic and cook for 3 minutes. Add the chipotle powder, roasted vegetables, salt, black pepper and stock. Bring to a boil, then reduce to a simmer and cook for 10 minutes until the flavours are blended.

6. Ladle one-third of the hot soup into the Vitamix container and secure the lid. Turn the machine on and slowly increase the speed to Variable 10, then to High. Blend for 1 minute.

7. Pour the hot soup into a clean pan. Repeat for 2 more batches. Stir together all three batches to combine. Add the rice to the soup and mix thoroughly.

8. Serve hot, garnished with avocado and herbs (or spring onions).

AMOUNT PER 240 ML SERVING: calories 190, total fat 7 g, saturated fat 1 g, cholesterol 0 mg, sodium 270 mg, total carbohydrate 29 g, dietary fibre 5 g, sugars 9 g, protein 5 g

Curried Corn and Coconut Soup

Sweet from corn and apple, creamy from low-fat coconut milk, and gently spiced from curry powder, Madras curry paste and cayenne, this brilliantly yellow soup is sure to please. Garnish with a little coriander or cooked sweetcorn. Add sautéed prawns to turn this into a main-dish soup. Always serve it with lime wedges, as the acidity from the lime brightens up the soup.

Preparation: **15 minutes**   Processing: **2 minutes**   Cook time: **25 minutes**   Yield: **2.8 litres**

1 tablespoon olive oil

135 g chopped onion

1 medium apple, cored and cut into pieces

1 teaspoon curry powder

60 ml red curry paste

½ teaspoon sea salt

¼ teaspoon ground black pepper

Pinch of cayenne pepper

900 g frozen sweetcorn kernels

960 ml low-sodium vegetable stock

240 ml canned light coconut milk

Lime wedges, for squeezing

OPTIONAL GARNISHES:

Sweetcorn kernels

Fresh coriander leaves

1. Heat the olive oil in a large stock pot. Add the onion and apple and cook until they just begin to soften, 2–3 minutes. Add the curry powder, curry paste, salt, black pepper and cayenne and stir to coat.

2. Add the sweetcorn and cook for 2–3 minutes, stirring frequently. Add the stock and coconut milk and bring to a boil. Reduce to a simmer, cover and cook for 15 minutes or until slightly softened.

3. Ladle half of the hot soup into the Vitamix container and secure the lid. Select Variable 1. Turn the machine on and slowly increase the speed to Variable 10, then to High. Blend for 1 minute.

4. Pour the puréed soup into a clean pan. Repeat with the remaining soup. Stir together both batches until combined.

5. Serve hot, with lime wedges for squeezing. If desired, garnish with sweetcorn and coriander. Recipe may easily be halved.

AMOUNT PER 240 ML SERVING (WITHOUT GARNISHES): calories 120, total fat 3.5 g, saturated fat 1.5 g, cholesterol 0 mg, sodium 170 mg, total carbohydrate 20 g, dietary fibre 3 g, sugars 5 g, protein 2 g

Earthy, Smoky Grilled Asparagus Soup

This silky-smooth soup shows nutrient-rich asparagus in a whole new light. Lightly smoky and a little garlicky, this soup is the perfect dish to serve when spring has officially arrived, but the nights are still chilly. Garnish with a little 0% fat Greek yoghurt and thin slices of the reserved asparagus spears.

Preparation: **15 minutes**   Processing: **40 seconds**   Cook time: **30 minutes**   Yield: **1.6 litres**

680 g asparagus spears, trimmed

3 tablespoons olive oil

¼ teaspoon ground black pepper

250 g diced red onion

2 garlic cloves, peeled and halved

2 teaspoons chopped fresh rosemary

960 ml low-sodium vegetable stock

½ teaspoon sea salt

1 tablespoon fresh lemon juice

120 ml natural 0% Greek yoghurt, stirred

1. Pre-heat a grill or griddle pan to a medium-high heat.

2. Toss the asparagus with 1½ tablespoons olive oil to coat in a large bowl.

3. Grill the asparagus, working in small batches, until tender and lightly charred.

4. Cut one-third of the asparagus into small pieces on the diagonal and set aside for garnish. Cut the remaining asparagus into 2.5-cm pieces.

5. Heat the remaining oil in a large pan. Add the onion and garlic and cook until the onion is translucent, about 5 minutes. Add the rosemary and cook for 1 minute. Add the stock and salt and bring to a boil. Reduce to a simmer and cook for 10 minutes. Add the asparagus pieces and lemon juice and cook for 5 minutes longer.

6. Ladle the mixture into the Vitamix container and secure the lid. Select Variable 1. Turn the machine on and slowly increase the speed to Variable 10, then to High. Blend for 40 seconds.

7. Serve the soup hot garnished with yoghurt and reserved asparagus.

AMOUNT PER 240 ML SERVING: calories 110, total fat 6 g, saturated fat 1 g, cholesterol 0 mg, sodium 260 mg, total carbohydrate 11 g, dietary fibre 3 g, sugars 5 g, protein 4 g

Carrot with Fennel Soup

More than a few of us have been told, 'Eat your carrots! They are good for your eyes!' This popular advice is actually the by-product, in part, of some clever British propaganda during World War II. During the war, the British Air Force ran an ad campaign that claimed that their pilots' accuracy was the result of the pilots eating lots of carrots. Truthfully, a new radar system was responsible for the Air Force's success, but the Air Force wanted to hide this truth from the German government. There is truth in the advertisement, though. The lutein and beta-carotene in carrots are known to be beneficial for eye health, particularly in preventing glaucoma. This flavourful soup, with its beautiful and bright orange colour, will be a feast for your eyes, and it may help keep them healthy too!

Preparation: **20 minutes**   Processing: **2 minutes**   Cook time: **20–25 minutes**   Yield: **2.2 litres**

1 tablespoon olive oil

170 g coarsely chopped onion

1 fennel bulb (312 g), cut into pieces

680 g carrots, cut into pieces

1 teaspoon sea salt

½ teaspoon ground fennel, lightly toasted

1 teaspoon ground coriander

1.4 litres low-sodium vegetable stock

½ teaspoon grated orange zest

OPTIONAL GARNISHES:

Cardamon-spiced Greek yoghurt

Chopped toasted pistachios

Ground fennel

1. Heat the olive oil in a large stock pot. Add the onion and fresh fennel and cook until the onion just begins to soften, 4–6 minutes.

2. Add the carrots, salt, ground fennel and coriander and cook for 1 minute. Add the stock, bring to a boil, then reduce to a simmer, cover and cook until the carrots are tender, 15–20 minutes. Remove from the heat and stir in the orange zest.

3. Ladle half of the hot mixture into the Vitamix container and secure the lid. Select Variable 1. Turn the machine on and slowly increase the speed to Variable 10, then to High. Blend for 1 minute.

4. Pour the puréed soup into a clean pan. Repeat with the remaining soup. Stir together both batches of soup.

5. Serve hot. If desired, garnish with the yoghurt, pistachios or fennel.

AMOUNT PER 240 ML SERVING (WITHOUT GARNISHES): calories 70, total fat 2 g, saturated fat 0 g, cholesterol 0 mg, sodium 400 mg, total carbohydrate 12 g, dietary fibre 4 g, sugars 5 g, protein 1 g

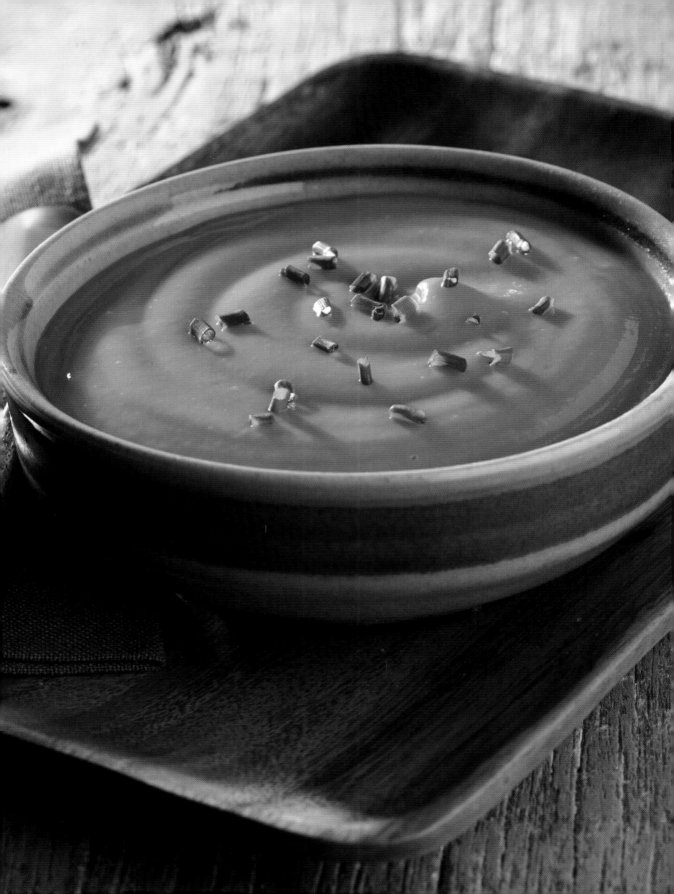

Carrot-Ginger Soup

This marigold-orange soup will brighten even the dreariest of days. The mellow sweetness of the carrots and parsnips is brightened by the warm spice of the fresh ginger. With the aid of your Vitamix, the soup will have the silky smooth texture of a restaurant-made soup, too!

Preparation: **10 minutes**   Processing: **8 minutes**   Yield: **1.2 litres**

3 tablespoons olive oil

380 g chopped carrots

1 tablespoon chopped onion

50 g chopped parsnips

720 ml low-sodium vegetable stock

1 thin slice fresh ginger

½ teaspoon sea salt

¼ teaspoon ground black pepper

1 tablespoon snipped fresh chives

Place the olive oil, carrots, onion, parsnips, stock, ginger, salt and pepper into the Vitamix container in the order listed and secure the lid. Select Variable 1. Turn the machine on and slowly increase the speed to Variable 10, then to High. Blend for 8 minutes or until heavy steam escapes from the vented lid. Serve garnished with the chives.

AMOUNT PER 240 ML SERVING: calories 120, total fat 9 g, saturated fat 1 g, cholesterol 0 mg, sodium 370 mg, total carbohydrate 11 g, dietary fibre 3 g, sugars 5 g, protein 1 g

Black Bean Tortilla Soup

Most of us aren't eating nearly enough fibre (just 15 grams per day, when we should get closer to 25 grams for women, 30–38 grams for men), and eating beans is a great way to close the gap. One cup of black beans contains 12 grams of fibre, and a serving of this soup contains 6 grams of fibre (24% of the recommended daily allowance for women).

Preparation: **10 minutes**   Processing: **7 minutes 20 seconds**   Yield: **1.4 litres**

3 tablespoons olive oil

1 garlic clove, peeled

60 g chopped red onion

125 g chopped red pepper

1 x 440 g can no-salt-added black beans, rinsed and drained

1½ teaspoons ground cumin

½ teaspoon dried oregano

¼ teaspoon chipotle powder

⅓ teaspoon ground cinnamon

½ teaspoon sea salt

¼ teaspoon ground black pepper

1.2 litres low-sodium chicken stock

80 g shelled edamame

135 g seeded, diced Roma (plum) tomatoes

OPTIONAL GARNISHES:

Diced avocado

Fresh coriander leaves

Tortilla chips (regular or blue corn)

1. Place the olive oil, garlic, 1 tablespoon of the onion, half the red pepper, half the black beans, all the spices and the stock into the Vitamix container in the order listed and secure the lid. Select Variable 1. Turn the machine on and slowly increase the speed to Variable 10, then to High. Blend for 7 minutes or until heavy steam escapes from the vented lid.

2. Reduce the speed to Variable 5 and remove the lid plug. Through the lid plug opening, add the edamame, tomatoes and the remaining onion, red pepper and black beans; blend for a further 20 seconds.

3. Serve hot. If desired, garnish with avocado, coriander leaves and tortilla chips.

AMOUNT PER 240 ML SERVING (WITHOUT GARNISHES): calories 160, total fat 8 g, saturated fat 1 g, cholesterol 0 mg, sodium 290 mg, total carbohydrate 16 g, dietary fibre 5 g, sugars 2 g, protein 9 g

Tastes Like Spring Pea Soup

The naturally occurring sugars in peas turn to starch as soon as they are picked. Peas that you buy frozen have been picked and frozen when they are very ripe, so they are often sweeter than the fresh peas you can buy. And frozen peas allow you to make this vibrantly green soup and dream of spring, even when snow still covers the ground!

Preparation: **15 minutes**   Processing: **1 minute**   Cook time: **20 minutes**   Yield: **1.6 litres**

2 tablespoons olive oil

140 g chopped fennel

95 g chopped onion

25 g chopped celery

960 ml fat-free low-sodium chicken stock

1 x 454-g bag frozen peas, thawed slightly

3 tablespoons fresh tarragon leaves

1 tablespoon fresh lemon juice

¾ teaspoon sea salt

75 g spinach

Greek yoghurt mixed with grated lemon zest or fresh herbs, for garnish (optional)

1. Heat the oil in a large pan over a medium heat. Add the fennel, onion and celery and cook just until soft, 4–6 minutes.

2. Add the stock and bring to a boil. Reduce to a simmer and cook for 10 minutes. Stir in the peas.

3. Ladle the hot mixture into the Vitamix container. Add the tarragon, lemon juice, salt and spinach and secure the lid. Select Variable 1. Turn the machine on and slowly increase the speed to Variable 10, then to High. Blend for 1 minute.

4. Wipe out the inside of the pan and pour the puréed soup back into the pan.

5. Serve hot. If desired, garnish with a dollop of lemon or herb Greek yoghurt.

AMOUNT PER 240 ML SERVING (WITHOUT GARNISH): calories 80, total fat 0 g, saturated fat 0 g, cholesterol 0 mg, sodium 440 mg, total carbohydrate 13 g, dietary fibre 4 g, sugars 4 g, protein 7 g

Easy 'Cheesey' Vegan Broccoli Soup

This simple vegan soup comes together in a flash with just the Vitamix, no hob required! Using cashews, you can create a creamy texture without adding any dairy. And the nutritional yeast has a nutty, cheese-like flavour and is a good source of vitamin B12.

Preparation: **15 minutes**   Processing: **8 minutes**   Yield: **1.4 litres**

600 ml water

50 g roasted red pepper (page 91)

1 teaspoon sea salt

35 g nutritional yeast

½ teaspoon onion powder

½ teaspoon garlic powder

½ teaspoon dried dill leaves

180 g unsalted roasted cashew pieces

450 g broccoli florets, steamed and cooled (or use thawed frozen)

Place all the ingredients into the Vitamix container in the order listed and secure the lid. Select Variable 1. Turn the machine on and slowly increase the speed to Variable 10, then to High. Blend for 8 minutes, or until heavy steam escapes from the vented lid. Serve hot.

AMOUNT PER 240 ML SERVING: calories 220, total fat 14 g, saturated fat 2.5 g, cholesterol 0 mg, sodium 500 mg, total carbohydrate 17 g, dietary fibre 5 g, sugars 1 g, protein 12 g

Fennel Spinach Soup

You will need 3 or 4 fennel bulbs for this recipe. If you buy fennel with the feathery green fronds still attached, consider adding a small handful to the soup when you add the spinach. The fronds have a lovely fennel flavour all their own and will add a little more green to the soup.

Preparation: **15 minutes**   Processing: **1 minute 15 seconds**   Cook time: **25–30 minutes**   Yield: **1.2 litres**

GARNISH:

120 ml natural 0% Greek yoghurt, stirred

½ lemon (with peel), halved

Dash of cayenne pepper

2 red peppers, roasted (page 91)

SOUP:

2 tablespoons extra virgin olive oil

480 g chopped fennel

165 g roughly chopped leeks

130 g chopped shallots

1 tablespoon fresh thyme leaves

¼ teaspoon sea salt

480 ml fat-free low-sodium chicken stock

240 ml water

1 bay leaf

115 g spinach leaves

¼ teaspoon ground black pepper

1. For the garnish: Place the ingredients into the Vitamix container in the order listed and secure the lid. Select Variable 1. Turn the machine on and slowly increase the speed to Variable 10, then to High. Blend for 15 seconds. Transfer to a bowl, cover and chill until ready to serve.

2. For the soup: Heat the olive oil in large pan over a medium heat. Add the fennel, leeks, shallots, thyme and salt. Cover and cook, stirring occasionally, for 10 minutes or until slightly softened. Add the stock, water and bay leaf and bring to a boil. Reduce to a simmer, cover and cook for 10 minutes or until the flavours are blended. Discard the bay leaf. Stir in the spinach and pepper and remove from the heat.

3. Ladle the hot mixture into the Vitamix container and secure the lid. Select Variable 1. Turn the machine on and slowly increase the speed to Variable 10, then to High. Blend for 1 minute.

4. Serve the soup hot dolloped with 2 tablespoons of the garnish.

AMOUNT PER 240 ML SERVING (WITH GARNISH): calories 130, total fat 6 g, saturated fat 1 g, cholesterol 0 mg, sodium 360 mg, total carbohydrate 19 g, dietary fibre 5 g, sugars 5 g, protein 4 g

Garlicky Leek and Artichoke Soup

Chefs love Vitamix, in part because of its ability to make silky, smooth purées and soups. Making this pale green soup gives you a chance to get restaurant-quality results at home! Vitamix Chef Bev Shaffer loves this soup for its clean, vibrant artichoke flavour with hints of thyme. Garnish with pesto (as here) or just a drizzle of extra virgin olive oil.

Preparation: **10 minutes**   Processing: **1 minute**   Cook time: **25–30 minutes**   Yield: **1.8 litres**

2 tablespoons olive oil

3 medium leeks, white parts only, chopped

9 garlic cloves, peeled

10 thyme sprigs

2 medium russet (baking) potatoes (511 g), peeled and cut into 2.5-cm pieces

1 x 396-g can water-packed artichoke hearts, rinsed and drained

480 ml low-sodium vegetable stock

½ lemon, peeled

½ teaspoon fine sea salt

6 tablespoons basil pesto

1. Heat the olive oil in a large pot over a medium-high heat. Add the leeks and garlic. Cook, stirring frequently, until the leeks soften, about 5 minutes. Do not brown. Add the thyme and cook for 1 minute.

2. Add the potatoes, artichokes and stock and bring to a boil. Reduce to a simmer, cover and cook over a low heat until the potatoes are tender, about 20 minutes.

3. Transfer the mixture to the Vitamix container with the lemon and salt and secure the lid. Select Variable 1. Turn the machine on and slowly increase the speed to Variable 10, then to High. Blend for 1 minute.

4. Serve hot topped with a dollop of pesto.

AMOUNT PER 240 ML SERVING: calories 140, total fat 4 g, saturated fat 0.5 g, cholesterol 0 mg, sodium 380 mg, total carbohydrate 23 g, dietary fibre 3 g, sugars 2 g, protein 3 g

Lemon Soup with Rice

This soup takes simple ingredients – vegetable stock, brown rice, tofu, turmeric, lemon and dill – and makes something extraordinary. Silky and filling and yet also bright with lemon and herbs.

Preparation: **15 minutes**   Processing: **1 minute**   Cook time: **35–45 minutes**   Yield: **1.5 litres**

960 ml low-sodium vegetable stock

60 g uncooked brown rice

1 tablespoon extra virgin olive oil

340 g soft silken tofu

¼ teaspoon ground turmeric

½ lemon, peeled

2 tablespoons fresh dill leaves

¼ teaspoon ground black pepper

OPTIONAL GARNISHES:

Kalamata olives, rinsed to remove excess salt

Chopped fresh flatleaf parsley

Diced tomato

1. Bring the stock to a boil in a large pan. Add the rice, reduce to a simmer and cover. Cook until the rice is just tender, 30–40 minutes.

2. Transfer the rice/stock mixture to the Vitamix container. Add the olive oil, tofu, turmeric, lemon, dill and pepper and secure the lid. Select Variable 1. Turn the machine on and slowly increase the speed to Variable 10, then to High. Blend for 1 minute.

3. Serve hot. If desired, garnish with olives, parsley and tomato.

AMOUNT PER 240 ML SERVING (WITHOUT GARNISHES): calories 90, total fat 3.5 g, saturated fat 0 g, cholesterol 0 mg, sodium 85 mg, total carbohydrate 10 g, dietary fibre 1 g, sugars 1 g, protein 3 g

Maple Sweet Potato Soup

The next time you find yourself with a couple of leftover baked sweet potatoes, use them to make this soup. Perfect for autumn, consider garnishing the soup with a little cranberry sauce or chopped spiced pecans.

Preparation: **10 minutes**   Processing: **2 minutes**   Cook time: **30–35 minutes**   Yield: **2.4 litres**

2 tablespoons olive oil

125 g chopped onion

140 g diced celery

1.4 litres fat-free low-sodium chicken stock

165 g chopped red potatoes

80 ml pure maple syrup

¼ teaspoon ground black pepper

900 g sweet potatoes, baked, cooled, peeled and quartered

1. Heat the olive oil in a large pan over a medium heat. Add the onions and celery and cook until just tender, 4–6 minutes. Add the stock and red potatoes and bring to a boil. Reduce to a simmer and cook until the potatoes are tender, 15–20 minutes.

2. Add the pepper, maple syrup and sweet potatoes and simmer for 5 minutes longer.

3. Ladle half of the mixture into the Vitamix container and secure the lid. Select Variable 1. Turn the machine on and slowly increase the speed to Variable 10, then to High. Blend for 1 minute.

4. Pour the puréed soup into a clean pan. Repeat with the remaining soup. Stir together both batches to combine.

5. Serve hot (reheat if necessary).

AMOUNT PER 240 ML SERVING: calories 140, total fat 3 g, saturated fat 0 g, cholesterol 0 mg, sodium 320 mg, total carbohydrate 28 g, dietary fibre 3 g, sugars 11 g, protein 2 g

Mushroom Lovers' Soup

Low-fat milk, potatoes and 0% Greek yoghurt give this mushroom soup a delightfully creamy flavour without adding too many calories or completely masking the mushroom flavour. A little champagne vinegar adds a lovely little punch of acidity, brightening the smooth soup.

Preparation: **20 minutes**   Processing: **7 minutes 15 seconds**   Yield: **1.4 litres**

1 tablespoon olive oil

400 g white button mushrooms, thinly sliced

1 tablespoon chopped onion

1 garlic clove, peeled

1 tablespoon sweet paprika

15 g fresh dill

480 ml low-sodium beef stock

480 ml low-fat (1%) milk

1 russet (baking) potato (180 g), baked, peeled and cut into 1-cm pieces

½ teaspoon sea salt

½ teaspoon ground black pepper

120 ml natural 0% Greek yoghurt, stirred

1½ tablespoons champagne vinegar

1. Place the oil, mushrooms, onion, garlic, paprika, dill, stock, milk, potato, salt and pepper into the Vitamix container and secure the lid. Select Variable 1. Turn the machine on and slowly increase the speed to Variable 10, then to High. Blend for 7 minutes or until heavy steam escapes from the vented lid.

2. Reduce the speed to Variable 5 and remove the lid plug. Through the lid plug opening, add the yoghurt and vinegar and blend for another 15 seconds.

3. Serve hot.

AMOUNT PER 240 ML SERVING: calories 180, total fat 3 g, saturated fat 1 g, cholesterol 5 mg, sodium 270 mg, total carbohydrate 29 g, dietary fibre 2 g, sugars 7 g, protein 8 g

Piquant Peanut Soup

This spicy, stick-to-your-ribs soup may be the best grown-up way to get your peanut butter fix. Red onion, carrots and ginger are cooked with sesame oil and a little water until tender. Sweet potatoes are added, and the veggies are cooked in chicken stock and Sriracha until they are tender. Add the peanut butter and a little lime juice and buzz in the Vitamix until smooth. Garnish with thinly sliced spring onions and chopped peanuts.

Preparation: **20 minutes**   Processing: **2 minutes**   Cook time: **25–35 minutes**   Yield: **2.6 litres**

1 tablespoon water

1 tablespoon sesame oil

240 g chopped red onion

140 g chopped carrots

1 tablespoon chopped fresh ginger

1.4 litres low-sodium chicken stock

520 g peeled, diced sweet potatoes

2 teaspoons Sriracha sauce

240 ml peanut butter

2 tablespoons fresh lime juice

GARNISHES:

30 g thinly sliced spring onion greens (cut at an angle)

50 g chopped unsalted, dry roasted peanuts

1. Heat the water and sesame oil in a large pan over a medium-high heat. Add the onion, carrots and ginger and cook until aromatic, 2–3 minutes. Add the stock, sweet potatoes and Sriracha and bring to a boil. Reduce to a simmer, cover and cook until the potatoes are tender, 20–25 minutes. Stir in the peanut butter and lime juice.

2. Ladle half of the hot soup into the Vitamix container and secure the lid. Select Variable 1. Turn the machine on and slowly increase the speed to Variable 10, then to High. Blend for 1 minute.

3. Pour the puréed soup into a clean pan. Repeat with the remaining soup. Stir together both batches to combine.

4. Serve hot, garnished with spring onion greens and peanuts.

AMOUNT PER 240 ML SERVING: calories 250, total fat 15 g, saturated fat 2 g, cholesterol 0 mg, sodium 410 mg, total carbohydrate 20 g, dietary fibre 4 g, sugars 6 g, protein 8 g

Red Pepper Soup with Hazelnuts

This flavourful red pepper soup is bursting with vitamin C as well as a number of phytochemicals. You will be able to taste the sweet peppers, maybe even get a hint of tomato or Hungarian paprika, but will you guess the secret ingredient? The hazelnuts add a subtle richness, even a little nuttiness, which rounds out the flavour of this stellar soup.

Preparation: **15 minutes**   Processing: **30 seconds**   Cook time: **35–40 minutes**   Yield: **1.2 litres**

2 tablespoons extra virgin olive oil

3 large red peppers (400 g), cut into pieces

5 tablespoons (50 g) chopped onion

2 medium tomatoes (225 g), quartered

60 ml dry sherry

2 garlic cloves, peeled

480 ml low-sodium vegetable stock

35 g skinned hazelnuts

1 teaspoon Hungarian sweet paprika

½ teaspoon sea salt

¼ teaspoon ground black pepper

1. Combine the olive oil, red peppers, onion, tomatoes, sherry and garlic with 2 tablespoons water in a large pan. Bring to a simmer and cook, covered, until the tomatoes soften and release their juices, 15–20 minutes.

2. Add the stock, hazelnuts, paprika, salt and black pepper and simmer 10 minutes longer.

3. Ladle the hot mixture into the Vitamix container and secure the lid. Select Variable 1. Turn the machine on and slowly increase the speed to Variable 10, then to High. Blend for 30 seconds.

4. Serve hot.

AMOUNT PER 240 ML SERVING: calories 160, total fat 10 g, saturated fat 1 g, cholesterol 0 mg, sodium 300 mg, total carbohydrate 11 g, dietary fibre 3 g, sugars 6 g, protein 3 g

Mushroom Leek Soup

Mushrooms, a solid source of vitamin D and some B vitamins, have a rich, almost meaty taste. This deeply satisfying soup has savoury mushroom flavour and lovely notes of rosemary and thyme. The combination of chicken and beef stock gives the soup a rich, silky depth. Consider garnishing the soup with sautéed mushrooms and fresh herbs.

Preparation: **20 minutes**   Processing: **1 minute**   Cook time: **35 minutes**   Yield: **2.1 litres**

2 tablespoons olive oil

145 g chopped leeks

130 g chopped celery

2 garlic cloves, peeled

65 g chopped fennel

1 teaspoon fresh thyme leaves

½ teaspoon fresh rosemary leaves, very finely chopped

1 teaspoon sea salt

½ teaspoon ground black pepper

450 g cremini mushrooms, stemmed and sliced

225 g white button mushrooms, stemmed and sliced

960 ml fat-free low-sodium chicken stock

240 ml low-sodium beef stock

1. Heat the olive oil in a large pan. Add the leeks, celery, garlic and fennel and cook until the leeks soften, 4–6 minutes. Add the thyme, rosemary, salt and pepper and cook 1 minute.

2. Add the mushrooms, tossing well to combine. Cover and cook, stirring occasionally, until the mushrooms have released most of their liquid, 8–10 minutes.

3. Add both stocks and bring to a boil. Reduce to a simmer, cover and cook for 20 minutes.

4. Ladle the hot mixture into the Vitamix container and secure the lid. Select Variable 1. Turn the machine on and slowly increase the speed to Variable 10, then to High. Blend for 1 minute.

5. Serve hot.

AMOUNT PER 240 ML SERVING: calories 60, total fat 3.5 g, saturated fat 0 g, cholesterol 0 mg, sodium 500 mg, total carbohydrate 7 g, dietary fibre 1 g, sugars 2 g, protein 3 g

Summer Courgette Soup with Herb Yoghurt

This soup, which calls for over a kilo of chopped courgettes, is the perfect solution to a garden overflowing with courgettes. Baby spinach, added just before the soup is finished in the Vitamix, gives the soup a lovely green hue.

Preparation: **15 minutes**   Processing: **2 minutes**   Cook time: **30 minutes**   Yield: **2.1 litres**

120 ml natural 0% Greek yoghurt, stirred

Grated zest of 1 lemon

4 teaspoons chopped fresh basil

4 teaspoons chopped fresh oregano

2 tablespoons olive oil

140 g chopped onion

1 garlic clove, peeled and halved

1.1 kg courgettes, diced

½ teaspoon sea salt

¼ teaspoon ground black pepper

720 ml fat-free low-sodium chicken stock

65 g baby spinach

1. Stir together the yoghurt, lemon zest and 2 teaspoons each of the basil and oregano in a bowl. Set aside for garnish.

2. Heat the olive oil in a large pan over a medium heat. Add the onion and garlic and cook, stirring frequently, for 4 minutes or until softened. Do not brown. Add the courgettes, salt, pepper and remaining basil and oregano. Cook until the courgette starts to release its liquid, 10–12 minutes.

3. Add the stock and bring to a boil. Reduce to a simmer and cook for 15 minutes until hot.

4. Ladle half of the hot mixture into the Vitamix container, add half the spinach, and secure the lid. Select Variable 1. Turn the machine on and slowly increase the speed to Variable 10, then to High. Blend for 1 minute.

5. Pour the puréed soup into a clean pan. Repeat with the remaining soup. Mix together both batches to combine, reheating if necessary.

6. Serve hot dolloped with yoghurt garnish.

AMOUNT PER 240 ML SERVING: calories 70, total fat 3.5 g, saturated fat 0.5 g, cholesterol 0 mg, sodium 310 mg, total carbohydrate 8 g, dietary fibre 2 g, sugars 4 g, protein 4 g

Chicken Potato Soup

The next time you roast a chicken and bake potatoes, save extra of both items, and whip up this delicious and hearty soup the next day without ever turning on the stove! Deeply comforting and simple to assemble, you will make this soup again and again.

Preparation: **15 minutes**   Processing: **5–6 minutes**   Yield: **1.2 litres**

240 ml low-sodium or no-salt-added chicken or vegetable stock

360 ml skimmed milk

½ small onion, peeled and chopped

3 medium russet (baking) potatoes (400 g), baked or boiled, with skin

⅛ teaspoon dried rosemary

1 tablespoon spinach, cooked or frozen

1 boneless skinless chicken breast (140 g), cooked and cut up

Salt (optional, to taste)

1. Place the stock, milk, onion, 2 of the potatoes and the rosemary into the Vitamix container and secure the lid. Select Variable 1. Turn the machine on and slowly increase the speed to Variable 10, then to High. Blend for 5–6 minutes, until heavy steam escapes from the vented lid.

2. Reduce the speed to Variable 3 and remove the lid plug. Through the lid plug opening, add the spinach and remaining potato and blend until the potato is chopped, about 10 seconds.

3. Drop in the chicken and blend for an additional 5 seconds.

4. Serve hot.

AMOUNT PER 240 ML SERVING: calories 180, total fat 5 g, saturated fat 1 g, cholesterol 15 mg, sodium 360 mg, total carbohydrate 24 g, dietary fibre 2 g, sugars 5 g, protein 9g

Roasted Broccoli, Garlic and Lemon Soup

You may have roasted both broccoli and garlic before, but roasting lemon slices? Yes! The lemon caramelises, concentrating the juices and adding mellow, sweet notes to balance the sourness of the fruit and the bitterness of the peel. Combined with chicken stock and Greek yoghurt, these roasted ingredients create a broccoli soup unlike any you have ever had before.

Preparation: **15 minutes**   Processing: **6 minutes 30 seconds**   Bake time: **55 minutes**   Yield: **1.4 litres**

6 garlic cloves, peeled

4 tablespoons olive oil

800 g broccoli florets

1 lemon, sliced

960 ml low-sodium chicken stock

120 ml natural 0% Greek yoghurt, stirred

¼ teaspoon ground black pepper

½ teaspoon sea salt

1. Pre-heat the oven to 200°C.

2. Wrap the garlic in foil and drizzle with 1 tablespoon of the oil. Seal well and roast on a baking sheet for 25 minutes.

3. Meanwhile, toss together the broccoli florets and remaining oil in a large bowl. Spread the broccoli on a foil-lined baking sheet in a single layer. Top with the lemon slices and roast for 30 minutes.

4. Place the stock, yoghurt, pepper, salt, roasted garlic, roasted broccoli and lemon slices into the Vitamix container in the order listed and secure the lid. Select Variable 1. Turn the machine on and slowly increase the speed to Variable 10, then to High. Blend for 6 minutes 30 seconds, or until heavy steam escapes from the vented lid.

5. Serve hot.

AMOUNT PER 240 ML SERVING: calories 160, total fat 10 g, saturated fat 1.5 g, cholesterol 0 mg, sodium 360 mg, total carbohydrate 11 g, dietary fibre 5 g, sugars 1 g, protein 10 g

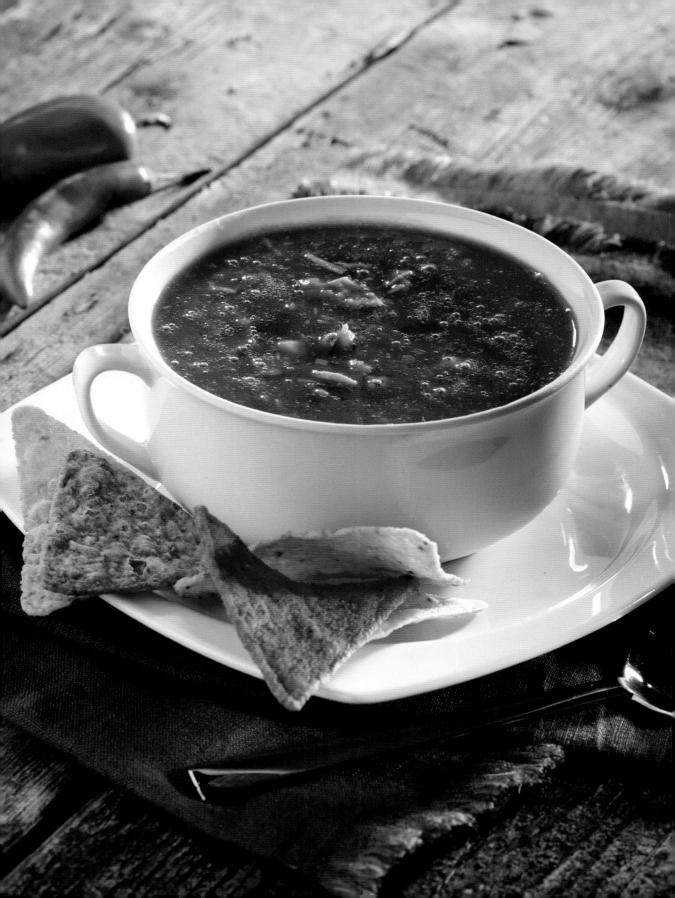

Tortilla Soup

Hungry for a healthy meal but short on time (or the desire to cook)? Drop the soup base ingredients into your Vitamix, and let it do its magic while you cut up cooked chicken, drain canned sweetcorn, slice a jalapeño and some olives and get out tortilla chips. In 15 minutes, you have a steaming hot, vegetable-packed soup, and dinner is served!

Preparation: **15 minutes**   Processing: **6–7 minutes**   Yield: **1.2 litres**

SOUP BASE:

720 ml low-sodium chicken, beef or vegetable stock

1 Roma (plum) tomato, halved

1 medium carrot, halved

1 celery stick, halved

1 thinly sliced onion

1 garlic clove, peeled

1 thinly sliced yellow squash

1 thinly sliced red pepper

1 thinly sliced cabbage

1 white button mushroom

Salt and ground black pepper to taste

1 teaspoon taco seasoning

Dash of ground cumin

OPTIONAL INGREDIENTS:

70 g chunked cooked chicken

½ jalapeño pepper

30 g sliced olives

50 g no-salt-added canned sweetcorn, drained

25 g tortilla chips

1. For the soup base: Place all the ingredients into the Vitamix container in the order listed and secure the lid. Select Variable 1. Turn the machine on and slowly increase the speed to Variable 10, then to High. Blend for 6–7 minutes or until heavy steam is released from the vented lid.

2. If adding optional ingredients, reduce the speed to Variable 2 and remove the lid plug. Through the lid plug opening, drop in the chicken, jalapeño, olives, sweetcorn and chips and blend for an additional 10 seconds.

AMOUNT PER 240 ML SERVING (WITH OPTIONAL INGREDIENTS): calories 90, total fat 2.5 g, saturated fat 0 g, cholesterol 10 mg, sodium 190 mg, total carbohydrate 10 g, dietary fibre 2 g, sugars 2 g, protein 8 g

Chilled Cucumber and Avocado Soup

This light, refreshing soup is the perfect antidote to the hottest summer day. Delicious as an appetizer or a light supper.

Preparation: **15 minutes**   Processing: **1 minute plus pulsing**   Yield: **1.7 litres**

240 g cucumber, peeled and chopped

2 Hass avocados, halved, pitted and peeled

2 spring onions, halved

2 tablespoons fresh lime juice

240 ml natural 0% Greek yoghurt, stirred

720 ml cold water

1 teaspoon sea salt

¼ teaspoon cracked black pepper

2 tablespoons fresh coriander leaves

OPTIONAL GARNISHES:

Lump crabmeat

Pico de gallo

Crème fraîche

1. Place all the ingredients except the coriander into the Vitamix container in the order listed and secure the lid. Select Variable 1. Turn the machine on and slowly increase the speed to Variable 10, then to High. Blend for 1 minute.

2. Stop the machine and remove the lid plug. Add the coriander through the lid plug opening. Select Variable 8. Use the On/Off switch to quickly pulse 2 times.

3. Chill well before serving. If desired, garnish with crab meat, pico de gallo or crème fraîche.

AMOUNT PER 240 ML SERVING (WITHOUT GARNISHES): calories 90, total fat 6 g, saturated fat 1 g, cholesterol 0 mg, sodium 360 mg, total carbohydrate 6 g, dietary fibre 3 g, sugars 2 g, protein 4 g

Barley and Vegetable Soup with Chicken and Pesto

This hearty soup, almost a stew, is chock-full of whole grains, veggies and chicken. Instead of using flour or another thickener, a portion of the cooked soup base is puréed before the chard leaves, barley and cooked chicken breast are added. The walnut and garlic pesto, an elegant finishing touch, adds a little richness and a garlicky punch.

Preparation: **45 minutes**   Processing: **15 seconds plus pulsing**   Cook time: **20–25 minutes**
Yield: **1.7 litres soup; 180 ml pesto**

PESTO:

2 tablespoons olive oil

1 garlic clove, peeled

60 g walnuts, toasted

30 g freshly grated Parmesan

SOUP:

2 tablespoons olive oil

180 g chopped onion

2 tablespoons grated garlic

2 x 10-cm portobello mushroom caps, gills removed and cut into pieces (see note)

160 g peeled, cubed butternut squash

80 g chopped carrot

70 g chopped celery

45 g Swiss chard stem, thinly sliced at an angle

1 thyme sprig

1 teaspoon finely chopped fresh rosemary

1.4 litres low-sodium chicken stock

¾ teaspoon sea salt

¼ teaspoon ground black pepper

2 boneless skinless chicken breasts (320 g), cooked and cut into large pieces

325 g cooked barley

75 g Swiss chard leaves, coarsely chopped

1. For the pesto: Place all the ingredients into the Vitamix container in the order listed and secure the lid. Select Variable 5. Use the On/Off switch to quickly pulse 3 times. Remove the lid, scrape down the sides and around the blades, secure the lid and pulse 3 times. Repeat this procedure 3 more times, or until the desired consistency is reached.

2. For the soup: Heat the olive oil in a large pan over a medium heat. Add the onion and garlic and cook until aromatic and the onion begins to soften, about 2 minutes.

3. Add the mushrooms, squash, carrot, celery, chard stems, thyme and rosemary. Cook for 2 minutes. Add the stock, salt and pepper and bring to a boil. Reduce to a simmer and cook until the vegetables are tender, 15–20 minutes.

4. Transfer one-third of the cooked mixture to the Vitamix container and secure the lid. Select Variable 1. Turn the machine on and slowly increase the speed to Variable 10, then to High. Blend for 15 seconds.

5. Stop the machine and remove the lid. Add the chicken to the container and secure the lid. Select Variable 6. Use the On/Off switch to quickly pulse 2 to 3 times to chop.

6. Add the contents of the Vitamix, the barley and Swiss chard leaves back to the pan. Mix well and heat to warm.

7. Ladle into bowls and garnish with a dollop of pesto. Store leftover pesto in the fridge for up to 1 week, covering the surface with clingfilm to prevent browning. Stir before using.

To gill the mushrooms: Gently remove the stems from the mushrooms, and using a spoon, go around the underside of the mushroom cap, removing as many of the 'gills' as possible by scraping them away. This should result in a smooth underside and create a nice, clean mushroom cap.

AMOUNT PER 240 ML SERVING WITH 1 TABLESPOON PESTO: calories 290, total fat 14 g, saturated fat 2.5 g, cholesterol 30 mg, sodium 500 mg, total carbohydrate 23 g, dietary fibre 4 g, sugars 3 g, protein 19 g

Garden-Fresh Tomato Soup

Few soups are as cosy or as nostalgic as good old tomato soup. In our version, you simply put stock, onion, celery, basil, tomato paste and whole tomatoes in a pot and simmer until the tomatoes are tender. Put the soup – tomato skins, seeds and all – in the Vitamix and purée to silky, smooth perfection. Garnish with Greek yoghurt and basil. This is delicious served with grilled cheese sandwiches.

Preparation: **10 minutes**   Processing: **7 minutes**   Yield: **1.2 litres**

480 ml fat-free low-sodium chicken stock

1 tablespoon chopped onion

2 tablespoons fresh basil leaves, plus more for garnish

2 tablespoons tomato paste

450 g Roma (plum) tomatoes, quartered

½ teaspoon sea salt

¼ teaspoon ground black pepper

6 tablespoons natural 0% Greek yoghurt, stirred

1. Place the stock, onion, 2 tablespoons of the basil, the tomato paste, tomatoes, salt and pepper into the Vitamix container in the order listed and secure the lid. Select Variable 1. Turn the machine on and slowly increase the speed to Variable 10, then to High. Blend for 7 minutes or until heavy steam escapes from the vented lid.

2. Serve hot. Garnish with a dollop of yoghurt and basil leaves.

AMOUNT PER 240 ML SERVING: calories 80, total fat 6 g, saturated fat 1 g, cholesterol 0 mg, sodium 450 mg, total carbohydrate 6 g, dietary fibre 2 g, sugars 4 g, protein 3 g

Roasted Aubergine and Tomato Soup

You may have roasted aubergine and tomatoes together to toss on pasta or layered them together for ratatouille or aubergine Parmesan, but a soup? Once you have tried this wonderful soup, you will have no doubts. The mellow roasted aubergine and caramelised roasted tomatoes are brightened by feta and a generous spoonful of lemon. The cream adds a little richness, and the oregano adds a gentle, herby note. You will make this soup again and again!

Preparation: **15 minutes**   Processing: **30 seconds**   Bake time: **30 minutes**   Yield: **1.8 litres**

680 g aubergine

¾ teaspoon sea salt

450 g Roma (plum) tomatoes, quartered

1 tablespoon olive oil

2 garlic cloves, peeled and halved

960 ml low-sodium vegetable stock

95 g crumbled feta

1 tablespoon fresh lemon juice

2 tablespoons single cream

1 tablespoon fresh oregano leaves, for garnish (optional)

1. Peel the aubergines and cut lengthwise into 1-cm planks. Salt both sides with the sea salt. Arrange on a wire rack and let drain for 30 minutes to remove the bitterness.

2. Pre-heat the oven to 220°C. Line a baking sheet with foil or a silicone baking mat.

3. Wipe the moisture from the aubergine planks. Cut the aubergine into 1-cm dice and place in a large bowl. Add the tomatoes, olive oil and garlic and toss to coat.

4. Spread the vegetables on the baking sheet and roast for 30 minutes, or until lightly caramelised.

5. Scrape the roasted vegetable mixture into the Vitamix container. Add half the stock and half the feta and secure the lid. Select Variable 1. Turn the machine on and slowly increase the speed to Variable 10, then to High. Blend for 30 seconds.

6. Pour the puréed aubergine mixture into a large pan. Add the remaining stock, the lemon juice and cream.

7. Heat and serve hot. Garnish each serving with remaining feta and oregano leaves, if desired.

AMOUNT PER 240 ML SERVING: calories 90, total fat 4.5 g, saturated fat 2 g, cholesterol 10 mg, sodium 450 mg, total carbohydrate 10 g, dietary fibre 4 g, sugars 5 g, protein 4 g

Spiced Butternut Squash Soup

Lots of people love kale these days, but if you need to sneak some greens to a less enthusiastic kale eater, try this quintessential autumn soup. Butternut squash, apple and carrot juice offer a sweetness that balances the bitterness of the greens. Almond milk and raw almonds give the soup a little creaminess, and the spices make it smell like autumn in a bowl.

Preparation: **15 minutes**   Processing: **2 minutes**   Cook time: **40 minutes**   Yield: **2.1 litres**

475 g peeled, chunked butternut squash

2 medium Gala apples (320 g), cored and cut into small pieces

90 g finely cut-up kale leaves (stems removed)

130 g diced onion

2 tablespoons apple cider vinegar

1.2 litres carrot juice

120 ml unsweetened almond milk

75 g raw almonds

1 teaspoon ground cinnamon

½ teaspoon ground nutmeg

1. Combine the squash, apples, kale, onion, vinegar, carrot juice, almond milk, almonds and spices in a large pan. Bring to a boil. Reduce to a simmer, cover and cook until the squash is tender, about 30 minutes.

2. Ladle half of the hot mixture into the Vitamix container and secure the lid. Select Variable 1. Turn the machine on and slowly increase the speed to Variable 10, then to High. Blend for 1 minute.

3. Pour the puréed soup into a clean pan. Repeat with the remaining soup. Stir together both batches to combine.

4. Serve hot.

AMOUNT PER 240 ML SERVING: calories 160, total fat 4.5 g, saturated fat 0 g, cholesterol 0 mg, sodium 110 mg, total carbohydrate 27 g, dietary fibre 4 g, sugars 6 g, protein 5 g

Thai Tempeh Soup

Hailing from Indonesia, tempeh is made from fermented cooked soybeans and has a firm texture and nutty flavour. A popular vegetarian source of protein, tempeh adds heartiness to this full-flavoured, veggie-packed, Thai-inspired vegan soup.

Preparation: **20 minutes**   Processing: **1 minute**   Cook time: **35 minutes**   Yield: **1.9 litres**

3 tablespoons toasted sesame oil

2 garlic cloves, chopped

1 tablespoon chopped fresh ginger

2 tablespoons thinly sliced lemon grass

1 jalapeño pepper, thinly sliced

170 g julienned shiitake mushrooms caps

1 teaspoon coriander seeds

1 teaspoon sweet paprika

1 teaspoon ground turmeric

960 ml white miso broth (see note)

1 x 400 ml can light coconut milk

135 g chopped carrots

65 g thinly sliced spring onions

135 g thinly sliced Chinese cabbage

225 g tempeh, steamed and finely diced

8 g chopped coriander leaves

OPTIONAL GARNISHES:

Beansprouts

Lime wedges

1. Heat half the sesame oil in a large pan over a medium heat. Add the garlic, ginger, lemon grass and jalapeño, and cook for 2 minutes. Add half of the shiitake mushrooms and cook until soft, 4–6 minutes.

2. Add the coriander seeds, paprika, turmeric, miso broth and coconut milk and bring to a boil. Reduce to a simmer and cook for 10 minutes.

3. Ladle the hot mixture into the Vitamix container and secure the lid. Select Variable 1. Turn the machine on and slowly increase the speed to Variable 10, then to High. Blend for 1 minute.

4. Heat the remaining sesame oil in a clean pan over a medium heat Add the carrots, spring onions, cabbage and remaining shiitakes and cook until the mushrooms are soft, 3–4 minutes.

5. Add the puréed broth and tempeh and bring to a boil. Reduce to a simmer and cook for 10 minutes. Stir in the coriander.

6. Serve hot. If desired, garnish with beansprouts and serve lime wedges for squeezing.

To make miso broth, mix 1 tablespoon shiro miso with 960 ml water

AMOUNT PER 240 ML SERVING (WITHOUT GARNISHES): calories 150, total fat 10 g, saturated fat 2.5 g, cholesterol 0 mg, sodium 80 mg, total carbohydrate 10 g, dietary fibre 4 g, sugars 2 g, protein 7 g

Creamy Celeriac Soup

Celeriac – beige and knobby looking – is unlikely to win any beauty contests, but this starchy root vegetable has a wonderfully green flavour that is very much like parsley and celery. This creamy soup can be simply garnished with a few celery or parsley leaves or dressed up with some wild mushrooms sautéed with fresh herbs. Did your celeriac come with stems and leaves attached? These stems have a more bitter flavour than regular celery, so while you can add them to a soup, they are not good for snacking.

Preparation: **20 minutes**   Processing: **2 minutes**   Cook time: **35–40 minutes**   Yield: **1.8 litres**

1 tablespoon olive oil

35 g chopped white onion

60 g chopped celery, leaves reserved for garnish

70 g chopped parsnips

500 g chopped peeled celeriac

3 tablespoons chopped shallot

1 garlic clove, peeled

1.4 litres low-sodium chicken stock

½ teaspoon sea salt

⅓ teaspoon cayenne pepper

240 ml single cream

OPTIONAL GARNISHES:

Sautéed wild mushrooms with fresh herbs

Parsley leaves

1. Heat the olive oil in a large pan over a medium heat. Add the onion, celery, parsnips and celeriac. Cook until softened, 4–6 minutes. Add the shallot and garlic and cook for 1 minute. Do not brown.

2. Add the stock and bring to a boil. Reduce to a simmer, cover and cook until the celeriac is tender, about 15 minutes.

3. Add the cream, salt and cayenne pepper, and simmer for an additional 5 minutes.

4. Ladle half of the hot mixture into the Vitamix container and secure the lid. Select Variable 1. Turn the machine on and slowly increase the speed to Variable 10, then to High. Blend for 1 minute.

5. Pour the puréed soup into a clean pan. Repeat with the remaining soup. Stir together both batches to combine.

6. Serve hot. If desired, garnish with sautéed mushrooms and parsley or celery leaves.

AMOUNT PER 240 ML SERVING (WITHOUT GARNISHES): calories 120, total fat 5 g, saturated fat 2.5 g, cholesterol 15 mg, sodium 370 mg, total carbohydrate 12 g, dietary fibre 2 g, sugars 3 g, protein 6 g

Tomato Fennel Soup

Gone are the days of peeling and seeding tomatoes before you make fresh tomato soup! Here, you simply chop whole tomatoes and cook them down with onions, fennel and herbs. By using low-sodium vegetable stock you control the sodium in your soup too. Easy, healthy and full of flavour, what soup could be better?

Preparation: **10 minutes**   Processing: **35 seconds**   Cook time: **25–30 minutes**   Yield: **1.6 litres**

2 tablespoons olive oil

190 g chopped white onion

135 g chopped fennel

2 garlic cloves, peeled

500 g chopped tomatoes

1 tablespoon grated lemon zest

1 tablespoon chopped fresh rosemary

½ teaspoon dried basil

170 g tomato paste

720 ml low-sodium vegetable stock

1 teaspoon light brown sugar

1 teaspoon sea salt

1 tablespoon fresh flatleaf parsley leaves

1 teaspoon fresh thyme leaves

1. Heat the olive oil in a large pan over a medium heat. Add the onion and fennel and cook until the onion begins to soften, 4–6 minutes. Add the garlic and cook for an additional 2 minutes. Do not brown.

2. Add the tomatoes, lemon zest, rosemary, basil and tomato paste and cook, stirring occasionally, until the tomatoes have released most of their liquid, about 5 minutes.

3. Stir in the stock, brown sugar and salt and bring to a boil. Reduce to a simmer, cover and cook for 15–20 minutes.

4. Ladle the hot mixture into the Vitamix container and secure the lid. Select Variable 1. Turn the machine on and slowly increase the speed to Variable 10, then to High. Blend for 30 seconds.

5. Reduce to Variable 6 and remove the lid plug. Through the lid plug opening, add the parsley and thyme and blend for an additional 5 seconds.

6. Serve hot.

AMOUNT PER 240 ML SERVING: calories 110, total fat 4.5 g, saturated fat 0.5 g, cholesterol 0 mg, sodium 510 mg, total carbohydrate 16 g, dietary fibre 4 g, sugars 8 g, protein 2 g

Garden-Fresh Minestrone

Here, the vegetable stock, tomatoes and a little less than half of the kidney beans are puréed to make a thick, flavourful base for the soup. Then nine vegetables (yes, nine!) are cooked until tender, simmered with nutrient-rich stock, and finished with ditalini pasta to make a delicious, stick-to-your-ribs soup.

Preparation: **20 minutes**   Processing: **7 minutes 20 seconds**   Yield: **2 litres**

225 g ditalini pasta

960 ml low-sodium vegetable stock

225 g Roma (plum) tomatoes, quartered

3 tablespoons extra virgin olive oil

40 g chopped carrots

40 g chopped onion

1 garlic clove, peeled

½ teaspoon sea salt

¼ teaspoon ground black pepper

½ teaspoon chopped fresh thyme

½ teaspoon chopped fresh oregano

1 x 200-g can kidney beans, rinsed and drained

40 g peeled and chopped fennel

35 g chopped red pepper

70 g chopped courgette

75 g chopped yellow squash

40 g thinly sliced escarole, outer leaves removed

OPTIONAL GARNISHES:

Pesto

Shaved Parmesan

1. Cook the pasta in a pot of boiling water according to the package directions. Drain.

2. Meanwhile, place the stock, tomatoes, olive oil, carrots, onion, garlic, salt, pepper, herbs and half the beans into the Vitamix container in the order listed and secure the lid. Select Variable 1. Turn the machine on and slowly increase the speed to Variable 10, then to High. Blend for 7 minutes or until heavy steam escapes the vented lid.

3. Reduce the speed to Variable 5 and remove the lid. Add the fennel, red pepper, courgette, squash, escarole and remaining beans through the lid plug and blend for another 20 seconds.

4. Portion into bowls and add warm pasta. If desired, garnish with pesto and/or Parmesan.

AMOUNT PER 240 ML SERVING (WITHOUT GARNISHES): calories 150, total fat 6 g, saturated fat 1 g, cholesterol 0 mg, sodium 260 mg, total carbohydrate 20 g, dietary fibre 4 g, sugars 2 g, protein 5 g

Tuscan Bean Soup with Whole Grains

Barley, like a number of other whole grains, freezes well. Make this hearty soup – full of beans, vegetables and nutty barley – and then stash any leftovers in the freezer for a quick lunch or dinner on a busy day.

Preparation: **20 minutes**   Processing: **7 minutes 30 seconds**   Yield: **1.5 litres**

3 tablespoons olive oil

1 tablespoon chopped onion

40 g coarsely chopped carrot

1 garlic clove, peeled

225 g coarsely chopped tomatoes

10 fresh sage leaves

1 thyme sprig

½ teaspoon sea salt

¼ teaspoon ground black pepper

700 ml fat-free low-sodium chicken stock

60 g spinach leaves

1 tablespoon flatleaf parsley leaves

1 x 425-g can no-salt-added white navy beans, rinsed and drained

2 teaspoons grated lemon zest

470 g cooked pearl barley

1. Place the olive oil, onion, carrot, garlic, tomatoes, sage, thyme, salt, pepper and stock into the Vitamix container and secure the lid. Select Variable 1. Turn the machine on and slowly increase the speed to Variable 10, then to High. Blend for 7 minutes or until heavy steam escapes the vented lid.

2. Reduce speed to Variable 5 and remove the lid plug. Through the lid plug opening, add the spinach, parsley, beans and lemon zest and blend an additional 30 seconds.

3. To serve, spoon half a cup of cooked barley into soup bowls and top with 1 cup of hot soup.

AMOUNT PER 240 ML SERVING: calories 220, total fat 7 g, saturated fat 1 g, cholesterol 0 mg, sodium 420 mg, total carbohydrate 34 g, dietary fibre 8 g, sugars 2 g, protein 6 g

One Potato, Two Tomato Soup

In this wonderful variation on the classic tomato soup, cinnamon and black pepper add a gentle heat to its flavour, and coconut oil and coconut water complement the spices. Using both canned and fresh tomatoes gives this soup a bright, rich tomato taste. A little Greek yoghurt and agave balance the tomatoes' natural acidity.

Preparation: **20 minutes**   Processing: **30 seconds**   Cook time: **30 minutes**   Yield: **1.6 litres**

1½ teaspoons coconut oil

1 tablespoon whole grain flour, preferably home-made (page 64)

1 small to medium yellow onion (125 g), cut into pieces

2 garlic cloves, peeled

320 g cherry tomatoes

1 x 425-g can no-salt-added diced tomatoes, with liquid

960 ml low-sodium vegetable stock

1 large russet (baking) potato (255 g), cut into pieces

½ teaspoon ground cinnamon

½ teaspoon sea salt

½ teaspoon ground black pepper

½ lemon, peeled

1 tablespoon agave nectar

60 ml natural 0% Greek yoghurt, stirred

1½ teaspoons chopped fresh basil

1 teaspoon fresh thyme leaves

60 ml unsweetened coconut water

1. Heat the coconut oil in a large stock pot over a medium heat. Stir in the flour and cook just until golden. Add the onion and garlic and cook over a medium heat until slightly browned, about 5 minutes. Add the cherry tomatoes and canned tomatoes (with juice) and cook for 5 minutes.

2. Add the stock, potato, cinnamon, salt and pepper and bring to a boil. Reduce to a simmer, partially cover and cook until the potatoes are very tender, about 20 minutes. Add the lemon juice, agave, yoghurt, basil, thyme and coconut water.

3. Ladle half of the soup into the Vitamix container and secure the lid. Select Variable 1. Turn the machine on and slowly increase the speed to Variable 10, then to High. Blend for 30 seconds.

4. Pour the puréed soup into a clean pan. Repeat with the remaining soup. Stir together both batches to combine.

5. Serve hot.

AMOUNT PER 240 ML SERVING: calories 100, total fat 1 g, saturated fat 1 g, cholesterol 0 mg, sodium 290 mg, total carbohydrate 20 g, dietary fibre 3 g, sugars 8 g, protein 3 g

Roasted Root Vegetable Soup for a Crowd

The perfect soup to start your Christmas dinner! Full of roasted root vegetables, this soup is simple to prepare. It can be made in advance and kept up to 4 days in the fridge or 1 month in the freezer.

Preparation: **20 minutes**   Processing: **2 minutes**   Bake time: **35–40 minutes**
Cook time: **20–30 minutes**   Yield: **3 litres**

900 g carrots, diced

225 g parsnips, diced

225 g turnips, diced

½ teaspoon fresh thyme leaves

2 tablespoons olive oil

170 g white onion, cut into pieces

2 garlic cloves, coarsely chopped

2.4 litres low-sodium vegetable stock

1 teaspoon fresh rosemary leaves, finely chopped

1 teaspoon sea salt

1. Pre-heat the oven to 200°C.

2. Combine the carrots, parsnips, turnips, thyme and 1 tablespoon of the olive oil in a large bowl. Mix thoroughly, divide between 2 foil-lined baking sheets and roast for 35–40 minutes, until the vegetables just begin to brown. Remove from the oven and set aside.

3. Heat the remaining 1 tablespoon oil in a large stock pot over a medium heat. Add the onion and cook until just beginning to soften, 4–6 minutes. Add the garlic and cook for 2 minutes.

4. Scrape the roasted vegetables into the pot. Add the stock and rosemary and bring to a boil. Reduce to a simmer and cook for 15 minutes until flavours are blended.

5. Ladle half of the hot soup into the Vitamix container and secure the lid. Select Variable 1. Turn the machine on and slowly increase the speed to Variable 10, then to High. Blend for 1 minute.

6. Pour the puréed soup into a clean pan. Repeat with the remaining soup. Stir together both batches to combine, reheating only if necessary.

7. Serve hot.

AMOUNT PER 240 ML SERVING: calories 90, total fat 2.5 g, saturated fat 0 g, cholesterol 0 mg, sodium 370 mg, total carbohydrate 15 g, dietary fibre 4 g, sugars 7 g, protein 1 g

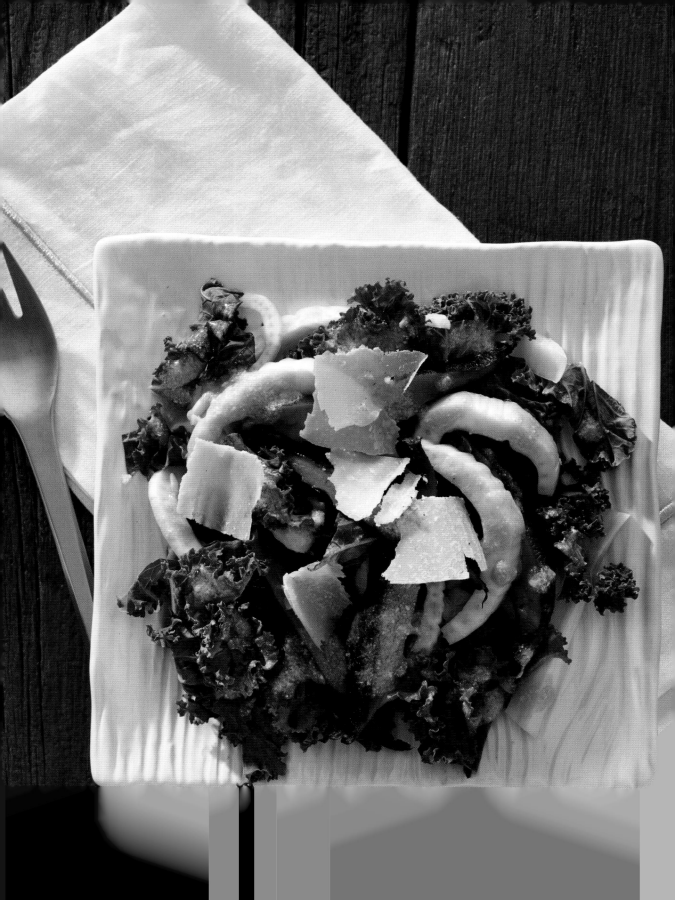

Fennel, Kale and Portobello Salad

Kale is something of a darling among vegetables at the moment. Nutrient-dense, full of vitamins A, C and K as well as a number of antioxidants, it is as delicious and nutritious as it is versatile. Here, we toss it with a balsamic vinaigrette, roasted portobello mushrooms and thinly sliced fennel for a hearty and healthy salad.

Preparation: **15 minutes** Processing: **20 seconds** Bake time: **20–30 minutes** Yield: **8 servings**

6 portobello mushrooms, stems removed

5–6 tablespoons olive oil

3 tablespoons balsamic vinegar

¼ teaspoon sea salt

⅓ teaspoon ground black pepper

1 garlic clove, peeled

45 g finely grated Parmesan

1 fennel bulb, trimmed and thinly sliced

200 g stemmed, washed, dried, and thinly sliced Tuscan (black) kale

1. Pre-heat the oven to 190°C.

2. Gently remove the stems from the mushrooms, and using a spoon, go around the underside of the mushroom cap, removing as many of the 'gills' as possible by scraping them away. This should result in a smooth underside and create a nice, clean mushroom cap. Brush the mushrooms with 2–3 tablespoons of the oil and roast for 20–30 minutes, or until tender. When cool enough to handle, slice them.

3. Place the vinegar, 1½ tablespoons water, the remaining 3 tablespoons oil, salt, pepper, garlic and half of the Parmesan into the Vitamix container in the order listed and secure the lid. Select Variable 1. Turn the machine on and slowly increase the speed to Variable 10, then to High. Blend for 20 seconds.

4. Combine the mushrooms, fennel and kale in a large bowl. Add dressing and some of the remaining Parmesan and toss to coat. Top with remaining Parmesan as desired.

AMOUNT PER SERVING: calories 150, total fat 13 g, saturated fat 2.5 g, cholesterol 5 mg, sodium 180 mg, total carbohydrate 8 g, dietary fibre 2 g, sugars 2 g, protein 4 g

Barley and Sweetcorn Salad with Yoghurt Chive Dressing

Toothsome pearl barley and sweetcorn are cooked together to form the base of this delicious salad. (You can also use hulled barley, sold at many health food stores. This form of barley has more fibre, but also takes longer to cook, closer to 40–50 minutes.) The barley is cooked until just tender, and the sweetcorn is added and cooked briefly. The grains are tossed with creamy yoghurt chive dressing. Sliced tomatoes and cucumbers add a welcome crunch. This salad is wonderful as a side or as a hearty meatless main dish.

Preparation: **10 minutes**   Processing: **20 seconds**   Cook time: **35 minutes**   Yield: **6 servings**

240 ml low-sodium or no-salt-added chicken stock

300 ml water

100 g pearl barley

290 g fresh or frozen sweetcorn kernels

80 ml natural 0% Greek yoghurt, stirred

1 tablespoon plus 1 teaspoon red wine vinegar

½ teaspoon sea salt

⅓ teaspoon ground black pepper

2 tablespoons chopped shallot

2 tablespoons snipped fresh chives

1 medium tomato, halved and thinly sliced

½ medium cucumber, thinly sliced

1. Combine the stock and water in a medium pan. Bring to a boil over a high heat. Stir in the barley and return to a boil. Reduce the heat to low, cover and simmer just until the barley is tender but still slightly firm to the bite, about 25 minutes.

2. Stir in the sweetcorn, cover and simmer for 5 minutes longer. Drain off any remaining liquid and transfer the mixture to a large serving bowl. Allow the mixture to cool to room temperature.

3. Place the yoghurt, vinegar, salt, pepper, shallot and chives into the Vitamix container in the order listed and secure the lid. Select Variable 1. Turn the machine on and slowly increase the speed to Variable 6. Blend for 20 seconds, using the tamper to press the ingredients into the blades.

4. Add the dressing, tomatoes and cucumber to the barley mixture and stir gently to combine. Serve chilled or at room temperature.

AMOUNT PER SERVING: calories 120, total fat 1 g, saturated fat 0 g, cholesterol 0 mg, sodium 240 mg, total carbohydrate 25 g, dietary fibre 4 g, sugars 4 g, protein 6 g

Kale Chips Salad with Spicy Dressing

A kale salad unlike any you have ever had before! Tons of herbs, shredded crunchy veggies, greens and a delightfully spicy dressing are crowned with crispy kale chips. The texture of kale chips made with black kale is more delicate – not unlike seaweed chips – than chips made with green curly kale.

Preparation: **20 minutes**   Processing: **30 seconds**   Bake time: **30 minutes**   Yield: **8 servings**

SPICY DRESSING:

2 tablespoons dark brown sugar

1 teaspoon grated lime zest

4 tablespoons fresh lime juice

2 tablespoons fish sauce

2 tablespoons olive oil

2 garlic cloves, peeled

½ red Thai chilli or ¼ red jalapeño pepper, seeded and cut into pieces

SALAD:

30x12-cm pieces of Tuscan (black) kale leaves (about 115 g)

1 tablespoon olive oil

½ teaspoon coarse sea salt

¼ teaspoon ground black pepper

45 g mixed fresh herb leaves, e.g., flatleaf parsley, mint, basil

315 g mixed shredded veggies, e.g., carrots, red pepper, daikon radish

70 g rocket or baby spinach

1. For the spicy dressing: Place all the ingredients into the Vitamix container in the order listed and secure the lid. Select Variable. Turn the machine on and slowly increase the speed to Variable 10, then to High. Blend for 30 seconds.

2. For the salad: Pre-heat the oven to 140°C. Brush the tops of the kale leaves with the oil. Sprinkle with the salt and pepper. Spread the kale on baking sheets. Bake for 30 minutes, or until the kale is crisp, rotating the sheets front to back halfway through the cooking time and watching carefully so the kale doesn't burn Transfer to a wire rack to cool.

3. Combine the herbs, shredded veggies and rocket in a large bowl. Toss with half of the dressing (save the remainder, covered in the fridge, for another use.) Serve the salad topped with a generous portion of kale chips. Store leftover kale chips in an airtight container to enjoy later.

AMOUNT PER SERVING: calories 70, total fat 4 g, saturated fat 0.5 g, cholesterol 0 mg, sodium 360 mg, total carbohydrate 9g, dietary fibre 2 g, sugars 3 g, protein 2 g

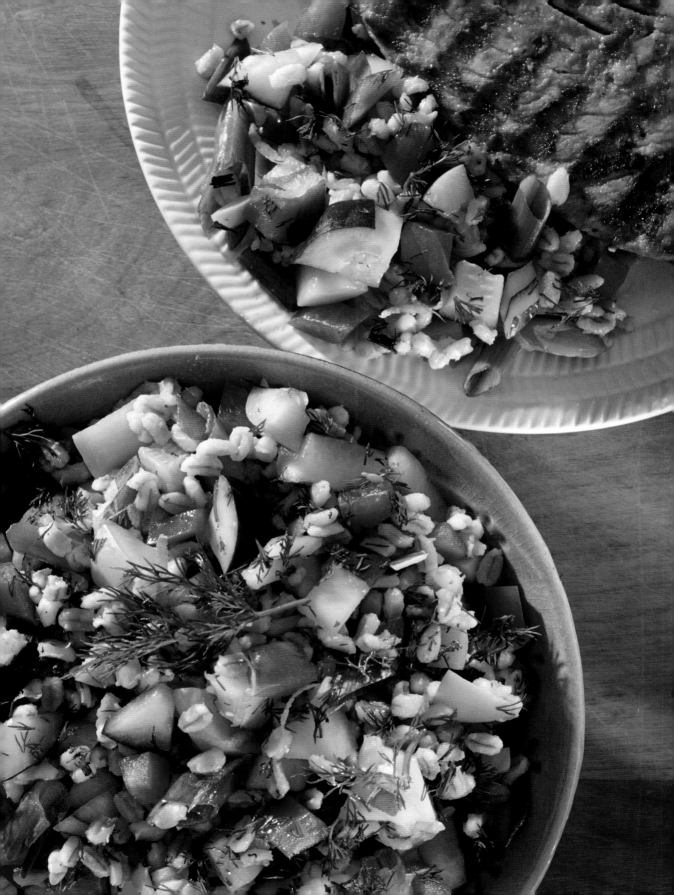

Festive Barley Salad

If you want a salad with your lunch or dinner, but want something heartier than a simple bowl of mixed greens, try this tasty, veggie-packed barley salad. Chop the vegetables and whip up the vinaigrette while the barley cooks. Steam the squash, courgette and red onion while the barley cools. Toss everything together and enjoy!

Preparation: **20 minutes**   Processing: **15 seconds**   Cook time: **45 minutes**   Yield: **4 servings**

200 g pearl barley

¾ teaspoon sea salt

1 small yellow squash, finely diced (about 140 g)

1 medium courgette, finely diced (about 210 g)

40 g finely diced red onion

120 ml olive oil

2 tablespoons red wine vinegar

½ large lemon, peeled

4 tablespoons chopped fresh dill

½ teaspoon ground black pepper

1 cucumber, finely diced (about 260 g)

1 medium red pepper, finely diced (about 110 g)

2 tablespoons thinly sliced spring onions

1. Rinse barley in a fine-mesh sieve until water runs clear.

2. In a medium pan, combine 1.4 litres water with ½ teaspoon salt and bring to a boil. Add the barley and bring back to a simmer. Reduce the heat to medium-low, cover, and cook until the barley is tender and all of the water has been absorbed, about 20 minutes.

3. Rinse the cooked barley in a sieve under cool running water to cool completely. Drain well.

4. Set up a large bowl of ice and water. In a steamer basket, combine the squash, courgette and red onion. Cover and steam until just tender, 3–4 minutes. Cold-shock the vegetables in the bowl of ice water. Drain well.

5. Place the oil, vinegar, lemon, 2 tablespoons of the dill, the black pepper and remaining ¼ teaspoon salt into the Vitamix container in the order listed and secure the lid. Select Variable 1. Turn the machine on and slowly increase the speed to Variable 10, then to High. Blend for 15 seconds.

6. Combine the barley, steamed vegetables, cucumber, pepper, spring onions and the remaining 2 tablespoons dill in a large bowl. Add the dressing and toss to mix well.

AMOUNT PER SERVING: calories 220, total fat 1.5 g, saturated fat 0 g, cholesterol 0 mg, sodium 470 mg, total carbohydrate 47 g, dietary fibre 10 g, sugars 5 g, protein 7 g

Greens and Berries Salad

This fresh, summery salad packs a double punch of strawberry flavour. Some of the strawberries are puréed into the dressing, while the remaining sliced fruit is tossed with greens, blueberries and toasted nuts.

Preparation: **15 minutes**   Processing: **20 seconds**   Yield: **6 servings**

STRAWBERRY DRESSING:

2 tablespoons fresh lemon juice

1 tablespoon extra virgin olive oil

75 g halved fresh strawberries

SALAD:

200 g combination of baby spinach, rocket, watercress

145 g fresh strawberries, sliced

75 g fresh blueberries

40 g coarsely chopped lightly toasted walnuts or pecans

1. For the strawberry dressing: Place the lemon juice, olive oil and strawberries into the Vitamix container in the order listed and secure the lid. Select Variable 1. Turn the machine on and slowly increase the speed to Variable 6. Blend for 20 seconds.

2. For the salad: Combine the greens and berries in a large serving bowl. Pour the dressing over the salad mixture and toss gently to combine. Scatter the nuts over the top.

AMOUNT PER SERVING: calories 100, total fat 7 g, saturated fat 0.5 g, cholesterol 0 mg, sodium 55 mg, total carbohydrate 9 g, dietary fibre 3 g, sugars 3 g, protein 2 g

Kale Salad with Avocado Tahini Dressing

Hearty greens like kale pair well with creamy dressings. In this case, our delicious Avocado Tahini Dip (page 87) gets a second, wonderful life as dressing for a kale salad. Packed with veggies and herbs, this salad makes an excellent main dish for lunch or a light supper.

Preparation: **10 minutes**   Processing: **35–40 seconds**   Yield: **6 servings**

285 g kale, torn into bite-sized pieces

1 medium cucumber, sliced

110 g grated carrots

30 g finely chopped fresh flatleaf parsley

2 tablespoons chopped fresh basil leaves

2 spring onions, thinly sliced

¾ cup Avocado Tahini Dip (page 87)

Combine the kale, cucumber, carrots, parsley, basil and spring onions. Add the dressing and toss well.

AMOUNT PER SERVING: calories 90, total fat 4 g, saturated fat 0.5 g, cholesterol 0 mg, sodium 50 mg, total carbohydrate 12 g, dietary fibre 3 g, sugars 2 g, protein 4 g

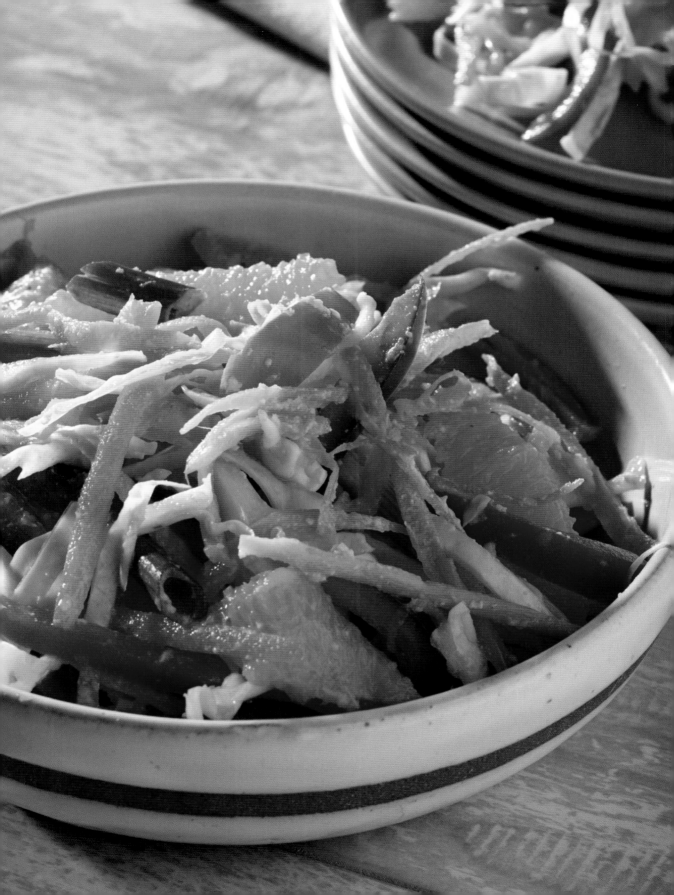

Lime-Dressed Ginger Carrot Slaw

What better way to get a bigger variety of veggies into your next BBQ than to whip up this colourful, vibrant slaw! This salad is a brightly coloured tangle of green, red and orange all tossed in a tangy, slightly spicy dressing. The salad uses about half the vinaigrette, and the remainder can and should be used to marinate meat or veggies.

Preparation: **20 minutes**   Processing: **30 seconds**   Yield: **8 servings**

LIME DRESSING:

4 tablespoons olive oil

1 teaspoon sesame oil

1 lime, peeled

2 tablespoons honey

2.5-cm cube fresh ginger

½ orange, peeled

½ teaspoon sea salt

¼ teaspoon red pepper flakes

SALAD:

1 small head cabbage (700 g), shredded

1 medium red pepper, cut into strips

1 medium green pepper, cut into strips

6 medium carrots, shredded

2 oranges, peeled and segmented

4 spring onions, sliced

Grated zest of 1 lime

1. For the lime dressing: Place all the ingredients into the Vitamix container in the order listed and secure the lid. Select Variable 1. Turn the machine on and slowly increase the speed to Variable 10, then to High. Blend for 30 seconds.

2. For the salad: Combine all the ingredients in a large bowl. Add half the dressing (keep the remainder in the fridge for another use) and toss well.

AMOUNT PER SERVING: calories 110, total fat 4 g, saturated fat 0.5 g, cholesterol 0 mg, sodium 125 mg, total carbohydrate 19 g, dietary fibre 5 g, sugars 12 g, protein 2 g

Fiesta Salad

A little sweet and a little spicy, this fabulously crunchy salad will brighten even the simplest meal. Its flavour would be a perfect complement to tacos or chilli, and you are sure to find yourself making it again and again.

Preparation: **20 minutes**   Processing: **30 seconds**   Yield: **8 servings**

VINAIGRETTE:

290 g diced mango

120 ml grapefruit juice

4 tablespoons fresh lime juice

½ dried chilli, seeded

2 tablespoons chopped shallot

1½ tablespoons vegetable oil

½ teaspoon sea salt

⅓ teaspoon ground black pepper

1 garlic clove, peeled

SALAD:

210 g shredded cabbage

140 g thinly sliced romaine lettuce

250 g diced mango

130 g diced peeled jicama
(Mexican yam)

120 g red onion pieces

1 x 200-g jar roasted red peppers,
drained and diced

40 g pumpkin seeds, toasted

1 tablespoon fresh coriander leaves

1. For the vinaigrette: Place all the ingredients into the Vitamix container in the order listed and secure the lid. Select Variable 1. Turn the machine on and slowly increase the speed to Variable 10, then to High. Blend for 30 seconds.

2. For the salad: Combine all the ingredients in a very large serving bowl. Add the vinaigrette and toss to coat.

AMOUNT PER SERVING: calories 140, total fat 6 g, saturated fat 1 g, cholesterol 0 mg, sodium 260 mg, total carbohydrate 21 g, dietary fibre 4 g, sugars 12 g, protein 4 g

Pear and Apple Salad with Flax-Crusted Goats' Cheese

Alice Waters first offered her famous mesclun salad with warm goats' cheese in the 1970s at her famed restaurant Chez Panisse. Today, we like to make our own variation with poached fruit, a lightly sweet vinaigrette and goats' cheese rounds encrusted with flax seeds and thyme. This elegant salad makes a lovely first course or light lunch.

Preparation: **15 minutes**   Processing: **15 seconds**   Cook time: **10–12 minutes**   Yield: **8 servings**

POACHED FRUIT:

2 tablespoons fresh lemon juice

2 tablespoons light brown sugar

1 large red pear, sliced

1 large green apple, sliced

VINAIGRETTE:

1 tablespoon pure maple syrup

1 tablespoon apple cider vinegar

1 tablespoon flax oil

2 tablespoons olive oil

½ teaspoon fresh thyme leaves

¼ teaspoon ground cinnamon

½ teaspoon Dijon mustard

SALAD:

1 tablespoon whole golden flax seeds

1 tablespoon flax meal

1 tablespoon fresh thyme leaves

½ teaspoon ground black pepper

¼ teaspoon sea salt

85 g goats' cheese log

680 g assorted baby salad greens

1. For the poached fruit: Combine 480 ml water, lemon juice and brown sugar in a large frying pan and bring to a boil. Add the pear and apple slices and gently poach just until soft, about 4 minutes (depending on the thickness of the slices).

2. Carefully lift out the fruit with slotted spoon and set aside to cool. Reserve the poaching liquid.

3. For the vinaigrette: Measure out 60 ml of the poaching liquid and place in the Vitamix container, followed by the maple syrup, vinegar, oils, thyme, cinnamon and mustard in that order and secure the lid. Select Variable 1. Turn the machine on and slowly increase the speed to Variable 10, then to High. Blend for 15 seconds.

4. For the salad: Combine the whole flax seeds, flax meal, thyme, pepper and salt in a bowl and mix well.

5. Roll the goats' cheese in the flax mixture to coat, then slice crossways.

6. In a bowl, toss the greens with the dressing. Serve the dressed greens topped with pear and apple slices and goats' cheese rounds.

AMOUNT PER SERVING: calories 150, total fat 8 g, saturated fat 2 g, cholesterol 5 mg, sodium 190 mg, total carbohydrate 18 g, dietary fibre 4 g, sugars 11 g, protein 5 g

Southwestern Quinoa Salad

Quinoa is a nutritional powerhouse, offering a healthy dose of protein (8 grams), fibre (5 grams) and iron (15% of the recommended daily intake) per 170 g of cooked. Bring more of this naturally gluten-free seed (yes, a seed) into your diet by making this flavour- and nutrient-packed salad. This salad keeps and travels well and would be a welcome addition to a packed lunch.

Preparation: **20 minutes**   Processing: **15 seconds**   Cook time: **20 minutes**   Yield: **6 servings**

720 ml low-sodium vegetable stock

255 g quinoa, rinsed well and drained

⅓ teaspoon sea salt

80 ml fresh lime juice

2 teaspoons ground cumin

½ teaspoon chilli powder

⅓ teaspoon chipotle powder

2 tablespoons red wine vinegar

2 tablespoons olive oil

4 garlic cloves, cut into pieces

1 x 425-g can black beans, rinsed and well drained

75 g fresh or frozen sweetcorn kernels

80 g diced red onion

75 g diced yellow or orange pepper

1 tablespoon finely chopped jalapeño pepper

1 tablespoon finely chopped fresh coriander

1. Bring the stock to a boil in a pan. Add the quinoa and salt and simmer, uncovered, until the liquid is almost absorbed, about 15 minutes. Remove from the heat and fluff with a fork. Set aside to cool.

2. Place the lime juice, cumin, chilli powder, chipotle powder, vinegar, olive oil and garlic into the Vitamix container in the order listed and secure the lid. Select Variable 1. Turn the machine on and slowly increase the speed to Variable 5. Blend for 15 seconds.

3. Combine the black beans, sweetcorn, onion, pepper, jalapeño and coriander in a medium bowl.

4. When the quinoa is cooled, add to the black bean mixture along with the dressing, tossing gently to coat. Serve chilled or at room temperature.

AMOUNT PER SERVING: calories 270, total fat 8 g, saturated fat 1 g, cholesterol 0 mg, sodium 135 mg, total carbohydrate 41 g, dietary fibre 6 g, sugars 2 g, protein 9 g

Lebanese Tabbouleh

In many traditional tabbouleh recipes, the parsley and mint are chopped by hand. Here we whip the herbs with lemon, extra virgin olive oil and spring onions into a fresh, vibrantly green dressing that is tossed with the cooked bulghar. Tomatoes are quickly pulsed in the Vitamix to complete the dish. The presentation may be a little different, but the flavours are true to the original dish.

Preparation: **20 minutes**   Processing: **20 seconds plus pulsing**   Yield: **8 servings**

365 g cooked bulghar

Grated zest of 1 lemon

4 tablespoons fresh lemon juice

6 tablespoons extra virgin olive oil

120 g fresh flatleaf parsley leaves

110 g fresh mint leaves

2 spring onions, cut into pieces

1 medium to large tomato, cut into large pieces

1. Combine half the bulghar and 400 ml boiling water. Cover and soak for 1 hour, then drain, place into a serving bowl and let stand until cool.

2. Meanwhile, place the lemon zest, lemon juice, oil, parsley, mint and spring onions into the Vitamix container in the order listed and secure the lid. Select Variable 1. Turn the machine on and slowly increase the speed to Variable 5. Blend for 20 seconds, or until mixture is blended, using the tamper to press the ingredients into the blades.

3. Add the dressing to the bulghar, and stir to combine.

4. Rinse out the Vitamix container. Place the tomato pieces into the container and secure the lid. Select Variable 3. Use the On/Off switch to quickly pulse until desired consistency, while using the tamper to press the ingredients into the blades.

5. Gently stir the tomato mixture into the bulghar mixture and serve.

AMOUNT PER SERVING: calories 150, total fat 11 g, saturated fat 1.5 g, cholesterol 0 mg, sodium 15 mg, total carbohydrate 11 g, dietary fibre 3 g, sugars 1 g, protein 2 g

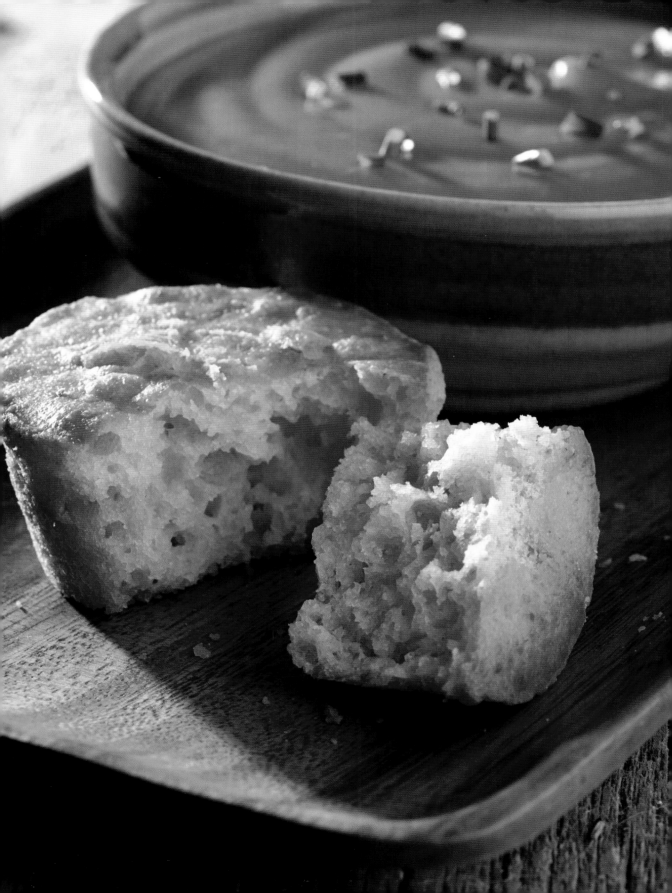

Gluten-Free Rolls

Few prepackaged gluten-free rolls can rival those that you make yourself. Once you have made your flour mix, these rolls will come together quickly. Unlike bread with gluten, you don't have to worry about overmixing – there isn't any gluten to overdevelop after all – so you can stir the batter until it is well combined.

Preparation: **10 minutes**   Processing: **20 seconds**   Yield: **12 rolls**

1 tablespoon fast-action dried yeast

1 tablespoon light brown sugar

228 g Gluten-Free Flour Mix (page 56)

30 g almond meal

1 teaspoon xanthum gum

½ teaspoon salt

1 teaspoon gluten-free baking powder

2 tablespoons olive oil

1 large egg

1. Pre-heat the oven to 180°C. Lightly coat 12 cups of a muffin tin with cooking spray.

2. Combine the yeast, 120 ml water and the brown sugar in a measuring jug. Stir lightly to combine and set aside for 5 minutes to prove.

3. Combine the flour mix, almond meal, xanthum gum, salt and baking powder in a medium bowl. Set aside.

4. Place the oil, 60 ml water and the egg into the Vitamix container in that order and secure the lid. Select Variable 1. Turn the machine on and slowly increase the speed to Variable and blend for 20 seconds.

5. Pour the egg mixture into the flour mixture and mix by hand to combine.

6. Fill each muffin cup half-full. Cover with lightly sprayed clingfilm and allow to rise until doubled in size, about 20 minutes.

7. Bake for 15 minutes, or until golden and puffed. Transfer to cooling racks immediately to prevent moisture from accumulating on the bottom. Serve warm.

AMOUNT PER SERVING: calories 130, total fat 4.5 g, saturated fat 0.5 g, cholesterol 15 mg, sodium 105 mg, total carbohydrate 21 g, dietary fibre 1 g, sugars 1 g, protein 2 g

Bulghar-Stuffed Baby Potatoes

Move over heavy and unhealthy stuffed baked potatoes, there is a new lighter option. Red potatoes are boiled, cooled and stuffed with a tempting filling of bulghar, sweetcorn, leeks and a home-made pecan pesto. Delicious as an appetizer or as a side alongside grilled chicken or fish.

Preparation: **15 minutes**   Processing: **2 minutes**   Cook time: **50 minutes**
Yield: **24 stuffed potato halves**

900 g red potatoes, at least 4 cm in diameter, boiled whole and cooled

1 tablespoon olive oil

45 g finely diced leeks

80 g fresh sweetcorn kernels

365 g cooked bulghar wheat

120 ml Parsley-Pecan Pesto (page 245)

½ teaspoon grated lemon zest

1. Trim a sliver off two opposite sides of each potato, to provide a flat surface on each end.

2. Cut each potato in half and using a 2.5-cm melon baller, scoop out almost the entire potato centre, resulting in a hollowed out potato 'cup'. Set the potatoes aside, cup side up.

3. Heat the oil in a large frying pan over a medium-high heat. Add the leeks and sweetcorn and cook until the leeks are soft, 2–4 minutes. Remove from the heat and cool completely.

4. Combine the bulghar, leek and sweetcorn mixture, pesto and lemon zest in a large bowl and mix well.

5. Fill each potato cup with about 1 tablespoon of the bulghar mixture.

AMOUNT PER 2 STUFFED HALVES: calories 180, total fat 8 g, saturated fat 1 g, cholesterol 0 mg, sodium 35 mg, total carbohydrate 25 g, dietary fibre 3 g, sugars 2 g, protein 4 g

Wild Rice Stuffing

Wild rice is not a grain like other rice, but rather is the seed of a long-grain marsh grass native to North America. Wild rice is wonderful plain, of course, but its nutty flavour really shines in this baked stuffing. Vegetables are quickly pulsed in the Vitamix, then sautéed with olive oil. The cooked veggies are folded into the cooked rice with chewy dried fruit and crunchy pumpkin seeds. Full of nutrients and wonderful flavours, this stuffing is the perfect winter side dish.

Preparation: **15 minutes**   Processing: **pulsing**   Cook time: **45 minutes**
Bake time: **20 minutes**   Yield: **8 servings**

400 g wild rice blend or wild rice

2 celery sticks, each cut into 4 pieces

1 large onion, peeled and quartered

2 garlic cloves, peeled

1 large jalapeño pepper, halved and seeded

2 tablespoons olive oil

¼ teaspoon sea salt

⅓ teaspoon ground black pepper

70 g roasted pumpkin seeds

40 g raisins

30 g unsweetened dried cherries

60 ml low-sodium vegetable stock

1½ teaspoons ground coriander

1 tablespoon apple cider vinegar

1. Pre-heat the oven to 190°C.

2. Cook the wild rice according to the packet instructions.

3. Fill the Vitamix container to the 720 ml mark with water. Add the celery, onion, garlic and jalapeño and secure the lid. Select Variable 8. Use the On/Off switch to quickly pulse 4 times. Drain well.

4. Heat the olive oil in a small frying pan over a medium heat. Add the chopped vegetables and cook until the onion is translucent. Season with the salt and black pepper.

5. Toss together the sautéed vegetables, cooked wild rice, pumpkin seeds, raisins, cherries, stock, coriander and vinegar in a large bowl.

6. Transfer the stuffing to a 20-cm square baking dish and bake for 20 minutes, or until heated through.

AMOUNT PER SERVING: calories 300, total fat 9 g, saturated fat 1.5 g, cholesterol 0 mg, sodium 100 mg, total carbohydrate 50 g, dietary fibre 5 g, sugars 7 g, protein 7 g

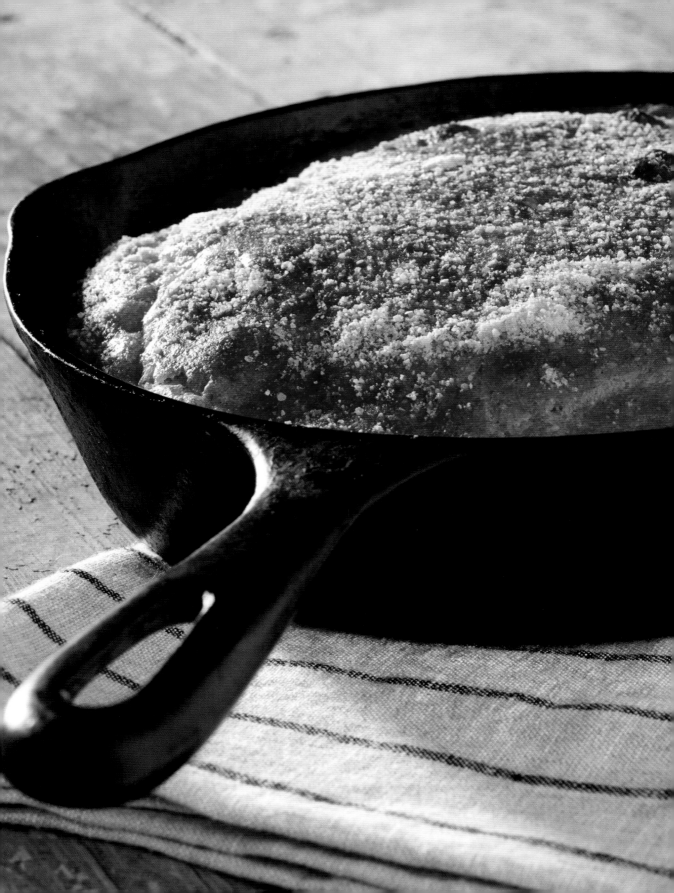

Cornbread

We included this simple, delicious cornbread to stuff the Cornbread-Stuffed Roasted Squash (page 197), but you may find yourself making it again to serve along with your favourite soup or chilli.

Preparation: **10 minutes**   Processing: **20 seconds**   Bake time: **15–18 minutes**   Yield: **8 servings**

120 ml skimmed milk

3 large egg whites

1 large egg

120 ml natural 0% Greek yoghurt, stirred

55 g best-quality vegan butter spread

3 tablespoons granulated sugar

125 g unbleached plain flour

105 g cornmeal, preferably home-made (page 60)

1½ teaspoons bicarbonate of soda

½ teaspoon salt

¼ teaspoon baking powder

1. Pre-heat the oven to 220°C. Lightly coat a 20-cm square tin with cooking spray.

2. Place the milk, egg whites, whole egg, yoghurt, vegan spread and sugar into the Vitamix container in the order listed and secure the lid. Select Variable 1. Turn the machine on and slowly increase the speed to Variable 8. Blend for 20 seconds.

3. Combine the flour, cornmeal, bicarbonate of soda, salt and baking powder in a medium bowl. Mix well.

4. Pour the egg mixture into the flour mixture and mix by hand until well combined.

5. Pour the batter into the pan and bake for 15–18 minutes, or until a toothpick inserted in the centre comes out with a few moist crumbs attached. Cool in pan and then slice.

AMOUNT PER SERVING: calories 220, total fat 8 g, saturated fat 2.5 g, cholesterol 25 mg, sodium 440 mg, total carbohydrate 29 g, dietary fibre 1 g, sugars 6 g, protein 6 g

ANNA KLINGER

CHEF AND CO-OWNER OF AL DI LA TRATTORIA, BAR CORVO, AND LINCOLN STATION, ALL IN BROOKLYN, NEW YORK

Vitamix machines appear in professional kitchens around the world. Often a Vitamix is the most loved tool in the kitchen. Why? A couple of reasons stand out. First, they are incredibly durable. They can purée, chop and emulsify day after day, often for long stretches at a time, and still keep working. The purées are silky, the vinaigrettes and sauces are well emulsified. Chefs with diverse culinary interests – ranging from modernist cuisine to raw foods to rustic Italian cooking – have found their Vitamix blenders indispensable.

Anna Klinger of al di la Trattoria, is one such chef. She first learned about the Vitamix about ten years ago. Five years later, she bought two Vitamix machines for her first restaurant, al di la, and she has never looked back. In fact, all three of her restaurants are equipped with the Vitamix. Klinger is impressed with the incredible durability of the machines and with the quality of the food that they produce. She notes that 'the Vitamix purées much more finely with much less effort than the simple bar blenders I've used in the past. I'm able to produce a silky velouté, for example, with that shiny quality that comes from being puréed very thoroughly, but in a fraction of the time and without the worry that I'm going to exhaust the motor. I have never had to replace mine and use it daily. I used to buy two little blenders a year'.

．．．．．．．．．．．．．．．．．．．．．．．．．．．．．．．．．．

Most Vitamix machines that are used in restaurant kitchens endure heavy use. Klinger's are no exception. She and her staff use the machines daily. The pastry staff at al di la use the Vitamix to blend whole fruits into smooth purées bursting with flavour for sorbets and to make French toast batter for brunch. The cooks, and Klinger herself, use the Vitamix to make a huge range of products. Tangy vinaigrettes, smooth sauces and delicious aiolis can be made quickly. Ingredients as diverse as sweetcorn, peas and sheeps' milk ricotta are transformed into smooth fillings for ravioli and tortelli. They purée soup, sometimes twenty-two quarts at a time, to a smooth and well-emulsified finish.

The whole foods success story? Klinger's many fans would say it is the exceptionally delicious food created in all three kitchens!

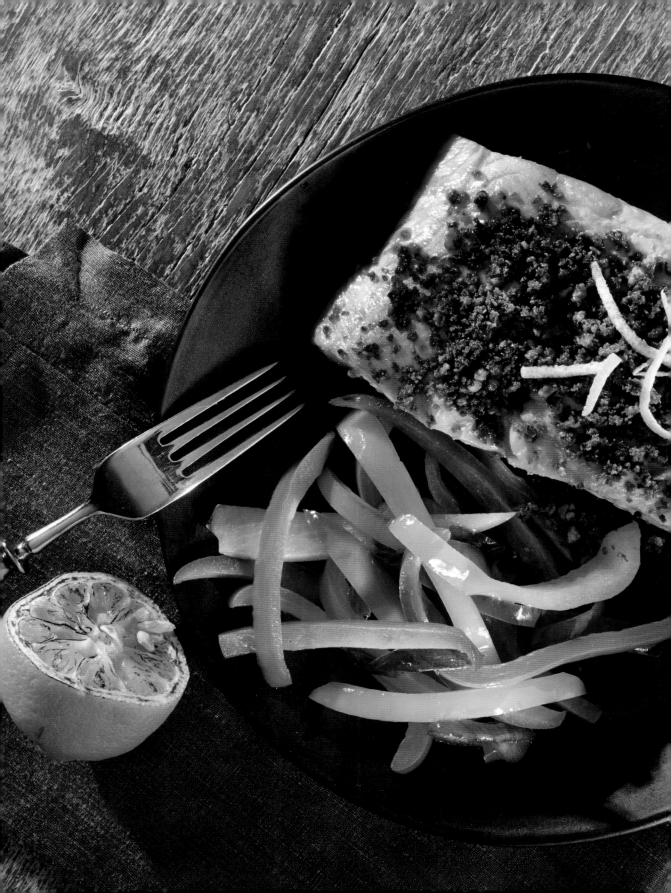

Chapter 5

Mains

I f our mornings often seem hectic, the nights are often just as busy – or worse. They certainly are in mine! There is dinner to prepare, homework to oversee, sports practice, chores, news to share – you name it – and we are tired and hungry to boot. In the midst of all this chaos, we try to sit down for a family meal as often as possible.

Some nights a soup that you can make right in the Vitamix is just perfect for dinner. On other nights, a delicious marinated meat that is ready to grill or a roasted vegetable sauce to toss with pasta will be what you crave. In this chapter, we will explore a whole bunch of healthy main courses that you can make with the help of your Vitamix. We will also discuss some of the different ways to chop vegetables in the Vitamix and ways you can organise yourself in the kitchen.

Before You Start Cooking

You don't have to be a professional cook to benefit from the habits of one. There are a number of simple steps that most cooks take when they get ready to work, and these habits can be invaluable to a home cook. By organising yourself before you start cooking and taking regular inventory of your fridge and store cupboard you will save both time and money.

Before any cook or chef begins a task in the kitchen, they organise their mise en place. Mise en place, or 'everything in its place', simply means getting everything ready before you start cooking: vegetables cut, spices out and measured, all necessary equipment set up. You will notice any missing ingredients and have a calm moment to either make a substitution or dash to the store. Taking time to organise yourself before you start cooking is ultimately a more efficient way to cook and so you will save time in the long run, too.

In a restaurant kitchen, the principle of 'first in, first out' or FIFO helps reduce waste. Simply put, the food that is purchased first is used first. Avoiding food waste helps restaurants and other food businesses save money and time, and this is true for the home cook as well. Once a week, take a quick inventory of what you have on hand. Make a note of everything that needs to be used first. Then think what meals or dishes you can make to use up these foods.

Here is a tip. Having trouble remembering which leftovers were cooked when? Invest in a roll of masking tape and a marker. Label and date containers before you put them in the fridge or freezer. You will know exactly what you have and how long you have had it.

Getting Organised

Some people are menu planners. Every week they write up a menu plan for the week and use this plan to write their grocery list. If this doesn't fit with your cooking style, you can still save yourself some time and avoid the temptation of takeaway. Any time you whip up a soup, or make a batch of salad dressing, nut milk or pasta sauce, make some extra. You can store it in the fridge to be used over the next couple of days or, for some foods, you can freeze it for later. Prepare more pork or fish than you need for dinner, and reinvent the leftovers in a main-dish salad or a wrap.

Look through your salad drawers and find the things that, as I like to say, 'must go!', then look through the recipes in this book and find a soup, smoothie or sauce that will use up this produce. You can also go ahead and make a big batch of your favourite smoothie to enjoy over the next few days, or whip up a tasty soup. You will use up all those good veggies and have a ready-to-go meal or snack, too!

It will be easier to ignore that takeaway menu when you know you have a quick-to-prepare dinner waiting at home. In the long run, cooking more whole foods at home will help you eat better, consume less salt and possibly save money as well. Now let's get cooking!

Dinner is Served

The previous chapters have focused on soups, appetizers and breakfast/brunch recipes. Here, we move on to savoury mains. Some of the dishes are meals in and of themselves. Cheese and Kale Ravioli (page 215), Cornbread-Stuffed Roasted Squash (page 197), Polenta Pizza (page 207) and Fish Tacos with Slaw (page 203) are all great examples.

Some mains are the beginning of a great meal, but you may want a salad from Chapter 4 or a simple sautéed or steamed vegetable to complete the meal. Baked Tofu, Two Ways (page 189), Marinated Sweet and Sour Tempeh (page 198) and Roasted Salmon with Coriander-Seed Pesto (page 211) are just a few of the dishes you could use to anchor your meal.

We will also show you how to make burgers – yes, burgers! Your Vitamix can help you whip up Turkey Burgers with Cherry Salsa (page 224), Courgette Burgers (page 227) and Quinoa and Black Bean Burgers (page 225) for your next barbecue. Healthy and delicious, too!

In this chapter, you will also find recipes that are vegetarian, vegan, gluten-free and kid-friendly. You will find lots of tasty dishes for every occasion and mood. You might just be amazed at all of the delicious, nutritious and different ways that the Vitamix can help you get dinner on the table!

Techniques used in this Chapter

If you have read any of the online Vitamix recipes or read one of our other cookbooks, you will be familiar with the two different ways that your machine can chop food. If you are new to Vitamix or just need to refresh your memory, let me just quickly explain dry-chopping and wet-chopping. Both of these techniques will be used in the recipes in this chapter. You can always chop ingredients by hand, of course, but if you are short on time or are not confident in your knife skills, you will find these methods helpful.

- Dry-chopping. Dry-chop with the Vitamix when you need to coarsely chop, and even-sized pieces are not important. For example, nuts that will be incorporated into a larger recipe do not need to be cut evenly. Place the ingredients in the container and run the machine on a low, variable speed. Or drop them through the lid plug opening while the Vitamix is running on low. Don't process the food too long! The ingredients will go from big chunks to purée faster than you might think. For instance, hard-boiled eggs can be chopped on a very low speed while carrots are chopped at a higher speed. Also, cheese is much easier to chop in a Vitamix machine if you freeze it first.

- Wet-chopping. This technique is used when the ingredients have a lot of moisture in them, e.g. cabbage for slaw. Add enough water to float the ingredients above the blades. The presence of the water will help pull the food down towards the blade, resulting in a more consistent chop. Pulse the Vitamix just a couple of times and chunks of produce will be shredded. Be careful not to pulse it too much or you will have cabbage soup instead of slaw. Drain the ingredients and proceed with the recipe as directed.

Let's get cooking!

Pork Tenderloin in Orange-Ginger Sauce

A zippy orange-ginger sauce brightens up pan-seared pork tenderloin slices cooked with peppers. Garnish with sliced spring onions and serve with brown rice if desired.

Preparation: **15 minutes**   Processing: **15–20 seconds**   Cook time: **13–15 minutes**   Yield: **6 servings**

680 g pork tenderloin

½ teaspoon salt

¼ teaspoon ground black pepper

1 strip orange peel

1 orange, peeled and halved

2 thin slices fresh ginger

1 teaspoon sesame oil

240 ml low-sodium or no-salt-added chicken stock

½ tablespoon honey

1 tablespoon cornflour

1 tablespoon vegetable oil

1 small red pepper, cut into thin bite-sized strips

2 tablespoons sliced spring onions

1. Cut the tenderloin crossways into 6 pieces. Place each piece cut side down between pieces of clingfilm and, starting at the centre, pound to a 5-mm thickness with a meat mallet or rolling pin. Season with the salt and pepper. Set aside.

2. Place the orange, ginger, sesame oil, stock, honey and cornflour into the Vitamix container and secure the lid. Select Variable 1. Turn the machine on and slowly increase the speed to Variable 10, then to High. Blend for 15–20 seconds.

3. Heat the vegetable oil in 30-cm non-stick frying pan over a medium-high heat. Add the pork and cook, turning once, until deep golden brown, 8–10 minutes. Transfer the pork to a plate.

4. Add the pepper to the frying pan and cook 2 minutes. Return the pork to the frying pan. Pour the orange mixture into the frying pan and cook, stirring occasionally, until the sauce is bubbling and thickened and the pork is no longer pink, about 3 minutes.

5. Serve the sauce over the pork and sprinkle with the spring onions.

AMOUNT PER SERVING: calories 190, total fat 7 g, saturated fat 1.5 g, cholesterol 65 mg, sodium 270 mg, total carbohydrate 7 g, dietary fibre 1 g, sugars 4 g, protein 25 g

Polenta with Flax and Tomato Sauce

Another great, naturally gluten-free dinner! Grind your own cornmeal and then transform it into a tasty polenta with flax, parsley and Parmesan. A fresh, herby tomato sauce is started on the hob and finished in the Vitamix. The polenta slices can be topped with sauce and baked or individually pan-seared in a little olive oil and finished with the warm sauce.

Preparation: **20 minutes**   Processing: **1 minute 30 seconds**   Cook time: **20–25 minutes**
Bake time: **15 minutes**   Yield: **8 servings**

POLENTA:

200 g coarse whole-grain cornmeal, preferably home-made (page 60)

35 g flax meal

15 g finely chopped fresh flatleaf parsley

32 g finely grated Parmesan

1 teaspoon golden flax seeds

TOMATO SAUCE:

2 tablespoons extra virgin olive oil

2 tablespoons chopped onion

1 garlic clove, peeled

680 g vine-ripened tomatoes, cut into pieces

1 teaspoon sea salt

¼ teaspoon ground black pepper

½ teaspoon finely chopped fresh basil leaves

¼ teaspoon fresh oregano leaves

¼ teaspoon fresh thyme leaves

1. For the polenta: Bring 540 ml water to a boil in a pan. Add the cornmeal, whisking constantly. Reduce to a simmer, cover and cook until thickened, about 5 minutes.

2. Remove from the heat and stir in the flax meal, parsley, Parmesan and flax seeds. Evenly spread the polenta into a greased 22 x 11 cm loaf tin. Let cool for 30 minutes.

3. For the tomato sauce: Heat the olive oil in a medium pan over a medium heat. Add the onion and garlic and cook until they're translucent, about 5 minutes. Stir in the tomatoes, salt, pepper and herbs and cover. Cook, stirring occasionally, until the tomatoes have broken down, 10–15 minutes.

4. Ladle the hot tomato mixture into the Vitamix container and secure the lid. Select Variable 1. Turn the machine on and slowly increase the speed to Variable 10, then to High. Blend for 30 seconds.

5. Remove the polenta from the loaf tin and slice into 8 pieces.

6. To bake the polenta: Pre-heat the oven to 180°C. Transfer the polenta slices into a baking dish, ladle the sauce over the polenta and bake for 15 minutes, or until heated through.

7. To pan-sear the polenta: Crisp the polenta slices on a non-stick griddle in a small amount of olive oil and serve topped with the warm tomato sauce.

AMOUNT PER SERVING: Calories 180, total fat 8 g, saturated fat 1.5 g, cholesterol 5 mg, sodium 360 mg, total carbohydrate 22 g, dietary fibre 6 g, sugars 3 g, protein 5 g

Baked Tofu, Two Ways

These two baked tofu preparations produced firm, flavourful tofu that can be tucked in a sandwich, served with rice and stir-fried vegetables or cubed and tossed in a salad. The possibilities are nearly endless!

Preparation: **15 minutes per marinade**   Processing: **20 seconds**
Bake time: **45 minutes**   Yield: **4 servings**

450 g firm tofu, drained

LEMON MARINADE WITH SPICE AND CORIANDER:

4 tablespoons fresh lemon juice

2 tablespoons low-sodium soy sauce

3 tablespoons olive oil

120 ml water

1 tablespoon fresh coriander leaves

1 tablespoon spring onion pieces

1 green chilli, halved and seeded

¼ teaspoon ground black pepper

LEMON MARINADE WITH ROSEMARY:

4 tablespoons fresh lemon juice

2 tablespoon low-sodium soy sauce

3 tablespoons olive oil

1 tablespoon lightly chopped fresh rosemary

¼ teaspoon ground black pepper

1. Make both marinades (see below).

2. Cut the tofu block into 8 even pieces. Pour half of each marinade into each of 2 baking dishes. Place 4 tofu slices in a single layer in each baking dish. Pour the remaining corresponding marinade over the tofu. Allow the tofu to absorb the flavours and marinate while the oven pre-heats.

3. Pre-heat the oven to 200°C.

4. Bake the tofu for 45 minutes, carefully turning the slices in the pan after 25 minutes. The baked tofu will be browned, bubbling and curling slightly at the edges.

5. Remove from the oven and transfer the slices to a serving platter. Serve tofu hot, warm, at room temperature or even chilled. (The tofu will keep in a covered container in the fridge for up to 3 days.)

For the marinade.

1. Place all the ingredients into the Vitamix container in the order listed and secure the lid. Select Variable 1. Turn the machine on and slowly increase the speed to Variable 7. Blend for 20 seconds or until well blended.

AMOUNT PER SERVING (MARINADE AND TOFU): calories 50, total fat 3 g, saturated fat 0 g, cholesterol 0 mg, sodium 130 mg, total carbohydrate 3 g, dietary fibre 0 g, sugars 1 g, protein 4 g

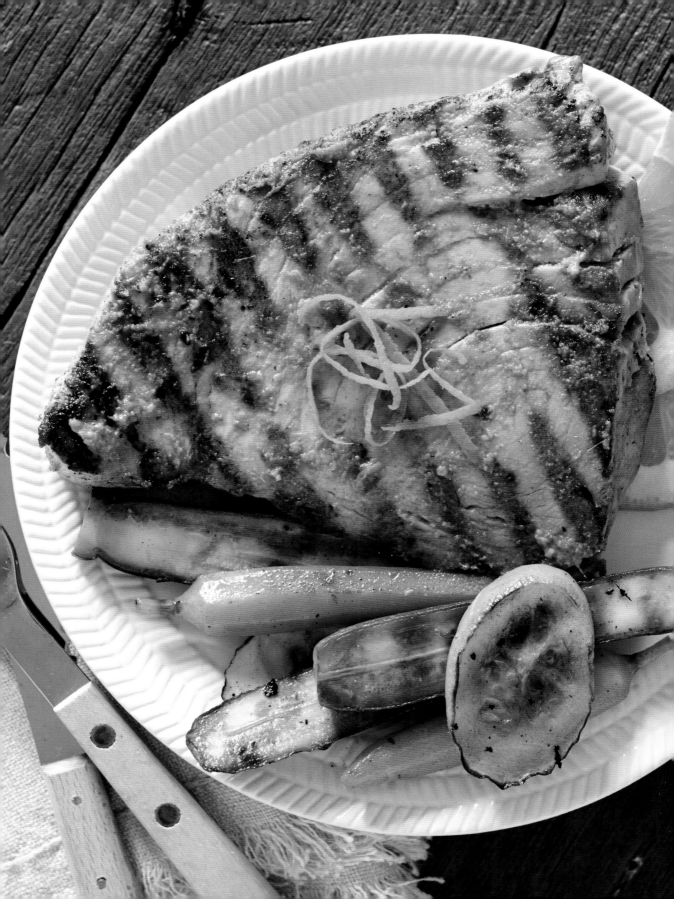

Citrus Ginger Marinated Tuna Steaks

A bright, sweet-savoury marinade makes simple tuna steaks something even more special. Be careful to marinate 2.5-cm-thick fish steaks for no longer than 1 hour; thinner steaks should only be marinated for 30 minutes. Fish is less dense than other proteins, and acidic marinades like this one will penetrate the steaks quickly.

Preparation: **1 hour**   Processing: **30 seconds**   Yield: **4 servings**

2 tablespoons low-sodium soy sauce

2 tablespoons olive oil

1 tablespoon sesame oil

1 teaspoon grated orange zest

1 orange, peeled and halved

2.5-cm slice of pineapple, peeled, with core intact

2 tablespoons chopped fresh ginger

1 garlic clove, peeled

2 spring onions, cut into pieces

⅓ teaspoon cayenne pepper

2 x 450-g tuna steaks, cut 2.5 cm thick

1. Place the soy sauce, olive oil, sesame oil, orange zest, orange, pineapple, ginger, garlic, spring onions and cayenne into the Vitamix container in the order listed and secure the lid. Select Variable 1. Turn the machine on and slowly increase the speed to Variable 10, then to High. Blend for 30 seconds, using the tamper as needed to push the ingredients into the blades.

2. Place the tuna in a shallow baking dish. Pour the marinade over the tuna and chill for 1 hour.

3. Remove the tuna from the marinade and griddle over a high heat to the desired amount of doneness.

AMOUNT PER SERVING: calories 390, total fat 14 g, saturated fat 3 g, cholesterol 85 mg, sodium 160 mg, total carbohydrate 10 g, dietary fibre 1 g, sugars 7 g, protein 54 g

Couscous Chicken Salad

In this colourful main-dish salad, a bright, citrus-filled vinaigrette is tossed with couscous, chicken, red peppers, onions and parsley. Take it to your next bring a dish lunch or make on Sunday evening for lunches during the week. (The salad will keep for 4 days.)

Preparation: **20 minutes**   Processing: **10 seconds**   Cook time: **30–40 minutes**   Yield: **6 servings**

SALAD:

110 g couscous

55 g slivered dried apricots

240 ml fat-free low-sodium or no-salt-added chicken stock

225 g boneless skinless chicken breast, cut into 1-cm chunks

1 medium red pepper, diced

40 g diced red onion

15 g chopped fresh flatleaf parsley

DRESSING:

3 tablespoons orange juice

2 tablespoons fresh lemon juice

1½ teaspoons ground cumin

¼ teaspoon granulated sugar

¼ teaspoon sea salt

¼ teaspoon ground black pepper

1 teaspoon grated orange zest

2 tablespoons extra virgin olive oil

1. For the salad: Bring 300 ml water to a boil in a medium pan. Stir in the couscous and apricots, then cover, remove from the heat and let stand for 5 minutes. Remove the lid and gently fluff with a fork. Cover loosely and set aside to cool until just warm.

2. Bring the stock to a boil in a high-sided frying pan. Stir in the chicken and simmer, stirring, until the chicken is no longer pink in the centre, about 10 minutes. With a slotted spoon, scoop out the chicken and cover to keep moist.

3. Return the stock in the frying pan to a high heat and boil rapidly until reduced to about 2 tablespoons, 5–8 minutes. Strain the liquid and set the reduced chicken stock aside.

4. Combine the chicken, couscous mixture, pepper, onion and parsley in a large salad bowl.

5. For the dressing: Place the reduced chicken stock and all of the dressing ingredients into the Vitamix container in the order listed and secure the lid. Select Variable 1. Turn the machine on and slowly increase the speed to Variable 5. Blend for 10 seconds.

6. Pour the dressing over the salad and toss all gently to combine.

AMOUNT PER SERVING: calories 200, total fat 7 g, saturated fat 1.5 g, cholesterol 20 mg, sodium 190 mg, total carbohydrate 25 g, dietary fibre 4 g, sugars 5 g, protein 12 g

Greek Chicken Pockets

Another great use for leftover rotisserie chicken! These tasty pitta pockets pair chicken with a cucumber yoghurt sauce, lettuce, cucumber, red onion and Kalamata olives. If you are packing these sandwiches for a picnic or packed lunch, pack the yoghurt sauce separately so the pitta doesn't get soggy.

Preparation: **20 minutes**   Processing: **3 seconds plus pulsing**   Yield: **4 sandwiches**

1 x 30-cm cucumber, halved lengthwise, seeds scooped out, cut into 4-cm chunks

340 g natural 0% Greek yoghurt, stirred

2 garlic cloves, peeled

1 teaspoon dried dill

Salt and ground black pepper

85 g red onion chunks

35 g pitted Kalamata olives

2 boneless skinless chicken breasts (125 g each), cut into 3

2 large multi-grain pitta breads, halved crossways, toasted

4 large leaf lettuce leaves

1. Place half of the cucumber chunks into the Vitamix container and secure the lid. Select Variable 2. Use the On/Off switch to pulse 3 times. Use the tamper to press the cucumber into the blades if necessary.

2. Add the yoghurt, garlic, dill and salt and pepper to taste to the Vitamix container and secure the lid. Select Variable 1. Turn the machine on and slowly increase the speed to Variable 3. Blend for 3 seconds. Scoop the mixture into a medium bowl and set aside.

3. Rinse the container. Place the remaining cucumber into the Vitamix container and secure the lid. Select Variable 2. Use the On/Off switch to pulse. If necessary, use a scraper to move larger pieces to the top. Cover and repeat. Drain and pour into another medium bowl.

4. Add the red onion to the Vitamix container and secure the lid. Select Variable 4. Use the On/Off switch to quickly pulse 3 times. Use a scraper to move larger pieces to the top and add the olives. Secure the lid and repeat the process 2 times. Scrape into the bowl with the cucumber.

5. Add the chicken to the Vitamix container and secure the lid. Select Variable 4. Use the On/Off switch to quickly pulse 3 times. Add to the vegetables in the bowl.

6. Line each pitta half with a lettuce leaf. Spoon the chicken mixture into the pitta and drizzle the yoghurt mixture over the top. Serve additional sauce on the side. (Store any leftover sauce, covered, in the fridge.)

AMOUNT PER SANDWICH: calories 270, total fat 5 g, saturated fat 1 g, cholesterol 55 mg, sodium 340 mg, total carbohydrate 25 g, dietary fibre 3 g, sugars 6 g, protein 31 g

Edamame and Sweetcorn Pot Pies

These delicious pot pies will take a little more time than your morning smoothie, but they are worth every minute. You start by making your own cornmeal – easy to do with the dry grains container of your Vitamix – and then cooking it with hot water and fresh thyme. This polenta, in turn, becomes the crust for a hearty pot pie with a sweetcorn and edamame filling. Enjoy!

Preparation: **15 minutes**   Processing: **2 minutes 30 seconds**   Bake time: **20–25 minutes**
Yield: **4 servings**

POLENTA CRUST:

1½ teaspoons fresh thyme leaves, finely chopped

150 g whole-grain cornmeal, preferably home-made (page 60)

FILLING:

180 ml low-fat (1%) milk

435 g fresh or thawed frozen sweetcorn kernels

2 teaspoons potato starch

½ teaspoon sea salt

⅓ teaspoon ground black pepper

1 teaspoon finely chopped fresh basil

¼ teaspoon finely chopped fresh rosemary

150 g shelled edamame

1. For the polenta crust: Pre-heat the oven to 190°C.

2. Bring 600 ml water and the thyme to a boil in a large pan. Slowly whisk in the cornmeal, reduce the heat and simmer, covered, until thickened, about 5 minutes. Remove the polenta from the heat.

3. Divide three-quarters of the polenta into 4 ramekins or ovenproof bowls that measure 11 cm across and 6 cm deep. Using damp hands, lightly press the polenta against the bottom and sides to form a crust.

4. Press or roll the remaining polenta between sheets of baking paper to 1-cm thickness. Cool completely.

5. Place the ramekins on a baking sheet and bake for 6 minutes to set the crust. Leave the oven on.

6. Meanwhile, for the filling: Place the milk and half of the sweetcorn into the Vitamix container and secure the lid. Select Variable 1. Turn the machine on and slowly increase the speed to Variable 10, then to High. Blend for 30 seconds.

7. Pour the sweetcorn purée into a large pan, place over a medium-high heat, and heat to a gentle simmer. Stir together the potato starch and 2 tablespoons water in a small bowl to make a paste. Whisk the paste into the sweetcorn purée and cook until thickened, 2–3 minutes.

8. Remove the sweetcorn purée from the heat and stir in the salt, pepper, basil, rosemary, edamame and the remaining sweetcorn. Mix well.

9. To assemble the pot pies: Divide the filling among the ramekins.

10. Cut the remaining polenta sheet into 1-cm strips. Carefully lay the strips in a criss-cross pattern across the top of each pot pie.

11. Return the ramekins to the oven to bake for 15–20 minutes, until heated thoroughly.

AMOUNT PER SERVING: calories 340, total fat 5 g, saturated fat 1 g, cholesterol 0 mg, sodium 360 mg, total carbohydrate 63 g, dietary fibre 10 g, sugars 10 g, protein 14 g

....

Mediterranean Tofu

Consider adding tofu to your diet, even if you are not a vegetarian. Tofu has over 8 grams of protein per 100-gram serving and contains all eight essential amino acids. Use this tasty baked tofu instead of feta cheese on a vegan Greek salad or slipped into a pitta with crunchy vegetables. This recipe can be served either hot or cold.

Preparation: **15 minute**s   Processing: **30 seconds**   Bake time: **35–45 minutes**   Yield: **4 servings**

450 g firm tofu

4 tablespoons olive oil

4 tablespoons red wine vinegar

½ lemon, peeled

1 garlic clove, peeled and halved

2 teaspoons fresh thyme leaves

1 teaspoon sea salt

Pinch of red pepper flakes

1. Drain the excess moisture from the tofu by wrapping it in two layers of kitchen paper and pressing it between two plates. Let stand overnight in the fridge, with a bowl or dish underneath the plates to catch any overflowing water.

2. The next day, pat the tofu dry and slice it 1 cm thick. Pre-heat the oven to 180°C.

3. Place the olive oil, vinegar, lemon, garlic, thyme, salt and red pepper flakes into the Vitamix container in the order listed and secure the lid. Select Variable 1. Turn the machine on and slowly increase the speed to Variable 10, then to High. Blend for 30 seconds.

4. Lay the tofu slices in a baking dish, in a single snug layer. Pour the marinade over the tofu.

5. Bake for 35–45 minutes, until the tofu is nearly dry and well browned.

AMOUNT PER SERVING: calories 130, total fat 9 g, saturated fat 1 g, cholesterol 0 mg, sodium 50 mg, total carbohydrate 4 g, dietary fibre 1 g, sugars 1 g, protein 10 g

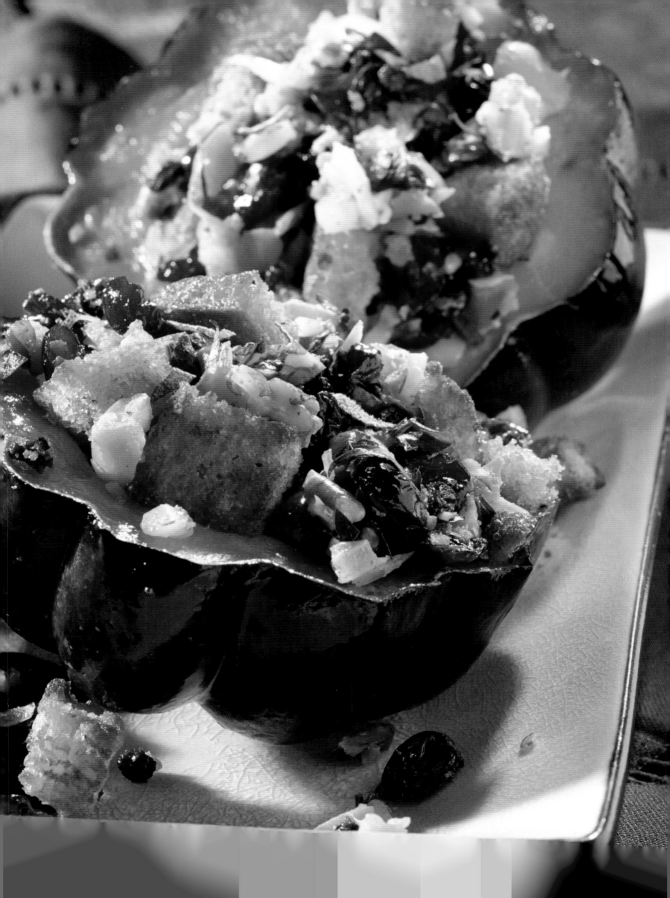

Cornbread-Stuffed Roasted Squash

Coming up with a scrumptious, satisfying vegetarian main dish for your guests can be tricky. Search no more! This stuffed squash is loaded with classic autumn flavours, and thanks in part to the Vitamix wet-chop, the prep for this dish is relatively simple.

Preparation: **30 minutes**   Processing: **pulsing**   Bake time: **1 hour 30 minutes**   Yield: **4 servings**

315 g finely cubed Cornbread (page 179)

20 g unsweetened dried cranberries

2 tablespoons dried currants

2 acorn squash (450 g each)

½ medium white onion, chopped

2 celery sticks

1 large carrot

2 teaspoons olive oil

1 tablespoon chopped fresh sage leaves

1 garlic clove, peeled

120 ml low-sodium vegetable stock

2 tablespoons chopped toasted pecans

1 tablespoon fresh flatleaf parsley leaves

½ teaspoon sea salt

¼ teaspoon ground black pepper

1. Pre-heat the oven to 200°C.

2. Spread the cornbread cubes on to a baking sheet and bake for 30 minutes, stirring halfway through, until golden brown and toasted. Set aside to cool on a wire rack. Leave the oven on but reduce the temperature to 180°C.

3. Meanwhile, combine the cranberries and currants with 240 ml boiling water in a heatproof bowl and let sit for 30 minutes to rehydrate. Drain well.

4. Halve each squash. Discard the seeds and membranes and place cut side down on a baking sheet lined with foil or a silicone baking mat. Roast for 30 minutes, or until the squash is just tender. Leave the oven on.

5. Meanwhile, wet-chop the vegetables: Fill the Vitamix container with water up to the 1.2-litre mark, add the onion and secure the lid. Select Variable 8. Use the On/Off switch to quickly pulse 3 times. Drain well and repeat the process with the celery (3 pulses) and carrot (4 pulses).

6. Heat the olive oil in a large frying pan over a medium-high heat. Add the onion, celery, carrot, sage and garlic and cook until the vegetables are softened and the onions are translucent, 3–5 minutes. Remove from the heat.

7. Mix together the toasted cornbread, cranberry-currant mixture, sautéed vegetables, the stock, pecans, parsley, salt and pepper in a large bowl.

8. Divide the stuffing among the squash halves. Place the squash in a large serving/baking dish, stuffing side up, and bake for 30 minutes, or until the squash is tender and the stuffing is golden brown.

Amount per serving: calories 370, total fat 12 g, saturated fat 3 g, cholesterol 20 mg, sodium 740 mg, total carbohydrate 60 g, dietary fibre 7 g, sugars 12 g, protein 9 g

Marinated Sweet and Sour Tempeh

A simple and speedy vegetarian dinner! Protein-packed tempeh simmers in a sweet and sour marinade while you cook brown rice and whip up a gently spicy peanut sauce. Sautéed greens or steamed snap peas would round out the meal.

Preparation: **20 minutes**   Processing: **1 minute 20 seconds**   Cook time: **15 minutes**   Yield: **6 servings**

450 g tempeh, cut into 2.5-cm cubes

MARINADE:

4 tablespoons olive oil

1 tablespoon sesame oil

4 tablespoons reduced-sodium tamari

4 tablespoons unseasoned rice vinegar

4 tablespoons mirin

1 tablespoon chopped fresh ginger

1 garlic clove, peeled

390 g cooked brown rice

PEANUT SAUCE:

260 g unsalted Peanut Butter (page 252)

4 tablespoons honey

3 tablespoons reduced-sodium tamari

3 tablespoons unseasoned rice vinegar

1 tablespoon chopped fresh ginger

2 garlic cloves, peeled

½ teaspoon cayenne pepper

1. For the marinade: Place 360 ml hot water into the Vitamix container, then add all the ingredients in the order listed and secure the lid. Select Variable 1. Turn the machine on and slowly increase the speed to Variable 10, then to High. Blend for 20 seconds.

2. Arrange the tempeh pieces in a single layer in a large frying pan. Pour the marinade over them and bring to a boil. Reduce to a simmer, cover and cook for 10 minutes. Remove from the heat.

3. For the peanut sauce: Place all the ingredients into the Vitamix container in the order listed and secure the lid. Select Variable 1. Turn the machine on and slowly increase the speed to Variable 10, then to High. Blend for 1 minute.

4. Serve the tempeh over the brown rice and top with a few tablespoons of peanut sauce. Keep the remaining peanut sauce in the fridge for another use.

AMOUNT PER SERVING: calories 395, total fat 19g, saturated fat 2.5 g, cholesterol 0 mg, sodium 400 mg, total carbohydrate 38 g, dietary fibre 8 g, sugars 6 g, protein 21 g

Falafel

A fried chickpea patty that is a staple in a number of Middle-Eastern countries, falafel may seem like the sort of dish that should be left to restaurants. How many of us want to deep-fry at home? Enter this flavour-packed baked falafel recipe! The filling comes together quickly in the Vitamix. The balls are then baked, not fried, saving on oil, calories and mess. Enjoy with Lebanese Tabbouleh (page 173).

Preparation: **15 minutes plus overnight soaking**   Processing: **35 seconds**   Bake time: **15 minutes**
Yield: **12 servings (2 balls per serving)**

350 g dried chickpeas, rinsed and picked over

100 g coarsely chopped onion

15 g fresh flatleaf parsley leaves

15 g fresh coriander leaves

8 garlic cloves, peeled

2 teaspoons ground cumin

1 teaspoon cayenne pepper

1½ teaspoons bicarbonate of soda

62 g unbleached plain flour

1. Place the chickpeas in a bowl and cover with cool water by about 2.5 cm. Cover and chill for 12–24 hours.

2. Drain the chickpeas. Place the chickpeas, onion, 60 ml water, parsley, coriander, garlic, cumin and cayenne into the Vitamix container and secure the lid. Select Variable 1. Turn the machine on and slowly increase the speed to Variable 10, then to High. Blend for 30 seconds, using the tamper to press the ingredients into the blades.

3. Sprinkle the bicarbonate of soda and 1 tablespoon of the flour over the mixture. Select Variable 4. Turn the machine on and blend for 4 seconds, using the tamper to press the ingredients into the blades until evenly combined. Scrape the mixture into a bowl. Add the remaining flour and mix by hand to combine. Chill overnight before cooking.

4. Pre-heat the oven to 200°C. Coat a large (28 x 43 cm) baking sheet with cooking spray.

5. Form the mixture into balls using 1½ tablespoons chickpea mixture for each. Place the balls on the baking sheet. Bake for 15 minutes, or until golden. Serve hot.

AMOUNT PER SERVING: calories 60, total fat 1 g, saturated fat 0 g, cholesterol 0 mg, sodium 70 mg, total carbohydrate 11 g, dietary fibre 3 g, sugars 2 g, protein 3 g

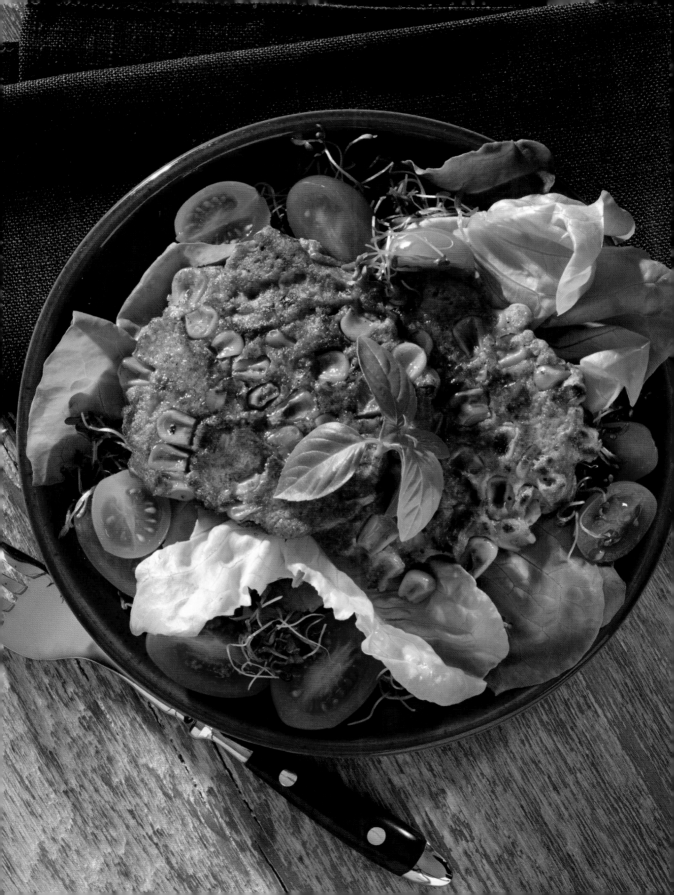

Summer Sweetcorn Cakes

Few foods are more quintessentially summery than sweetcorn. Corn on the cob should be eaten within 24 hours of being picked for the best flavour. If you have two ears that are a bit past their prime, transform them into these sweetcorn cakes, a delicious vegetarian main dish or side for your next dinner party.

Preparation: **20 minutes**   Processing: **25 seconds**   Cook time: **40 minutes**   Yield: **10 cakes**

62 g whole grain flour, preferably home-made (page 64)

½ teaspoon baking powder

120 ml whole milk

2 large eggs

2 tablespoons vegetable oil

½ teaspoon salt

¼ teaspoon ground black pepper

12 g fresh basil leaves

310 g fresh sweetcorn kernels (from 2 large ears)

1. Combine the flour and baking powder in a medium bowl. Set aside.

2. Place the milk, eggs, 1 tablespoon of the oil, salt and pepper into the Vitamix container and secure the lid. Select Variable 1. Turn the machine on and blend for 10 seconds.

3. Remove the lid plug and add the basil through the lid plug opening. Blend for an additional 10 seconds.

4. Stop the machine and remove the lid. Add the sweetcorn kernels and secure the lid. Select Variable 2. Turn the machine on and blend for 5 seconds. Pour the sweetcorn mixture into the flour mixture and mix by hand to combine.

5. Heat the remaining oil in a large non-stick frying pan over a medium heat. Pour 60 ml batter for each cake into the pan. Cook until the edges are dry, about 2 minutes. Flip and cook 2 minutes more, until golden brown.

AMOUNT PER CAKE: calories 90, total fat 4.5 g, saturated fat 1 g, cholesterol 40 mg, sodium 160 mg, total carbohydrate 11 g, dietary fibre 1 g, protein 3 g

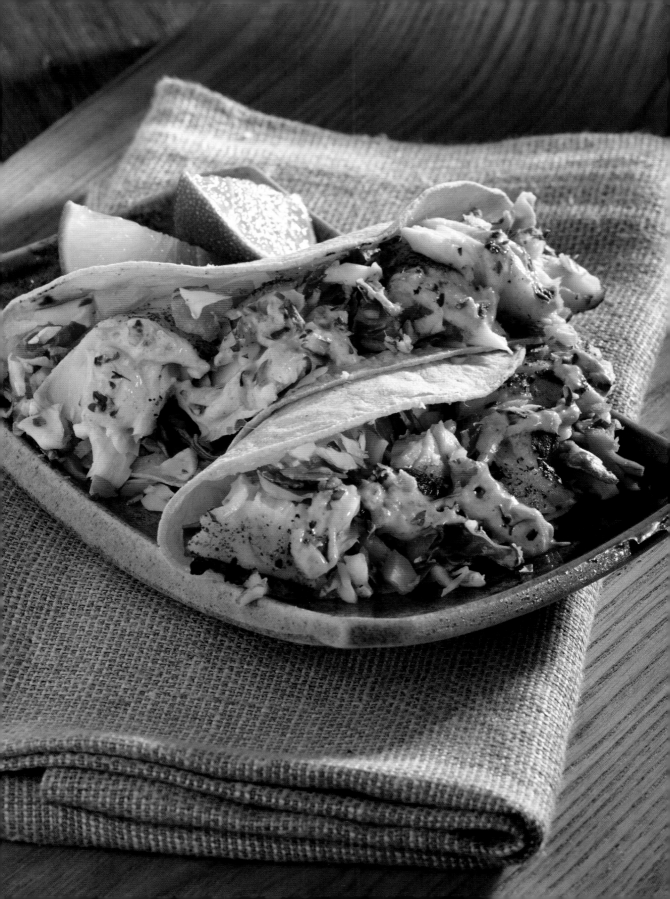

Fish Tacos with Slaw

Fish is generally a good source of protein and omega-3 fatty acids and is low in saturated fat. Make these tangy, crunchy tacos with cabbage slaw to get one of these servings. The Vitamix will do the bulk of the mixing and chopping for you.

Preparation: **20 minutes plus marinating time** Processing: **1 minute plus pulsing**
Cook time: **15 minutes** Yield: **8 servings**

900 g skinless white fish fillets (tilapia, walleye or snapper), cut into eight portions

MARINADE:

120 ml fresh lime juice
120 ml fresh orange juice (page 303)
240 ml olive oil
1 teaspoon honey
1½ teaspoons ground cumin
1 teaspoon sea salt
7 g fresh coriander leaves

DRESSING:

½ orange, peeled
240 ml natural 0% Greek yoghurt, stirred
½ teaspoon ground cumin
½ teaspoon sea salt
⅓ teaspoon chipotle powder
7 g fresh coriander leaves

SLAW:

115 g large chunks green cabbage
85 g large chunks red cabbage
1 medium carrot, halved
8 corn tortillas (15 cm)

OPTIONAL GARNISHES:

Lime wedges
Coriander leaves
Thinly sliced radish and jalapeños

1. For the marinade: Place all the ingredients into the Vitamix container in the order listed and secure the lid. Select Variable 1. Turn the machine on and slowly increase the speed to Variable 10, then to High. Blend for 30 seconds.

2. Place the fish fillets in a shallow pan, pour the marinade over the fish and marinate in the fridge for no longer than 30–40 minutes.

3. For the dressing: Place all the ingredients into the Vitamix container in the order listed and secure the lid. Select Variable 1. Turn the machine on and slowly increase the speed to Variable 6. Blend for 30 seconds. Pour the dressing into a squeezey bottle and set aside until serving.

4. For the slaw: Fill the Vitamix container with water up to the 960 ml mark. Add the green cabbage to the Vitamix container and secure the lid. Select Variable 6. Use the On/Off switch to quickly pulse 4 times. Drain well and transfer to a bowl. Repeat the process with the red cabbage (4 pulses) and the carrot (6 pulses), transferring them to the bowl with the green cabbage.

5. Wrap the tortillas in foil and put them in a warm oven until they're heated through.

6. Remove the fillets from the marinade and grill or pan-sear the fish until cooked through.

7. Fill each tortilla with a few tablespoons of slaw, the fish and 2 tablespoons of dressing and serve with garnishes, if you like.

AMOUNT PER SERVING: calories 240, total fat 10 g, saturated fat 1.5 g, cholesterol 55 mg, sodium 310 mg, total carbohydrate 14 g, dietary fibre 2 g, sugars 5 g, protein 26 g

Green Tea and Nut Crusted Salmon

Fatty fish like salmon are high in two kinds of omega-3 fatty acids: eicosapentaenoic acid (EPA) and docosahexaenoic acid (DHA), which have demonstrated benefits at reducing heart disease. Not only nutritious, this salmon dish, with its crunchy and flavourful topping, is delicious, too!

Preparation: **10 minutes**   Processing: **15 seconds plus pulsing**   Bake time: **14–16 minutes**
Yield: **4 servings**

1 tablespoon plus 1 teaspoon olive oil

40 g unsalted roasted pistachios

1½ teaspoons matcha green tea powder

1 teaspoon light brown sugar

3 tablespoons fine dried breadcrumbs

1 teaspoon finely grated lemon zest

450 g skinless salmon fillet, cut into 4 portions

1. Pre-heat the oven to 170°C. Line a baking sheet with baking paper.

2. Place the olive oil, 1 tablespoon water, pistachios, matcha, brown sugar, breadcrumbs and lemon zest into the Vitamix container in the order listed and secure the lid. Select Variable 1. Turn the machine on and slowly increase the speed to Variable 4. Blend for 15 seconds, using the tamper to press the ingredients into the blades.

3. Stop the machine, remove the lid and scrape the sides of the container to incorporate any unblended ingredients. Replace the lid. Select Variable 6. Use the On/Off switch to quickly pulse 6 times.

4. Place the salmon on the baking sheet and top with the crumb mixture. Bake for 14–16 minutes, or until the fish reaches an internal temperature of 60°C.

AMOUNT PER SERVING: calories 290, total fat 16 g, saturated fat 2.5 g, cholesterol 60 mg, sodium 170 mg, total carbohydrate 8 g, dietary fibre 1 g, sugars 3 g, protein 27 g

Spaghetti with Roasted Vegetable Sauce

Roasting vegetables for this pasta sauce deepens their flavours and helps to caramelise any naturally occurring sugars. (In addition, the lycopene in tomatoes is more easily absorbed by the body when the tomatoes are cooked.) The finished sauce has a deeply nuanced flavour and, thanks to the Vitamix, a silky smooth texture that will coat the spaghetti evenly.

Preparation: **20 minutes**   Processing: **1 minute 10 seconds**   Bake time: **20 minutes**   Yield: **6 servings**

900 g Roma (plum) tomatoes, halved

3 garlic cloves, peeled

½ large carrot

145 g white button mushrooms

1 wedge (4 cm thick) red onion

3 tablespoons extra virgin olive oil

Salt and ground black pepper

340 g whole wheat spaghetti

115 g Parmesan, cut into 2.5-cm chunks

1 x 170-g can tomato paste

6 g fresh basil leaves

6 g fresh oregano leaves

1. Pre-heat the oven to 230°C.

2. Place the tomatoes, garlic, carrot, mushrooms and onion on a large baking sheet. Drizzle with the olive oil and season with salt and pepper to taste. Roast for 20 minutes, or until the tomatoes are very tender, stirring the mushrooms and garlic once.

4. Meanwhile, cook the pasta according to the packet instructions. Drain well, reserving 120 ml of cooking water. Keep warm.

5. Place the cheese into the Vitamix container and secure the lid. Select Variable 1. Turn the machine on and slowly increase the speed to Variable 7. Blend until finely grated. Transfer to a small bowl.

6. Place the roasted vegetables (and any liquid from the pan) and tomato paste into the Vitamix container and secure the lid. Select Variable 1. Turn the machine on and slowly increase the speed to Variable 7. Blend for 1 minute, or until smooth, using the tamper to press the ingredients into the blades.

7. Stop the machine and remove the lid. Add the basil and oregano to the Vitamix container and secure the lid. Select Variable 1. Turn the machine on and slowly increase the speed to Variable 3. Blend for 5 seconds. If a thinner sauce is desired, add the pasta cooking water 1 tablespoon at a time.

8. Serve the sauce over the pasta. Sprinkle with the cheese.

AMOUNT PER SERVING: calories 400, total fat 14 g, saturated fat 3.5 g, cholesterol 15 mg, sodium 380 mg, total carbohydrate 55 g, dietary fibre 13 g, sugars 10 g, protein 18 g

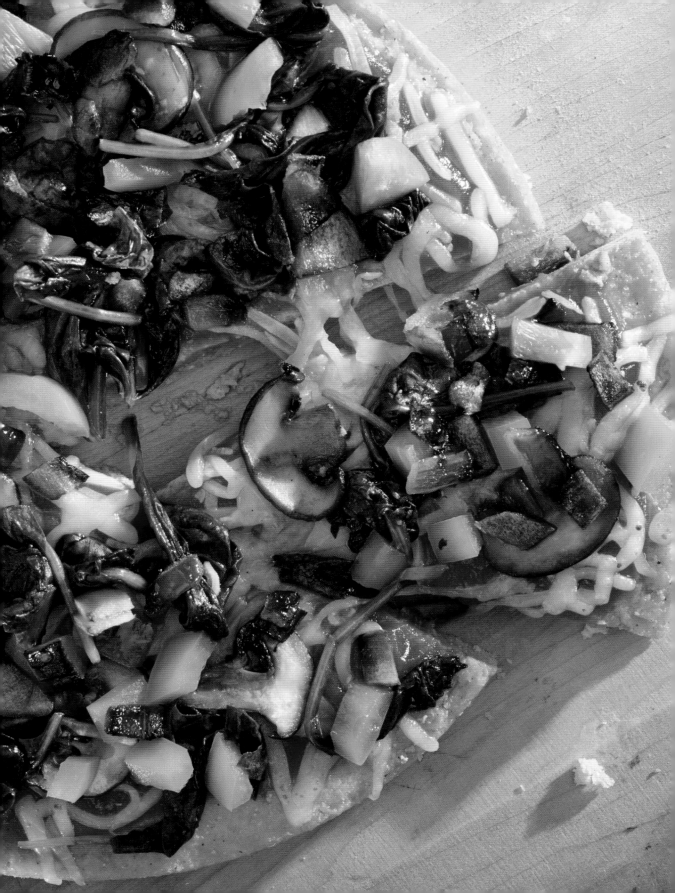

Polenta Pizza

A naturally gluten-free main course to add to your dinner rotation. Grind your own cornmeal and make a quick polenta. Top with a simple pizza sauce, low-fat mozzarella and veggies and bake to bubbly perfection. Enjoy!

Preparation: **20 minutes**   Processing: **1 minute**   Cook time: **10 minutes**
Bake time: **25 minutes**   Yield: **8 servings**

300 ml low-sodium vegetable stock

300 ml low-fat (1%) milk

2 tablespoons plus ½ teaspoon olive oil

¼ teaspoon sea salt

160 g coarse whole-grain cornmeal, preferably home-made (page 60)

120 ml Quick and Easy Pizza Sauce (page 243)

55 g grated reduced-fat mozzarella

2 tablespoons diced red onion

2 tablespoons diced orange pepper

2 tablespoons thinly sliced cremini mushrooms

2 tablespoons sautéed spinach

1. Pre-heat the oven to 200°C. Lightly coat a 23-cm round springform tin with cooking spray.

2. Combine the stock, milk, 2 tablespoons of the oil and the salt in a medium pan and bring to a boil. Reduce to a simmer and add the cornmeal, whisking constantly. Reduce the heat to low, cover and cook for 5 minutes to thicken.

3. Remove the polenta from the heat and immediately spread into the bottom of the springform tin. With a lightly greased spatula or spoon, gently push the polenta over the bottom and at least 5 mm up the sides of the pan to create a raised edge/crust.

4. Brush the remaining ½ teaspoon oil over the crust and bake for 12–15 minutes, until the crust is lightly browned. Remove from the oven and let cool for 5 minutes. Leave the oven on.

5. Top the polenta crust with the pizza sauce, mozzarella and vegetables.

6. Return to the oven and bake for 5 minutes, or until the cheese has melted.

7. Remove the sides of the springform pan, cut pizza into 8 wedges and serve hot.

AMOUNT PER SLICE: calories 180, total fat 8 g, saturated fat 2 g, cholesterol 5 mg, sodium 220 mg, total carbohydrate 21 g, dietary fibre 3 g, sugars 3 g, protein 6 g

Herb and Goats' Cheese Turkey

You may have made stuffed chicken breasts before, but perhaps you haven't ever thought about turkey. After you make these herb, cheese and walnut roasted turkey breasts, you will be hooked! Full of flavour and finished with a simple sauce, this dish is elegant enough for your next dinner party and quick enough for a weeknight supper.

Preparation: **15 minutes**   Processing: **pulsing**   Bake time: **8–10 minutes**
Cook time: **5 minutes**   Yield: **6 servings**

40 g walnut halves

28 g goats' cheese, softened

43 g Neufchâtel (⅓-less-fat cream cheese)

2 teaspoons grated lemon zest

2 garlic cloves, peeled and halved

⅓ teaspoon finely chopped fresh rosemary

Sea salt and ground black pepper

6 skinless turkey breast fillets (115 g each)

1 tablespoon olive oil

1 tablespoon fresh lemon juice

4 tablespoons fat-free low-sodium or no-salt-added chicken stock

1 tablespoon walnut oil

2 tablespoons fresh flatleaf parsley

1. Pre-heat the oven to 190°C.

2. Place the walnuts, goats' cheese, Neufchâtel, lemon zest, garlic, rosemary, ¼ teaspoon salt and ⅛ teaspoon pepper into the Vitamix container in the order listed and secure the lid. Select Variable 7. Use the On/Off switch to quickly pulse 3 times, using the tamper to press the ingredients into the blades. Stop the machine, remove the lid and scrape down the sides of the container. Secure the lid and pulse an additional 3 times. Transfer the goats' cheese filling to a small bowl.

3. Cut a small pocket into the side of each turkey breast. Evenly divide and stuff the filling into the turkey breast pockets. Gently press to flatten the turkey, making sure to keep the stuffing in. Lightly season the turkey with salt and pepper.

4. Heat the oil in a large ovenproof frying pan over a medium-high heat. Add the turkey breast and cook until golden brown, then carefully flip the turkey and transfer the pan to the oven. Roast for 8–10 minutes, or until the turkey reaches an internal temperature of 74°C.

5. Transfer the turkey to a platter to keep warm.

6. Place the pan back over a medium heat. Add the lemon juice and stock to the pan and cook, scraping up the browned bits from the bottom of the pan. Simmer for 4 minutes to slightly reduce. Stir in the walnut oil and parsley.

7. Spoon the sauce over the turkey and serve.

AMOUNT PER SERVING: calories 240, total fat 12 g, saturated fat 2.5 g, cholesterol 80 mg, sodium 210 mg, total carbohydrate 2 g, dietary fibre 1 g, sugars 1 g, protein 30 g

Herb-Marinated Pork Tenderloin

Thyme, basil, rosemary, oregano, citrus and spices make simple pork tenderloin something special. Pair with one or two of the salads in the Chapter 4 for a satisfying dinner. Leftover pork, cold and thinly sliced, makes wonderful sandwiches.

Preparation: **10 minutes plus marinating time**   Processing: **15 seconds**   Yield: **8 servings**

120 ml vegetable oil

4 tablespoons fresh lime juice

3 tablespoons fresh oregano leaves

3 tablespoons fresh thyme leaves

2 tablespoons fresh basil leaves

1 tablespoon fresh rosemary leaves

1 teaspoon grated lemon zest

1½ teaspoons onion powder

½ teaspoon sea salt

½ teaspoon ground black pepper

2 garlic cloves, peeled

900 g pork tenderloin, trimmed

1. Place the vegetable oil, lime juice, oregano, thyme, basil, rosemary, lemon zest, onion powder, salt and pepper into the Vitamix container in the order listed and secure the lid. Select Variable 1. Turn the machine on and slowly increase the speed to Variable 8. Blend for 10 seconds.

2. Stop the machine and scrape the sides of the container with a spatula. Add the garlic to the Vitamix container and secure the lid. Select Variable 6. Use the On/Off switch to quickly pulse 4 to 5 times.

3. Place the pork tenderloin in a large zip-lock plastic bag and pour the marinade into the bag. Chill for 1 hour, but not more than 1 hour 30 minutes.

4. Remove the pork from the marinade (discard the marinade). Grill to desired level of doneness.

AMOUNT PER SERVING: calories 160, total fat 6 g, saturated fat 1 g, cholesterol 75 mg, sodium 100 mg, total carbohydrate 2 g, dietary fibre 0 g, sugars 0 g, protein 24 g

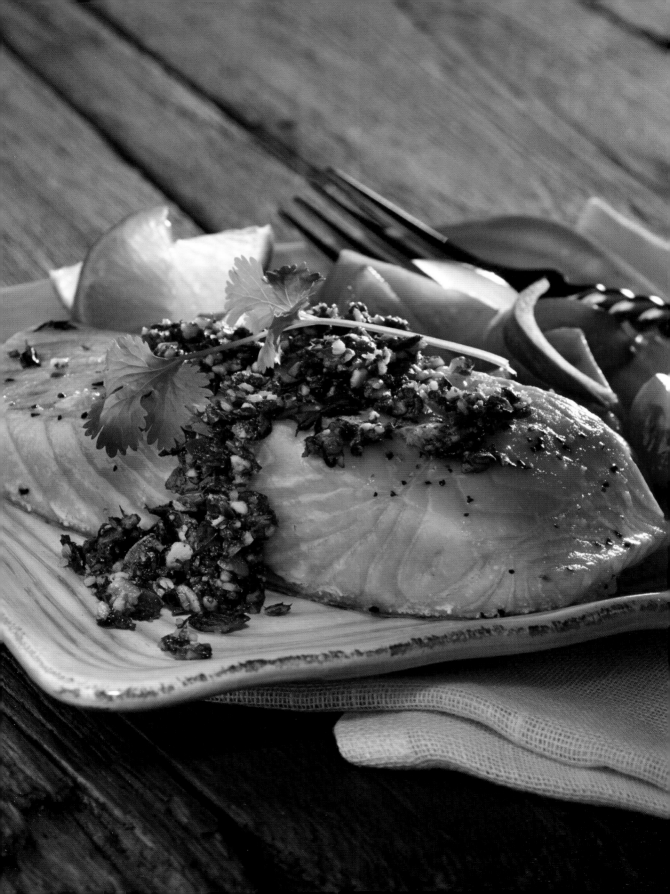

Roasted Salmon with Coriander-Seed Pesto

Not only is salmon chock-full of omega-3 fatty acids, it is quick to cook, too. While the salmon is roasting, you will have just enough time to whip up this unique pesto. The pesto, made from fresh coriander, coriander seeds, pumpkin seeds, garlic, lime and olive oil, provides a bright, tangy contrast to the rich fish.

Preparation: **15 minutes**   Processing: **45 seconds**   Bake time: **12–14 minutes**   Yield: **4 servings**

PESTO:

4 tablespoons extra virgin olive oil

60 g unsalted roasted pumpkin seeds

14 g fresh coriander leaves

¼ teaspoon coriander seeds

1 small garlic clove, peeled

1 tablespoon fresh lime juice

¼ teaspoon sea salt

⅓ teaspoon ground black pepper

SALMON:

680 g skin-on salmon fillet, cut into 6 portions

2 tablespoons olive oil

1 tablespoon fresh thyme leaves

Grated zest of 1 lemon

½ teaspoon ground black pepper

1. For the pesto: Place the ingredients into the Vitamix container in the order listed and secure the lid. Select Variable 1. Turn the machine on and slowly increase the speed to Variable 4. Blend for 15 seconds, using the tamper to press the ingredients into the blades. Stop, scrape and repeat twice.

2. For the salmon: Pre-heat the oven to 170°C. Line a baking sheet with foil or a silicone baking mat.

3. Place the salmon skin side down on the baking sheet. Brush with the olive oil and rub with the thyme, lemon zest and pepper. Roast salmon for 12–14 minutes, or until the salmon is opaque in the centre and reaches and internal temperature of 60°C.

4. Serve the pesto on top of the roasted salmon.

AMOUNT PER SERVING: calories 350, total fat 25 g, saturated fat 4 g, cholesterol 60 mg, sodium 230 mg, total carbohydrate 2 g, dietary fibre 1 g, sugars 0 g, protein 27 g

Yoghurt-Marinated Turkey Breast

This flavour-packed marinade gives lean turkey breasts a big boost of flavour. The recipe yields eight servings, and any leftovers will be the beginning of a pretty amazing turkey sandwich or wrap.

Preparation: **15 minutes**   Processing: **30 seconds**   Yield: **8 servings**

8 pieces boneless skinless turkey breast (about 170 g each)

80 ml olive oil

480 ml natural 0% Greek yoghurt, stirred

½ small lime, peeled

6 garlic cloves, peeled

5-cm piece fresh ginger, peeled and cut into pieces

1 tablespoon garam masala

1 teaspoon sea salt

1 teaspoon ground black pepper

16 g fresh coriander leaves

1 medium onion (170 g), cut into pieces

1. Place the turkey between sheets of greaseproof paper and gently pound to a 1-cm thickness.

2. Transfer the turkey to a sturdy zip-lock plastic bag.

3. Place the oil, yoghurt, lime, garlic, ginger, garam masala, salt, pepper, coriander and onion into the Vitamix container in the order listed and secure the lid. Select Variable 1. Turn the machine on and slowly increase the speed to Variable 10, then to High. Blend for 30 seconds.

4. Pour the marinade over the turkey, seal the bag and chill for at least 3 hours or overnight.

5. Remove the turkey from the marinade (discard the marinade). Griddle (or grill) over a medium-high heat until cooked through.

AMOUNT PER SERVING: calories 260, total fat 3.5 g, saturated fat 0.5 g, cholesterol 105 mg, sodium 180 mg, total carbohydrate 6 g, dietary fibre 1 g, sugars 3 g, protein 47 g

Fall Flavours Ravioli

The only thing better than a ravioli full of the flavours of autumn is how easy it can be to make this simple, savoury dish yourself. The ravioli are served in a parsley-flecked broth for a beautiful presentation.

Preparation: **20 minutes**   Processing: **30 seconds plus pulsing**   Yield: **30 ravioli (7–8 servings)**

280 g roasted pumpkin or butternut squash, cut into chunks

45 g grated Parmesan

⅓ teaspoon ground sage

Pinch of ground nutmeg

⅓ teaspoon sea salt

⅓ teaspoon ground black pepper

60 wonton wrappers

240 ml low-sodium vegetable stock

1½ teaspoons finely chopped fresh flatleaf parsley, plus more for garnish

1. Place the roasted pumpkin into the Vitamix container and secure the lid. Select Variable 1. Turn the machine on and slowly increase the speed to Variable 6. Blend for 15 seconds, using the tamper to press the ingredients into the blades. Stop the machine, remove the lid and scrape the sides of the container. Repeat the procedure.

2. Remove the lid. Add the Parmesan, sage, nutmeg, salt and pepper to the Vitamix container and secure the lid. Select Variable 4. Use the On/Off switch to quickly pulse 4 to 5 times, while using the tamper to press the ingredients into the blades. Scrape the filling into a bowl.

3. Place half of the wonton wrappers on to a lightly floured work surface. Spoon 2 teaspoons of filling into the centre of each wonton wrapper. Dip your finger in water and wet the edges of the wrappers. Place another wrapper over the mound of filling and press gently to seal the edges and work out any air bubbles between the wrappers.

4. Heat the stock and 1½ teaspoons parsley in a small pan to a simmer.

5. Meanwhile, cook the ravioli in a large pan of boiling water. Add them in small batches and gently cook until they float, about 4 minutes. Scoop out the ravioli with a slotted spoon and drain well, then place in the pan with the warmed vegetable stock and parsley.

6. Serve in wide shallow bowls garnished with parsley.

AMOUNT PER SERVING: calories 230, total fat 3 g, saturated fat 1 g, cholesterol 15 mg, sodium 510 mg, total carbohydrate 42 g, dietary fibre 2 g, sugars 1 g, protein 8 g

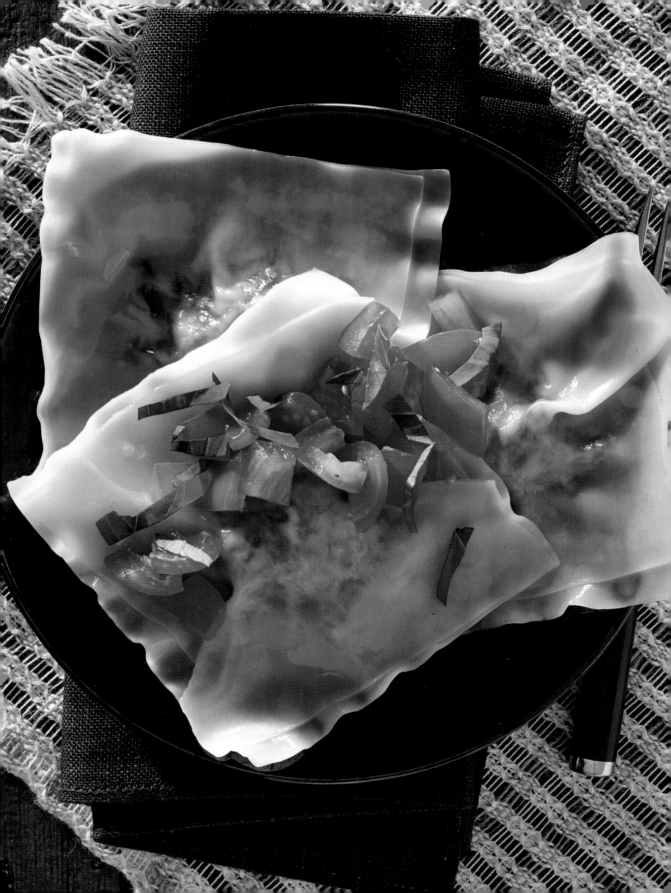

Cheese and Kale Ravioli

The filling for this cheese and kale ravioli comes together quickly in the Vitamix. As for assembling the ravioli? Many hands make light work! Get your kids, friends or even your dinner guests to help.

Preparation: **15 minutes**   Processing: **pulsing**   Cook time: **1 hour**   Yield: **30 ravioli**

1 tablespoon olive oil

3 tablespoons chopped shallots

1 bunch Tuscan (black) kale, stemmed and cut into small pieces (about 155 g)

125 g reduced-fat ricotta

55 g goats' cheese

80 ml natural 0% Greek yoghurt, stirred

½ teaspoon ground black pepper

1 teaspoon dried basil

810 g coarsely chopped tomatoes

2 tablespoons chopped fresh basil

60 wonton wrappers

1. Heat the oil in a large frying pan over a medium-high heat. Add the shallots and cook until just tender. Add the kale and cook until wilted, 3–4 minutes. Let cool completely.

2. Place the cheeses, yoghurt, pepper and basil into the Vitamix container and secure the lid. Select Variable 6. Use the On/Off switch to quickly pulse 4 to 6 times.

3. Add the cooled kale mixture to the Vitamix container and secure the lid. Select Variable 1. Use the On/Off switch to pulse 8 times. Remove the lid and scrape the sides of the container. Pulse an additional 8 times while using the tamper in between pulses to press the ingredients into the blades.

4. Combine the tomatoes and basil in a bowl and set aside.

5. Place half of the wonton wrappers on a lightly floured work surface. Spoon 2 teaspoons of the cheese mixture into the centre of each wrapper. Dip your finger in water and wet the edges of the wrappers. Place another wrapper over the mound of filling and press gently to seal the edges and work out any air bubbles between the wrappers.

6. Bring a large pan of water to a boil. Reduce to a simmer and place 6–8 of the ravioli at a time into the water. Gently cook for 4–5 minutes. Remove with a slotted spoon and drain well.

7. Serve the ravioli hot with the tomato mixture.

AMOUNT PER SERVING (4 RAVIOLI): calories 280, total fat 6 g, saturated fat 2.5 g, cholesterol 15 mg, sodium 430 mg, total carbohydrate 45 g, dietary fibre 3 g, sugars 4 g, protein 12 g

Spinach Couscous Patties

These bright spinach patties combine many of the flavours of Greek spinach pie – greens, feta, dill – in a healthier package with fewer calories than most purchased varieties of spinach pie. A great vegetarian dinner or a hot appetizer.

Preparation: **10 minutes**   Processing: **15 seconds plus pulsing**   Cook time: **30 minutes**
Yield: **12 patties**

45 g baby spinach

165 g whole wheat couscous

240 ml natural 0% Greek yoghurt, stirred

50 g crumbled feta

1 garlic clove

¼ teaspoon sea salt

½ teaspoon ground black pepper

40 g chopped red onion

9 g fresh dill

1 tablespoon olive oil

1. Heat 1 tablespoon water in a large pan, add the spinach, and cook until the spinach wilts and releases its liquid. Remove from the heat and transfer to a fine-mesh sieve. Let cool completely, pressing out any additional moisture.

2. Bring 300 ml water to a boil in a small pan. Stir in the couscous, remove from the heat, cover and set aside for 10 minutes. Uncover, fluff the couscous with a fork and transfer to a large bowl.

3. Place the yoghurt, feta, garlic, salt and pepper into the Vitamix container in the order listed and secure the lid. Select Variable 1. Turn the machine on and slowly increase the speed to Variable 4. Blend for 15 seconds.

4. Stop the machine, remove the lid and scrape down sides of the container. Add the spinach, onion, dill and oil. Secure lid. Select Variable 6. Use the On/Off switch to quickly pulse 10 times, using the tamper between pulses. You may need to scrape down the sides of the container with a spatula in between pulses.

5. Combine the yoghurt mixture with the cooked couscous and mix well. Form into 12 patties.

6. Working in batches, cook the patties in a non-stick frying pan coated with cooking spray over a medium heat until light golden brown, 3–4 minutes each side. Transfer the patties to a baking sheet.

7. Prior to serving, place the patties in a 150°C oven for 6 minutes, or until heated through.

AMOUNT PER PATTY: calories 80, total fat 2.5 g, saturated fat 1 g, cholesterol 5 mg, sodium 110 mg, total carbohydrate 13 g, dietary fibre 2 g, sugars 1 g, protein 4 g

Quinoa and Barley Sliders

A hearty, flavourful vegan burger for your next barbecue. Cook the barley and quinoa separately and then pulse the filling together in the Vitamix. These burgers are best cooked in a pan with hot oil. Searing creates a golden-brown crust that helps these delicate, grain-filled burgers hold together.

Preparation: **10 minutes**   Processing: **45 seconds**   Cook time: **1 hour**   Yield: **14 sliders**

660 ml low-sodium vegetable stock

85 g quinoa, rinsed well and drained

100 g pearl barley

200 g firm tofu

2 garlic cloves, peeled

4 g fresh coriander leaves

½ teaspoon chilli powder

½ teaspoon ground cumin

130 g panko breadcrumbs

2 tablespoons vegetable/olive oil blend

14 whole wheat slider buns, split and toasted

OPTIONAL GARNISHES:

Baby spinach

Tomato slices

Red onion slices

1. In a small pan, bring 240 ml of the vegetable stock to a boil. Add the quinoa and cook, simmering, for 10 minutes or until quinoa grains have puffed and are cooked through. Remove the pan from heat and cool completely.

2. In a small pan, cook the barley in the remaining 420 ml vegetable stock. Drain and cool completely.

3. Place the tofu, garlic, coriander, chilli powder, cumin, half the cooked barley and 2 tablespoons of the panko breadcrumbs into the Vitamix container in the order listed and secure the lid. Select Variable 1. Turn the machine on and slowly increase the speed to Variable 10, then to High. Blend for 45 seconds, using the tamper to press the ingredients into the blades.

4. Pour the tofu mixture into a large bowl. Add the quinoa and remaining barley and stir to combine. Form the mixture into 14 slider patties. Coat the patties with the remaining panko breadcrumbs.

5. Heat the oil in a large frying pan over a medium heat. Add the patties and cook until golden and heated through, 3–4 minutes per side.

6. Serve the sliders on toasted slider buns. If desired, garnish with baby spinach, tomato and red onion slices.

AMOUNT PER SLIDER: calories 230, total fat 7 g, saturated fat 0.5 g, cholesterol 0 mg, sodium 270 mg, total carbohydrate 36 g, dietary fibre 5 g, sugars 1 g, protein 8 g

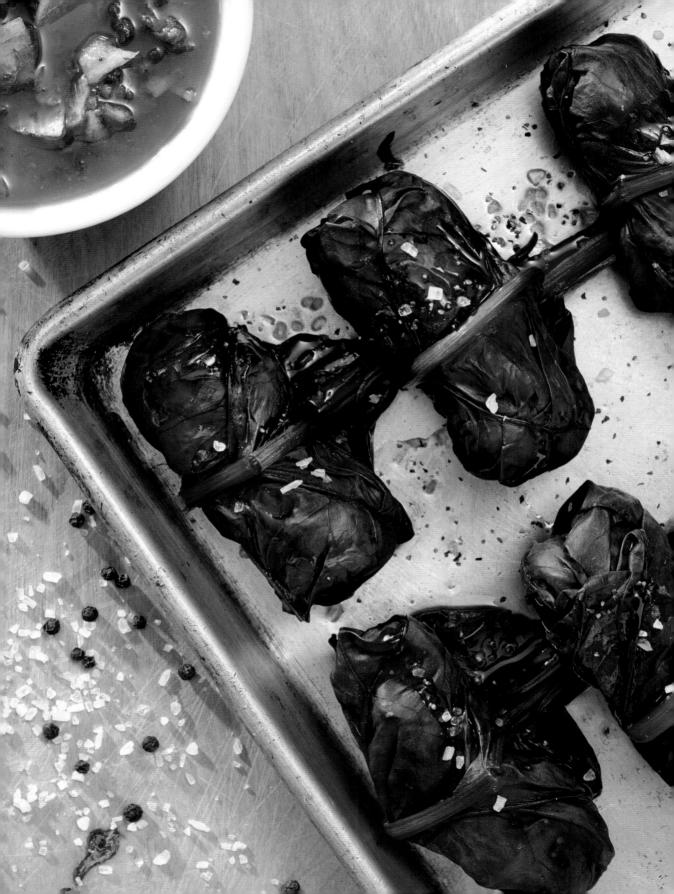

Stuffed Chard Leaves with Kalamata Olive Vinaigrette

The next time you need a special main course for a vegetarian guest or you simply want an elegant meatless meal, reach for this recipe. Swiss chard leaves are blanched and then filled with a satisfying mix of potato, Swiss chard stems, herbs and goats' cheese. The rolls are baked and then topped with flavourful Kalamata olive vinaigrette. Greens have never tasted so good!

Preparation: **20 minutes**   Processing: **15 seconds plus pulsing**   Cook time: **10 minutes**

Bake time: **15–20 minutes**   Yield: **12 servings**

12 ruby chard leaves, stemmed (about 2 bunches)

FILLING:
1 tablespoon extra virgin olive oil
4 garlic cloves, minced
75 g diced onion
90 g diced chard stems
2 medium russet (baking) potatoes (555 g), baked until tender and peeled
¾ teaspoon sea salt
½ teaspoon ground black pepper
¼ teaspoon ground nutmeg
115 g goats' cheese
2 tablespoons chopped fresh basil
2 tablespoons snipped fresh chives

VINAIGRETTE:
120 ml olive oil
6 tablespoons red wine vinegar
½ teaspoon sea salt
¼ teaspoon ground black pepper
75 g pitted Kalamata olives, rinsed
35 g finely chopped shallots

1. Pre-heat the oven to 190°C.

2. Bring a large pan of water to a boil. Set up a large bowl of ice and water. Carefully blanch each chard leaf and then cold-shock in ice water. Drain well and pat dry on kitchen paper.

3. For the filling: Heat the olive oil in a large frying pan over a medium-high heat. Add the garlic, onion and chard stems. Cook until the onions are tender, 4–6 minutes. Remove from the heat.

4. Transfer the sautéed vegetables to the Vitamix container and secure the lid. Select Variable 6. Use the On/Off switch to quickly pulse 4 times. Stop, remove the lid and scrape the sides of the container. Repeat the process 3 more times for a total of 12 pulses.

5. In a large bowl, mash the potatoes with a fork and then add the sautéed onion mixture, salt, pepper, nutmeg, goats' cheese, basil and chives. Mix well.

6. Lay out the blanched chard leaves on a clean work surface. Place about 3 tablespoons of the potato mixture in the centre of each leaf. Fold in the sides and, starting at the top of the leaf, roll up to enclose all filling. Place in a greased 20-cm square baking dish.

7. Bake the stuffed chard for 15–20 minutes, or until heated through.

8. Meanwhile, for the vinaigrette: Place the oil, vinegar, salt and pepper into the Vitamix container in the order listed and secure the lid. Select Variable 1. Turn the machine on and slowly increase the speed to Variable 10, then to High. Blend for 10 seconds.

9. Stop the machine and remove the lid. Add the olives and shallots to the Vitamix container and secure the lid. Select Variable 1. Turn the machine on and slowly increase the speed to Variable 4. Blend for 5 seconds.

10. To serve, top the warmed chard rolls with the vinaigrette.

AMOUNT PER SERVING: calories 200, total fat 14 g, saturated fat 3 g, cholesterol 5 mg, sodium 500 mg, total carbohydrate 14 g, dietary fibre 2 g, sugars 2 g, protein 4 g

Spicy Jerk Chicken

The wonderfully spicy flavour in this jerk marinade will transport you to the West Indies, brightening even the gloomiest days. Freshly ground spices and ginger really make the flavours pop. Serve with brown rice and garnish with thinly sliced spring onions.

Preparation: **15 minutes**   Processing: **45 seconds**   Yield: **8 servings**

MARINADE:

6 tablespoons olive oil

4 tablespoons fresh lime juice

4 spring onions, cut into pieces

1 small Scotch Bonnet or jalapeño pepper, halved and seeded

3 garlic cloves, peeled

2 tablespoons fresh thyme leaves

1-cm piece fresh ginger, peeled

1 tablespoon dark brown sugar

2 teaspoons allspice berries

1 teaspoon sea salt

¼ teaspoon ground black pepper

2 tablespoons distilled white vinegar

900 g boneless skinless chicken thighs

1. For the marinade: Place all the ingredients into the Vitamix container in the order listed and secure the lid. Select Variable 1. Turn the machine on and slowly increase the speed to Variable 10. Blend for 45 seconds.

2. Place the chicken in a glass dish and toss with the marinade. Cover and chill for 4 hours or overnight.

3. Bake or grill until cooked.

AMOUNT PER SERVING: calories 240, total fat 15 g, saturated fat 2.5 g, cholesterol 110 mg, sodium 400 mg, total carbohydrate 4 g, dietary fibre 0 g, sugars 2 g, protein 22 g

Tempeh Teriyaki with Slaw

Cabbage has just 22 calories per 85 g and tons of crunch. Here, in this refreshing, Asian-influenced slaw, the cabbage provides the perfect complement to the chewy, slightly salty tempeh.

Preparation: **15 minutes**   Processing: **pulsing**   Cook time: **20 minutes**   Yield: **4 servings**

SLAW:

255 g Chinese cabbage chunks

½ medium carrot

¼ small red onion, halved

1 teaspoon hoisin sauce

2 teaspoons unseasoned rice vinegar

⅛ teaspoon sea salt

TEMPEH:

225 g tempeh, cut into thin strips

1 teaspoon Chinese five-spice powder

1 tablespoon sesame oil

2 tablespoons reduced-sodium soy sauce

2 large whole wheat pitta breads, halved crossways, toasted

1. For the slaw: Fill the Vitamix container with 1.4 litres water. Add the cabbage and secure the lid. Select Variable 8. Use the On/Off switch to quickly pulse 3 times. Drain the cabbage well into a fine-mesh sieve, pressing out as much liquid as possible. Transfer to a large bowl.

2. Place the carrot and onion into the Vitamix container and secure the lid. Select Variable 6. Use the On/Off switch to quickly pulse 6 times. Stop, scrape down the sides of the container and pulse an additional 6 times.

3. Transfer the carrot-onion mixture to the bowl with the cabbage. Add the hoisin, vinegar and salt and mix well. Set aside.

4. For the tempeh: Bring 240 ml water to a simmer in a large, covered frying pan. Add the tempeh and cook until plump and just soft, 8–10 minutes. Remove the tempeh from the frying pan and immediately sprinkle with the five-spice powder.

5. Heat the sesame oil in a large frying pan over a medium heat. Add the tempeh strips and cook, turning once, until lightly browned, being careful not to burn the five-spice powder. Remove the pan from the heat and sprinkle the tempeh with the soy sauce.

6. To serve, divide the tempeh and slaw among the 4 pitta halves.

AMOUNT PER SERVING: calories 250, total fat 9 g, saturated fat 1.5 g, cholesterol 0 mg, sodium 450 mg, total carbohydrate 30 g, dietary fibre 8 g, sugars 2 g, protein 16 g

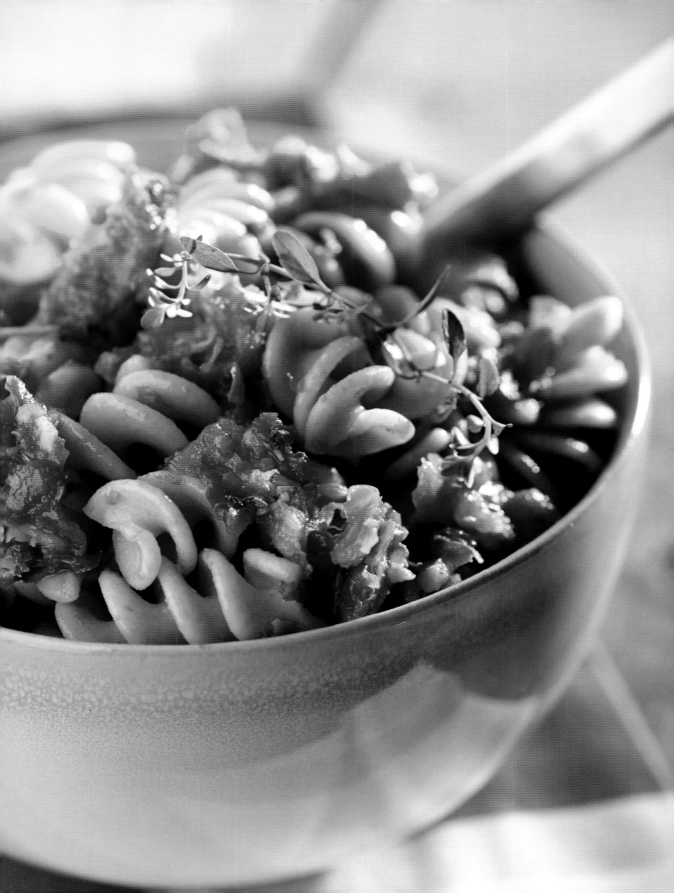

Whole Wheat Pasta with Dried Tomato and Caper Vinaigrette Sauce

Perhaps best described as a sun-dried tomato pesto, this delicious sauce will be the perfect finishing touch for your pasta when fresh tomatoes are not in season. Made of store cupboard staples, this is also a great go-to dinner on the nights when the fridge is on the empty side.

Preparation: **15 minutes**   Processing: **10–15 seconds**   Cook time: **15 minutes**   Yield: **6 servings**

450 g whole wheat pasta

3 tablespoons olive oil

2 tablespoons red wine vinegar

55 g sun-dried tomatoes in olive oil, rinsed, well drained and chopped into pieces

1 tablespoon small capers, rinsed and well drained

1 tablespoon fresh thyme leaves

1 garlic clove, peeled

¼ teaspoon ground black pepper

1. Cook the pasta according to the packet instructions. Drain and keep warm.

2. Meanwhile, place the olive oil, vinegar, tomatoes, capers, thyme, garlic and pepper into the Vitamix container in the order listed and secure the lid. Select Variable 5. Blend for 10–15 seconds.

3. Transfer the hot pasta to a large serving bowl, spoon the sun-dried tomato mixture on top and generously toss to coat pasta well. Serve hot.

AMOUNT PER SERVING: calories 350, total fat 10 g, saturated fat 1 g, cholesterol 0 mg, sodium 80 mg, total carbohydrate 55 g, dietary fibre 13 g, sugars 1 g, protein 13 g

Turkey Burgers with Cherry Salsa

Did you know you could mince meat in your Vitamix? It will be more of a very fine chop, rather than the mince you may be used to from the supermarket or butcher. The upside of mincing your own meat is that you know exactly what is in it. No mystery meat! Cutting and partially freezing the meat before you pulse it helps the Vitamix cut the meat instead of tearing or smearing it.

Preparation: **20 minutes**   Processing: **pulsing**   Yield: **4 servings**

SALSA:

1 navel orange, peeled and halved

1 jalapeño pepper, quartered and seeded

140 g fresh pitted or thawed frozen cherries

6 g fresh coriander leaves

1 tablespoon agave nectar

BURGERS:

½ medium onion, quartered

450 g frozen boneless turkey breast, partially thawed, cut into 2.5-cm cubes

1 large egg

1 tablespoon reduced-sodium soy sauce

¼ teaspoon ground black pepper

30 g fine dried breadcrumbs

2 tablespoons grated Parmesan

2 garlic cloves, finely chopped

2 whole wheat hamburger buns, split and toasted

1. For the salsa: Place all the ingredients into the Vitamix container in the order listed and secure the lid. Select Variable 6. Use the On/Off switch to quickly pulse 12–14 times, using the tamper to press the ingredients into the blades.

2. For the burgers: To wet-chop the onion, fill the Vitamix container with water up to the 960-ml mark. Add the onion and secure the lid. Select Variable 6. Use the On/Off switch to quickly pulse 4 times. Drain well and clean the container.

3. To mince the turkey, work in two batches, 225 g at a time. Add the partially thawed frozen turkey to the Vitamix container and secure the lid. Select Variable 8. Use the On/Off switch to pulse 8–10 times, until the mixture resembles minced meat. Use the tamper while pulsing to press the ingredients into the blades.

4. Place the minced turkey in a large bowl and add the onion, egg, soy sauce, pepper, breadcrumbs, Parmesan and garlic. Mix well.

5. Form into 4 patties and griddle over a medium-high heat until an internal temperature of 74°C is reached.

6. Serve the burgers open-face on a toasted bun half. Top with the cherry salsa.

AMOUNT PER SERVING: calories 310, total fat 4.5 g, saturated fat 1.5 g, cholesterol 95 mg, sodium 480 mg, total carbohydrate 33 g, dietary fibre 4 g, sugars 16 g, protein 35 g

Quinoa Black Bean Burgers

This is an amazing vegan burger! Packed with delicious and nutritious ingredients – black beans, quinoa, sweetcorn, roasted poblano peppers and lots of spices – these burgers will be a hit with vegetarians and meat-eaters alike. Serve with Guacamole (page 97) or California Salsa (page 100), sliced tomatoes, lettuce, sliced red onion and pickled jalapeños.

Preparation: **15 minutes**   Processing: **30 seconds**   Cook time: **12–20 minutes**   Yield: **8 patties**

1 x 425-g can no-salt-added black beans, rinsed and drained

95 g cooked quinoa

85 g frozen sweetcorn kernels, thawed

1 roasted poblano pepper, peeled, seeded, and chopped (about 55 g)

40 g panko breadcrumbs

4 g fresh coriander leaves

4 drops of Tabasco sauce

½ teaspoon chilli powder

½ teaspoon ground cumin

½ teaspoon garlic powder

½ teaspoon sea salt

½ teaspoon ground black pepper

4 tablespoons olive oil

1. Place 2 tablespoons water and half of the black beans into the Vitamix container and secure the lid. Select Variable 1. Turn the machine on and slowly increase the speed to Variable 4. Blend for 30 seconds, using the tamper to press the ingredients into the blades.

2. Transfer the bean purée to a large bowl and add the quinoa, sweetcorn, poblano, panko, coriander, Tabasco, chilli powder, cumin, garlic powder, salt and black pepper. Mix well to incorporate. Form into 8 small patties and transfer to a baking sheet. Place the baking sheet in the fridge for at least 15–20 minutes to firm up the patties.

3. Heat 2 tablespoons of the oil in a large frying pan over a medium heat. Add 4 of the patties and cook until golden brown and crispy, 3–5 minutes per side. Repeat with the remaining oil and patties.

AMOUNT PER PATTY: calories 130, total fat 7 g, saturated fat 1 g, cholesterol 0 mg, sodium 115 mg, total carbohydrate 14 g, dietary fibre 3 g, sugars 0 g, protein 3 g

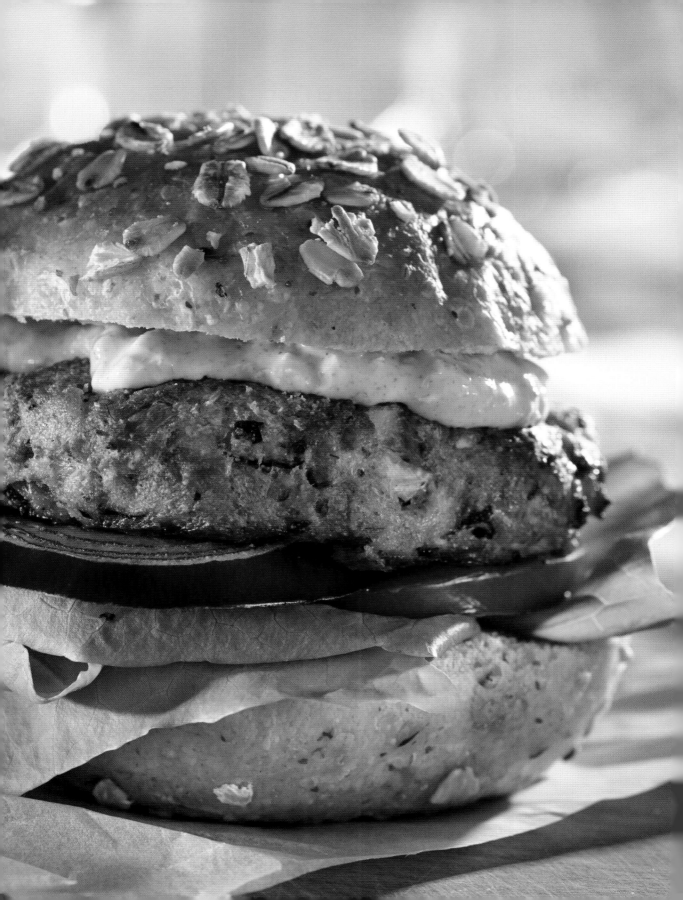

Courgette Burgers

When your garden is bursting with courgettes, and you have eaten all of the courgette bread you can manage, try making these delicious burgers. Packed with courgettes and spices, these burgers are baked instead of pan-seared. Serve on whole-grain buns with lettuce, tomato and red onion. Instead of ketchup, try the patties with California Salsa (page 100).

Preparation: **15 minutes**   Processing: **pulsing**   Bake time: **15 minutes**   Yield: **17 patties**

900 g courgettes, cut into large chunks

1 large onion (195 g), quartered

180 g Italian seasoned dried breadcrumbs

3 large eggs

50 g grated Parmesan

½ teaspoon garlic powder

½ teaspoon onion powder

½ teaspoon dried parsley

½ teaspoon dried basil

½ teaspoon dried oregano

1. Pre-heat the oven to 230°C. Coat a 28 x 43 cm baking sheet with cooking spray.

2. To wet-chop the courgettes, place into the Vitamix container and add enough water so the courgette floats off the blades. Secure the lid. Select Variable 4. Use the On/Off switch to quickly pulse. Repeat 4 times. Drain well and pat dry. Transfer to a large bowl.

3. Place the onion into the Vitamix container and secure the lid. Select Variable 3. Use the On/Off switch to quickly pulse. Repeat 4 times to evenly chop. Add to the courgette.

4. And the breadcrumbs, eggs, cheese and seasonings to the bowl and stir until evenly combined. Measure 60-g portions of the courgette mixture and place on the prepared baking sheet. Spread gently to form a patty.

5. Bake the patties for 15 minutes, or until hot through.

AMOUNT PER PATTY: calories 80, total fat 2.5 g, saturated fat 1 g, cholesterol 35 mg, sodium 240 mg, total carbohydrate 10 g, dietary fibre 1 g, sugars 2 g, protein 5 g

SUSAN AMICK

Many athletes at all performance levels enjoy smoothies and whole-food juices as part of their training diet, while others drink them to aid their after-workout recovery. Susan Amick, her boyfriend, Boris, and her son are a seriously active and athletic family and routinely make smoothies and juices. But prior to buying a Vitamix, they couldn't stop breaking blenders. 'We were making lots of smoothies,' Susan remembers. 'If we wanted to use frozen fruit or ice, anything that was still whole, be it a fruit or vegetable, [the blenders] just couldn't take it!' Susan bought a Vitamix in 2003 and she and her family have been using it non-stop ever since. The family is now using a new Vitamix, but their first machine is still going strong with new owners.

Today, Susan, a tai chi instructor, Boris, a triathlete coach and gym owner, and Susan's son, a professional cyclist in Europe, still use their Vitamix to power their busy, active lives. Susan says she frequently makes

....

healthy smoothies as well as soups. Susan's son likes to make quick recovery drinks of protein powder and fruit after hard workouts. (He even took a Vitamix when he went to college.) Susan said the family started using their Vitamix the moment it arrived. 'Our Vitamix,' Susan laughs, 'probably gets used more than in any other household with a Vitamix. We use it a couple of times a day!' Susan's son misses his Vitamix when he is racing in Europe and looks forward to buying one there so he can power his races with his favourite smoothies.

Using whole foods to power a healthy, very active life? A whole foods success story if ever there was one!

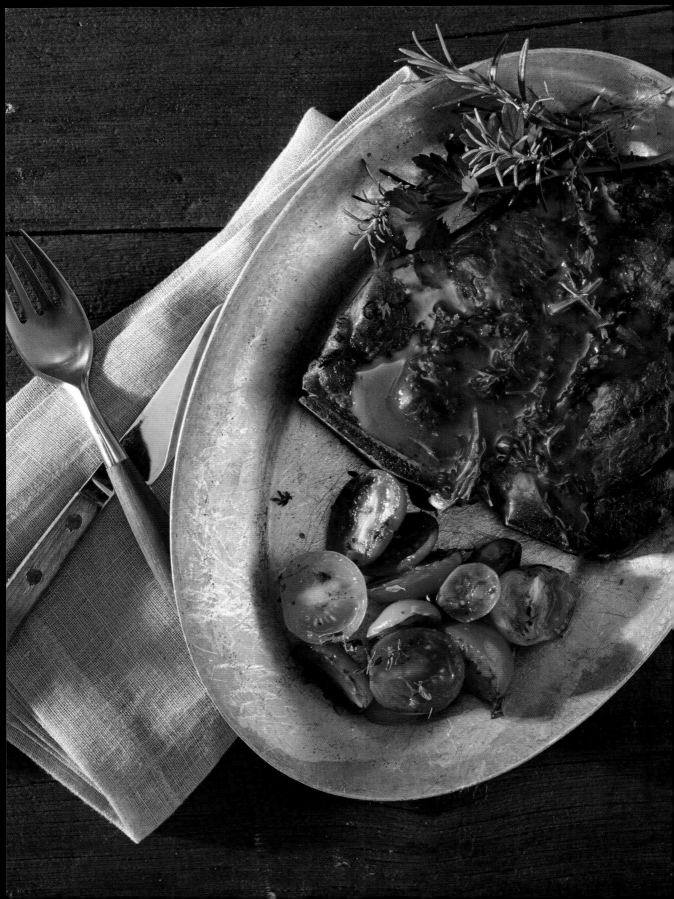

Chapter 6

Dressings, Sauces and Spreads

My grandma Ruth and grandpa Bill were quite a pair! Grandpa was a natural salesman, full of ideas and a genuine love of people, animals and laughter. Grandma brought order to the pandemonium that his gregarious style often created. My grandfather had a powerful presence but always joked, teased and made funny faces. He was larger than life. He had great ideas and the tenacity to pursue them. My grandmother would silently, quietly put things in place. They couldn't do it without each other.

How does this relate to sauces and dressings? Think of it like this. Plain vegetables are good. They are certainly healthy as they are, simple and pretty tasty. But a nutritious vinaigrette can really make a salad sing. And undressed pasta might be the perfect dish for many children, but a hearty tomato sauce makes it a more complete meal. The sauces and dressings, on the other hand, aren't really good to eat on their own. They need something to dress. A good partnership can be a wonderful presence in our lives and on our plates. Grandma and Grandpa worked together like pasta and tomato sauce, like a healthy salad dressing and a bowl full of fresh, crunchy vegetables. A perfect combination, an amazing team.

At Vitamix, we completely understand that we are more likely to want to eat healthy food if it tastes delicious. The sauces and dressings in this chapter add flavour, spice and sparkle to your food. Intense and rich flavour is achieved using whole foods, healthy fats and lots of spices and herbs, both dried and fresh. Making these sauces and dressings at home instead of buying them gives you the opportunity to know exactly what you are eating. You can avoid the additives and extra sodium often found in purchased products, and you might just save a little money in the process. Let's take a look at some of the recipes featured in this chapter.

Delectable Sauces

Both the classic Apple Sauce (page 247) and the pink-hued Berry Apple Sauce (page 249) burst with fresh fruit flavour and are so quick to make you may soon wonder why you ever bought the jarred stuff. Home-made apple sauce was a tradition in my grandpa and grandma's house, and it may become one in yours too. We put it on pancakes, bread (preferably 3-minute bread mixed in the Vitamix), oatmeal and cracked wheat cereal. YUM! Packed in small containers with tight-fitting lids, either sauce would be a welcome addition to your child's lunchbox.

There are two fantastic tomato sauces in this chapter. For Fresh Tomato Sauce (page 242), whole tomatoes, onions, carrots, garlic, spices, a little tomato paste and brown sugar are combined in the Vitamix and simmered until the juices reduce a little and the flavours come together. This sauce will freeze beautifully once it is a cooled. Spicy Tomato Cream Sauce (page 241) combines low-fat milk or soya milk, a cooked sweet potato, fresh tomatoes, garlic, sun-dried tomatoes and spices. The ingredients for this tasty sauce are cooked in the Vitamix, just like the soups in Chapter 4. Sauces containing low-fat dairy should not be frozen, because the dairy can separate when it is reheated. Instead, enjoy this sauce within 4 days of preparing it.

Not-So Cheese Sauce (page 242) would dress up any vegetable and provides tons of cheesey flavour without any dairy. Parsley-Pecan Pesto (page 245), a delicious riff on the traditional Genovese pesto, would be welcome mixed with cooked grains, tossed with steamed vegetables or as a spread on a sandwich. Cashew Crema (page 251), a decadent non-dairy cream, will transform a bowl of sliced fresh fruit into a simple and delicious dessert.

Flavourful Vinaigrettes

When you have a home-made salad dressing in your fridge, getting a healthy salad on the table is a little easier. Three of the vinaigrettes in this chapter – Fresh Apple and Pear Dressing (page 237), Tomato Vinaigrette (page 235) and Balsamic Orange Dressing (page 236) – call for whole fruits along with more traditional ingredients like oil, lemon juice or vinegar. Adding these whole foods adds nutrients as well as a fresh, vibrant flavour not often found in vinaigrettes.

Silky Miso Vinaigrette (page 239) uses tofu along with spices, herbs and other ingredients to create a creamy, bright salad dressing without any dairy.

Let's get saucy!

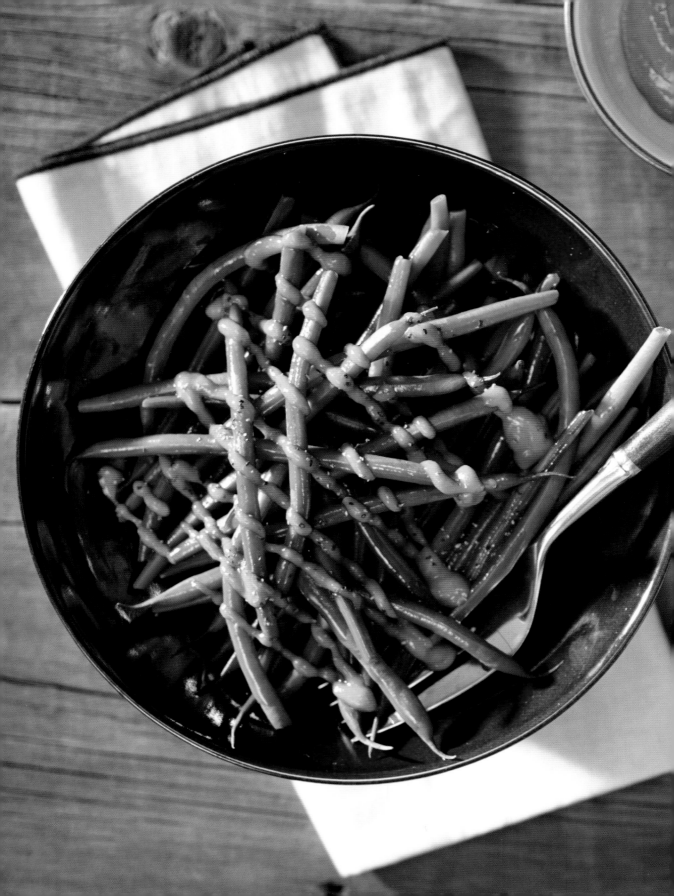

Tomato Vinaigrette

Toss this delicious dressing with steamed green beans or cauliflower and a little parsley to make a fantastic vegetable side.

Preparation: **10 minutes**   Processing: **30 seconds**   Bake time: **40 minutes**   Yield: **240 ml**

3 Roma (plum) tomatoes, quartered

2 garlic cloves, peeled and halved

1 shallot, peeled and quartered

5 tablespoons olive oil

½ teaspoon sea salt

¼ teaspoon ground black pepper

2 tablespoons sherry vinegar

1. Pre-heat the oven to 200°C.

2. Toss the tomatoes, garlic and shallot with 1 tablespoon of the olive oil, the salt and pepper. Evenly spread the vegetables on to a baking sheet lined with foil or a silicone baking mat. Roast for 40 minutes or until golden. Set the baking sheet on a wire rack to cool completely.

3. Transfer the roasted vegetables to the Vitamix container. Add the remaining oil and the vinegar and secure the lid. Select Variable 1. Turn the machine on and slowly increase the speed to Variable 10, then to High. Blend for 30 seconds.

AMOUNT PER 30 ML SERVING: calories 80, total fat 9 g, saturated fat 1.5 g, cholesterol 0 mg, sodium 150 mg, total carbohydrate 2 g, dietary fibre 0 g, sugars 1 g, protein 0 g

Balsamic Orange Dressing

Once you get the hang of making your own salad dressings, you may never buy a bottle of it again! This fresh, zippy dressing is the perfect finishing touch for a bowl of mixed greens, and it comes together in minutes.

Preparation: **10 minutes**   Processing: **30 seconds**   Yield: **300 ml**

4 tablespoons balsamic vinegar

2 teaspoons grated orange zest

½ orange, peeled

¼ teaspoon sea salt

¼ teaspoon ground black pepper

1 teaspoon Dijon mustard

150 ml extra virgin olive oil

½ teaspoon fresh thyme

1. Place 2 tablespoons water, the vinegar, orange zest, orange, salt, pepper and mustard into the Vitamix container in the order listed and secure the lid. Select Variable 1. Turn the machine on and slowly increase the speed to Variable 10, then to High. Blend for 10 seconds.

2. Reduce the speed to Variable 4 and remove the lid plug. Drizzle in the olive oil in a thin steady stream through the lid plug opening. Replace the lid plug and slowly increase the speed to Variable 10. Blend for 5 seconds.

3. Stop the machine, remove the lid, and add the thyme. Select Variable 1. Turn the machine on and slowly increase the speed to Variable 2. Blend for 5 seconds to mix.

AMOUNT PER 30 ML SERVING: calories 140, total fat 14 g, saturated fat 2 g, cholesterol 0 mg, sodium 75 mg, total carbohydrate 2 g, dietary fibre 0 g, sugars 2 g, protein 0 g

Fresh Apple and Pear Dressing

This fresh, lightly sweet dressing is delicious drizzled on salad greens or tossed with shredded cooked chicken, finely chopped celery and red onion and some fresh parsley for a tasty and slightly unconventional chicken salad.

Preparation: **15 minutes**   Processing: **20 seconds plus pulsing**   Cook time: **30 minutes**   Yield: **540 ml**

1 pear, cored and chopped

1 apple, cored and chopped

50 g granulated sugar

1 teaspoon fresh tarragon leaves or 2 teaspoons dried

2 tablespoons apple cider vinegar

2 tablespoons fresh lemon juice

1. Place the pear, apple, sugar, tarragon and 160 ml water in a medium pan. Cover and bring to a simmer over a medium heat. Cook until very soft, about 8 minutes. Remove lid and let the water evaporate. There should be about 420 ml fruit and liquid when finished cooking. Let cool for 15 minutes.

2. Ladle the warm mixture into the Vitamix container and secure the lid. Select Variable 1. Turn the machine on and slowly increase the speed to Variable 10, then to High. Blend for 20 seconds or until smooth.

3. Add the vinegar and lemon juice to the Vitamix container and secure the lid. Select Variable 1. Use the On/Off switch to quickly pulse 2 to 3 times to combine. Cool to room temperature before serving.

AMOUNT PER 30 ML SERVING: calories 30, total fat 0 g, saturated fat 0 g, cholesterol 0 mg, sodium 0 mg, total carbohydrate 8 g, dietary fibre 1 g, protein 0 g

Farmers' Market Marinara Sauce

Make this simple, flavourful marinara sauce when your garden or the local farmers' markets are bursting with red, ripe tomatoes. First, use the wet-chop method to dice the garlic, carrot and onion, and then use the dry-chop method to chunk up the tomatoes – seeds, skins and all. Once the sauce is cooked, use the Vitamix to purée it to your desired consistency. Enjoy now or, if you like, freeze for later. For more variety, add sautéed mushrooms or aubergine. Meat lovers can add turkey sausage.

Preparation: **15 minutes**   Processing: **30 seconds**   Cook time: **1 hour 10 minutes**   Yield: **1 litre**

2 garlic cloves, peeled

1 small carrot, cut into big pieces

1 small onion, peeled and quartered

3 tablespoons olive oil

80 ml dry red wine

2.2 kg tomatoes, quartered

10 g fresh basil leaves

1 tablespoon fresh oregano leaves

1 tablespoon fresh thyme leaves

1 teaspoon sea salt

½ teaspoon ground black pepper

1 teaspoon granulated sugar

1. For the wet-chop: Place the garlic, carrot and onion into the Vitamix container. Add water until the vegetables float above the blades. Secure the lid. Select Variable 1. Turn the machine on and slowly increase the speed to Variable 6. Turn off the machine. Repeat until your desired consistency is reached. Drain well.

2. Heat the oil in a large pan over a medium-low heat. Add the drained onion mixture and cook, stirring often, until soft but not browned, about 15 minutes.

3. Add the wine and stir well, loosening any bits stuck to the pot. Simmer and cook until slightly reduced, about 8 minutes.

4. Place one-third of the tomatoes into the Vitamix container and secure the lid. Select Variable 1. Turn the machine on and slowly increase the speed to Variable 4. Blend 5–10 seconds or until chopped, using the tamper to press the ingredients into the blades. Transfer to a bowl and repeat with the remaining tomatoes.

5. Add the tomatoes and their juices to the pan. Add the basil, oregano, and thyme and simmer for 45 minutes. Remove from the heat and let cool 10 minutes.

6. Ladle the hot tomato mixture into the Vitamix container. Add salt, pepper and sugar and secure the lid. Select Variable 1. Turn the machine on and slowly increase the speed to Variable 8. Blend for 20 seconds or until the desired consistency is reached.

7. Use right away or cool completely and chill or freeze.

AMOUNT PER 120 ML SERVING: calories 100, total fat 5 g, saturated fat 0.5 g, cholesterol 0 mg, sodium 280 mg, total carbohydrate 12 g, dietary fibre 3 g, sugars 8 g, protein 2 g

Silky Miso Vinaigrette

Umeboshi paste, made from Japanese pickled salt plums, adds a sour, briny note to this delicious vinaigrette. Spoon this sauce over steamed vegetables or toss it with crunchy romaine lettuce and thinly sliced radishes, carrots and spring onions.

Preparation: **15 minutes**   Processing: **1 minute 15 seconds**   Yield: **720 ml**

170 g firm tofu, drained

4 tablespoons apple cider vinegar

1 lemon, peeled and halved

1 tablespoon plus 1 teaspoon shiro (white) miso paste

1 tablespoon chopped fresh ginger

1 garlic clove, peeled

1 tablespoon umeboshi paste

2 teaspoons honey

120 ml extra virgin olive oil

180 ml olive oil

1. Place the tofu, vinegar, lemon, miso, ginger, garlic, umeboshi paste and honey into the Vitamix container in the order listed and secure the lid. Select Variable 1. Turn the machine on and slowly increase the speed to Variable 10, then to High. Blend for 15 seconds.

2. Reduce the speed to Variable 4 and remove the lid plug. Slowly drizzle the oil through the lid plug opening in a pencil-thin stream. Once all of the oil has been added, replace the lid plug and slowly increase the speed to Variable 10. Blend for an additional 15 seconds.

AMOUNT PER 30 ML SERVING: calories 110, total fat 12 g, saturated fat 1.5 g, cholesterol 0 mg, sodium 70 mg, total carbohydrate 1 g, dietary fibre 0 g, sugars 1 g, protein 1 g

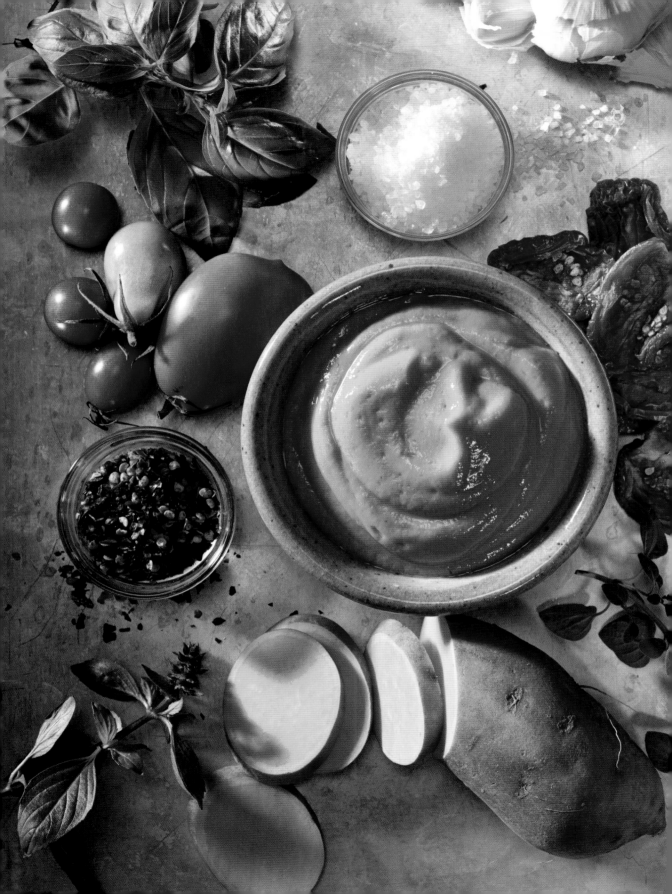

Spicy Tomato Cream Sauce

Ten ingredients are put into the Vitamix and 6 minutes later, a creamy, slightly spicy tomato sauce emerges. This sauce is delicious tossed with pasta or spooned over roasted chicken.

Preparation: **20 minutes**   Processing: **6 minutes**   Yield: **960 ml**

480 ml low-fat (1%) milk or soya milk

½ medium baked sweet potato, quartered

2 Roma (plum) tomatoes, quartered

½ teaspoon salt

1 garlic clove, peeled

1½ teaspoons chopped fresh basil or ½ teaspoon dried

1½ teaspoons chopped fresh oregano or ½ teaspoon dried

28 g sun-dried tomatoes

¼ teaspoon red pepper flakes

⅛ teaspoon ground white pepper

Place all the ingredients into the Vitamix container in the order listed and secure the lid. Select Variable 1. Turn the machine on and slowly increase the speed to Variable 10, then to High. Blend for 6 minutes, or until heavy steam escapes from the vented lid.

AMOUNT PER 60 ML SERVING: calories 60, total fat 0 g, saturated fat 0 g, cholesterol 0 mg, sodium 210 mg, total carbohydrate 6 g, dietary fibre 1 g, sugars 2 g, protein 2 g

Fresh Tomato Sauce

Instead of peeling, seeding and chopping the vegetables for this fresh, tasty tomato sauce, you simply pop them in the Vitamix and process them to silky, smooth perfection. Once the sauce has simmered and the flavours have come together, you can toss it over pasta or freeze it in containers with tight-fitting lids for another time.

Preparation: **15 minutes**   Processing: **1 minute**   Cook time: **35–40 minutes**   Yield: **480 ml**

6 medium Roma (plum) tomatoes, quartered

1 small onion, halved

1 small carrot, halved

2 tablespoons tomato paste

1 garlic clove, peeled

½ teaspoon dried basil

½ teaspoon dried oregano

½ teaspoon fresh lemon juice

½ teaspoon light brown sugar

½ teaspoon sea salt

1. Place all the ingredients into the Vitamix container in the order listed and secure the lid. Select Variable 1. Turn the machine on and slowly increase the speed to Variable 10, then to High. Blend for 1 minute, using the tamper to press the ingredients into the blades if necessary.

2. Pour into a pan and simmer for 35–40 minutes.

AMOUNT PER 60 ML SERVING: calories 25, total fat 0 g, saturated fat 0 g, cholesterol 0 mg, sodium 170 mg, total carbohydrate 6 g, dietary fibre 2 g, sugars 4 g, protein 1 g

Not-So Cheese Sauce

It is really kind of amazing to watch as 6 ingredients are put into a Vitamix and then, about 5 minutes later, a warm non-dairy cheese sauce emerges. This delicious, tangy sauce will dress up steamed broccoli or cauliflower and would not be out of place drizzled on a burrito.

Preparation: **15 minutes**   Processing: **3 minutes 15 seconds**   Yield: **420 ml**

2 tablespoons fresh lemon juice

50 g canned pimientos or 1 large roasted red pepper, peeled (page 91)

95 g cashews or almonds

1¼ teaspoons onion powder

30 g nutritional yeast

Sea salt (optional)

1. Place all the ingredients and 240 ml water into the Vitamix container in the order listed and secure the lid. Select Variable 1. Turn the machine on and slowly increase the speed to Variable 10, then to High. Blend for 3 minutes 15 seconds, or until heavy steam escapes from the vented lid.

2. Season to taste with salt, if desired.

AMOUNT PER 60 ML SERVING: calories 100, total fat 7 g, saturated fat 0.5 g, cholesterol 0 mg, sodium 25 mg, total carbohydrate 5 g, dietary fibre 3 g, sugars 1 g, protein 5 g

Quick and Easy Pizza Sauce

This simple pizza sauce, made with onions, garlic, herbs, canned tomatoes and tomato paste, yields a generous quantity of sauce. Freeze in small portions so you can whip up a pizza like Polenta Pizza (page 206) any time.

Preparation: **10 minutes**   Processing: **25–45 seconds**   Cook time: **1 hour**   Yield: **960 ml**

3 tablespoons olive oil

230 g onion, peeled and cut into chunks

1 tablespoon chopped fresh basil

1 tablespoon fresh oregano leaves

3 large garlic cloves, peeled and halved

2 tablespoons tomato paste

2 x 400-g cans crushed tomatoes (with added purée)

½ teaspoon sea salt

¼ teaspoon ground black pepper

1. Heat the olive oil in a pan over a medium heat. Add the onion, basil and oregano and cook, stirring occasionally, until the onion softens slightly, about 6 minutes. Stir in the garlic and cook 2 minutes.

2. Add the tomato paste and cook for 3 minutes, stirring occasionally. Add the crushed tomatoes and bring to a simmer. Simmer until the sauce thickens, about 30 minutes. Season with the salt and pepper and remove from the heat. Let cool for 15 minutes.

3. Ladle the hot sauce into the Vitamix container and secure the lid. Select Variable 1. Turn the machine on and slowly increase the speed to Variable 4. Blend for 25–45 seconds, until the desired consistency is reached.

AMOUNT PER 60 ML SERVING: calories 50, total fat 2.5 g, saturated fat 0 g, cholesterol 0 mg, sodium 160 mg, total carbohydrate 4 g, dietary fibre 0 g, sugars 2 g, protein 1 g

Garlic-Parsley Crème Sauce

Too long dismissed as merely a garnish, it's time to enjoy parsley in its own right. Tasting deeply green and just a little bitter, parsley really sings in this delicious sauce. Tangy with garlic, some red pepper flakes and red wine vinegar, this sauce will liven up grilled seafood or meats, portobello mushrooms or sautéed tofu.

Preparation: **10 minutes**   Processing: **30 seconds**   Yield: **240 ml**

120 ml olive oil

60 ml red wine vinegar

½ teaspoon sea salt

⅓ teaspoon red pepper flakes

1 garlic clove, peeled

55 g fresh flatleaf parsley leaves

1. Place all the ingredients into the Vitamix container in the order listed and secure the lid. Select Variable 1. Turn the machine on and slowly increase the speed to Variable 4. Blend for 15 seconds.

2. Stop the machine, remove the lid and scrape the sides of the container with a spatula. Secure the lid. Select Variable 1. Turn the machine on and slowly increase the speed to Variable 10. Blend for an additional 15 seconds.

AMOUNT PER 30 ML SERVING: calories 130, total fat 14 g, saturated fat 2 g, cholesterol 0 mg, sodium 150 mg, total carbohydrate 1 g, dietary fibre 0 g, sugars 0 g, protein 0 g

Tahini

When buying sesame seeds, you can often find larger containers of them at a less expensive price in the Asian food section of the supermarket instead of with the rest of the spices. Toasting the seeds at home gives the tahini a more intense flavour. To toast, bake at 180 degrees^0 C for about 5 minutes or until light brown. Do not overcook.

Preparation: **10 minutes**   Processing: **1–2 minutes**   Yield: **600 g**

640 g sesame seeds, lightly toasted

1. Place sesame seeds into the Vitamix container and secure lid. Select Variable 1. Turn machine on and quickly increase speed to Variable 10 then to High. Blend for 1–2 minutes, using the tamper to press the mixture into the blades. Blend until the consistency of peanut butter and until all the seeds are completely ground.

AMOUNT PER 30g SERVING: calories 170, total fat 15 g, saturated fat 2 g, cholesterol 0 mg, sodium 0 mg, total carbohydrate 7 g, dietary fibre 4 g, sugars 0 g, protein 5 g

Parsley-Pecan Pesto

When you think of pesto, the traditional Genovese pesto with basil and pine nuts may be the first thing that comes to mind. But what do you do when basil is out of season and the price of pine nuts goes through the roof? Whip up this delicious pesto made with readily available and often cheaper ingredients. Toss it on pasta and steamed green beans for a simple, delicious dinner.

Preparation: **10 minutes**   Processing: **1 minute**   Yield: **240 ml**

2 tablespoons olive oil

35 g fresh flatleaf parsley leaves

1 garlic clove, peeled

30 g unsalted roasted pecans

2 tablespoons grated Parmesan

1 tablespoon nutritional yeast

1 teaspoon fresh lemon juice

Pinch of sea salt

Pinch of ground black pepper

1. Place all the ingredients and 3½ tablespoons water into the Vitamix container in the order listed and secure the lid. Select Variable 1. Turn the machine on and slowly increase the speed to Variable 4. Blend for 30 seconds, using the tamper to press the ingredients into the blades.

2. Stop, remove the lid and scrape down the sides of the container. Secure the lid. Select Variable 1. Turn the machine on and slowly increase the speed to Variable 6. Blend for 30 seconds, using the tamper to press the ingredients into the blades.

AMOUNT PER 30 ML SERVING: calories 70, total fat 7 g, saturated fat 1 g, cholesterol 5 mg, sodium 30 mg, total carbohydrate 1 g, dietary fibre 1 g, sugars 0 g, protein 1 g

Pesto Sauce

Delicious as a pasta sauce or a great addition to other recipes, this pesto is fresh and easy to make in just a couple of minutes. Season to taste.

Preparation: **5 minutes**   Processing: **1 minute**   Yield: **360 ml**

120 ml olive oil

50 g grated Parmesan cheese

3 medium garlic cloves, peeled

80 g fresh basil leaves

25 g pine nuts

Salt and pepper, to taste

1. Place all ingredients, except salt and pepper, into the Vitamix container in the order listed and secure lid. Select Variable 1. Turn machine on and quickly increase speed to Variable 7. Blend for 1 minute, using the tamper to press the ingredients into the blades. Season to taste.

AMOUNT PER 30 ML SERVING: 172 calories, total fat 17 g, saturated fat 2 g, cholesterol 5 mg, sodium 96 mg, total carbohydrate 2 g, dietary fibre 1 g, sugars 0 g, protein 3 g

Red Pepper Paste

Once you have made this red pepper paste, bursting with wonderful, fragrant flavour, you will not be able to imagine your life without it. Slather on top of grilled chicken, meats or tofu for a guilt-free delight.

Preparation: **10 minutes**   Processing: **30 seconds**   Cook time: **15 minutes**   Yield: **120 ml**

60 ml dry red wine (Cabernet or Merlot)

1 teaspoon cayenne pepper

½ teaspoon sea salt

¼ teaspoon ground ginger

⅓ teaspoon ground cardamom

⅓ teaspoon ground cinnamon

⅓ teaspoon ground coriander

⅓ teaspoon ground cloves

⅓ teaspoon ground nutmeg

⅓ teaspoon ground black pepper

2 tablespoons diced onion

1 garlic clove, peeled

28 g sweet paprika

1. Place the wine, spices, onion and garlic into the Vitamix container and secure the lid. Select Variable 1. Turn the machine on and slowly increase the speed to Variable 10, then to High. Blend for 15 seconds.

2. Stop the machine, remove the lid and scrape the sides of the container. Secure the lid. Select Variable 1. Turn the machine on and slowly increase the speed to Variable 10, then to High. Blend for an additional 15 seconds.

3. Heat the paprika in a large pan over a medium heat, stirring frequently, for 1 minute. Gradually whisk in the wine mixture. Bring to a simmer and cook until thick and hot, about 4 minutes.

4. Cool completely.

AMOUNT PER 30 ML SERVING: calories 40, total fat 1 g, saturated fat 0 g, cholesterol 0 mg, sodium 300 mg, total carbohydrate 5 g, dietary fibre 3 g, sugars 1 g, protein 1 g

Apple Sauce

After you try this fresh, bright apple sauce, you may never crave cooked or purchased varieties again. Enjoy as a snack or on top of Apple Pancakes (page 48).

Preparation: **10 minutes**   Processing: **1 minute 45 seconds**   Yield: **900 ml**

900 g apples, seeded and cut into large pieces (with or without peel)

2 tablespoons fresh lemon juice

Place all the ingredients into the Vitamix container in the order listed and secure the lid. Select Variable 1. Turn the machine on and slowly increase the speed to Variable 7. Blend for 1 minute 45 seconds, using the tamper to press the ingredients into the blades.

AMOUNT PER 120 ML SERVING: calories 60, total fat 0 g, saturated fat 0 g, cholesterol 0 mg, sodium 0 mg, total carbohydrate 16 g, dietary fibre 3 g, sugars 12 g, protein 0 g

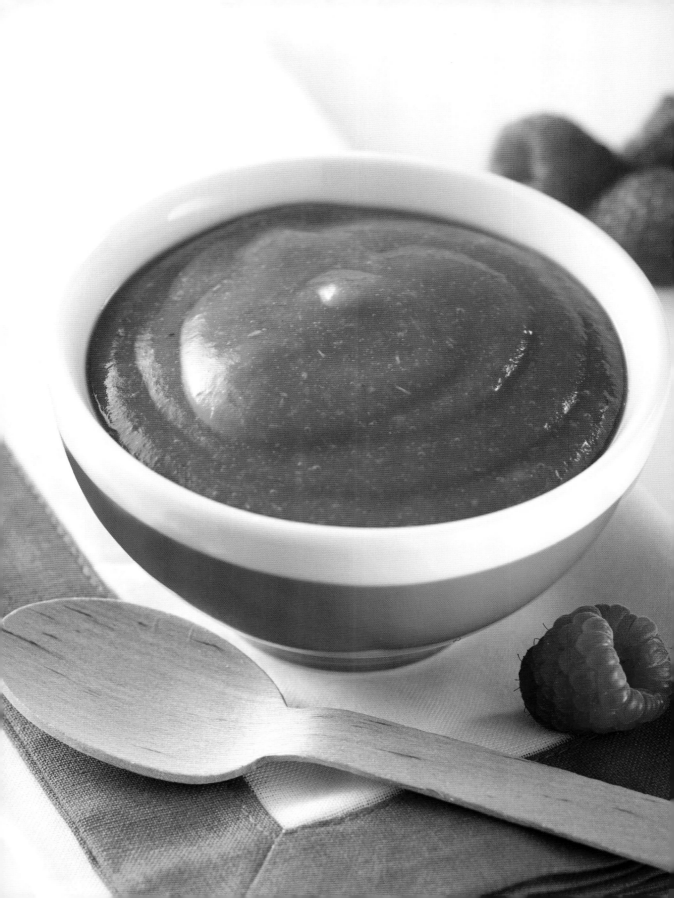

Berry Apple Sauce

A small cup of this beautifully pink and flavourful berry apple sauce would be a great addition to your child's packed lunch. Full of fruit but without any added sugar or food colouring, it is a tasty and healthy treat.

Preparation: **10 minutes**   Processing: **20 seconds**   Cook time: **20 minutes**   Yield: **1 litre**

4 medium crisp, sweet-tart apples (about 500 g), cored and cut into large pieces

1 tablespoon honey

1 teaspoon fresh lemon juice

190 g fresh or frozen red raspberries

1. Place the apples and 360 ml water in a large non-reactive pan and bring to a simmer over a high heat. Reduce the heat to medium and simmer for 10 minutes.

2. Add the honey and remove the pan from the heat. Let cool for 10 minutes.

3. Ladle the hot apple mixture into the Vitamix container. Add the lemon juice and raspberries and secure the lid. Select Variable 1. Turn the machine on and slowly increase the speed to Variable 10, then to High. Blend for 20 seconds or until smooth.

AMOUNT PER 120 ML SERVING: calories 50, total fat 0 g, saturated fat 0 g, cholesterol 0 mg, sodium 0 mg, total carbohydrate 13 g, dietary fibre 3 g, sugars 8 g, protein 0 g

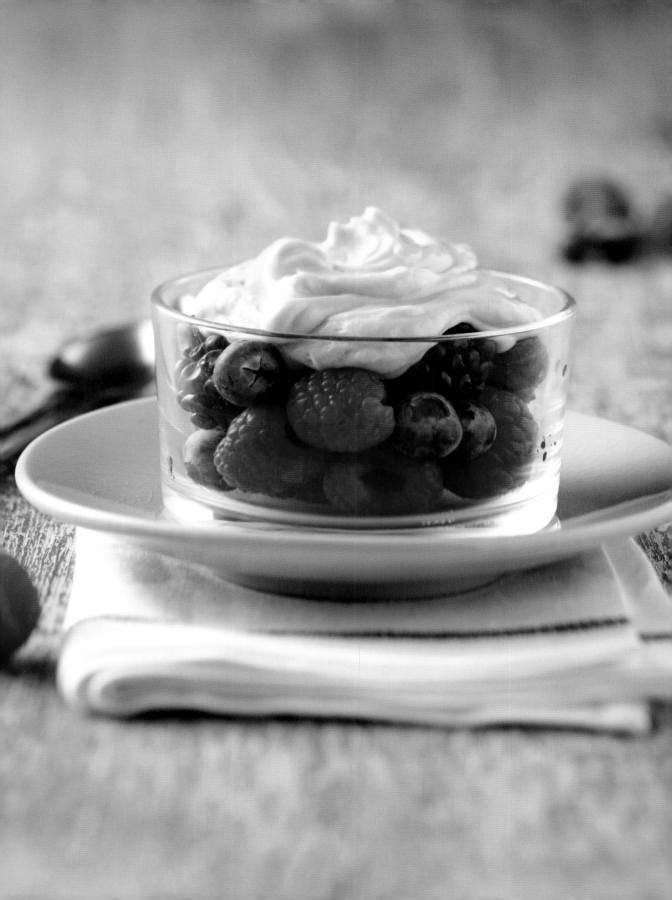

Cashew Crema

This lightly sweet, decadent cashew crema is a vegan's answer to whipped cream. Spoon this crema over fresh fruit or a slice of vegan cake for a delicious after-dinner treat.

Preparation: **15 minutes**   Processing: **1 minute**   Yield: **480 ml**

2 tablespoons fresh lemon juice

1 tablespoon fresh orange juice

1 tablespoon light olive oil

1 teaspoon vanilla extract

225 g extra-firm tofu, drained

60 ml agave nectar

115 g cashew pieces

½ teaspoon sea salt

Place all the ingredients into the Vitamix container in the order listed and secure the lid. Select Variable 1. Turn the machine on and slowly increase the speed to Variable 10, then to High. Blend for 1 minute, using the tamper to press the ingredients into the blades. Chill well before using.

AMOUNT PER 30 ML SERVING: calories 70, total fat 4 g, saturated fat 0.5 g, cholesterol 0 mg, sodium 50 mg, total carbohydrate 6 g, dietary fibre 0 g, sugars 4 g, protein 2 g

Peanut Butter

Once you taste freshly made peanut butter, you may never want to buy it again. As with the Cashew Peanut Butter (page 253), use the tamper to push the nuts towards the blades and don't be afraid to run the Vitamix on its top speed. The results are worth it!

Preparation: **5 minutes**   Processing: **2 minutes**   Yield: **360 ml**

440 g unsalted roasted peanuts

1. Place the nuts into the Vitamix container and secure the lid. Select Variable 1. Turn the machine on and slowly increase the speed to Variable 10, then to High. Use the tamper to press the ingredients into the blades.

2. In 1 minute you will hear a high-pitched chugging sound. Once the butter begins to flow freely through the blades, the motor sound will change and become low and labouring. Stop the machine.

3. Chill in an airtight container for up to 1 week. It can also be frozen for longer storage.

AMOUNT PER 30 ML SERVING: calories 210, total fat 18 g, saturated fat 2.5 g, cholesterol 0 mg, sodium 0 mg, total carbohydrate 8 g, dietary fibre 3 g, sugars 2 g, protein 7 g

Cashew Peanut Butter

The milder flavour of cashews combined with roasted peanuts creates a delicious nut butter. The flavour is decidedly peanut-y and the texture will stay smooth, even when it is chilled – unlike natural peanut butters bought in the store.

Preparation: **10 minutes**   Processing: **1 minute 30 seconds**   Yield: **420 ml**

290 g salted roasted peanuts

275 g salted roasted cashews

1. Place the nuts into the Vitamix container and secure the lid. Select Variable 1. Turn the machine on and slowly increase the speed to Variable 10 then to High. Use the tamper to press the ingredients into the blades.

2. In 1 minute you will hear a high-pitched chugging sound. Once the butter begins to flow freely through the blades, the motor sound will change from a high pitch to a low labouring sound. Stop the machine. Then blend for an additional 30 seconds or until it reaches the desired consistency.

3. Store in an airtight container in the fridge for up to 1 week. It can also be frozen for longer storage.

AMOUNT PER 30 ML SERVING: calories 180, total fat 15 g, saturated fat 2.5 g, cholesterol 0 mg, sodium 80 mg, total carbohydrate 7 g, dietary fibre 2 g, protein 7 g

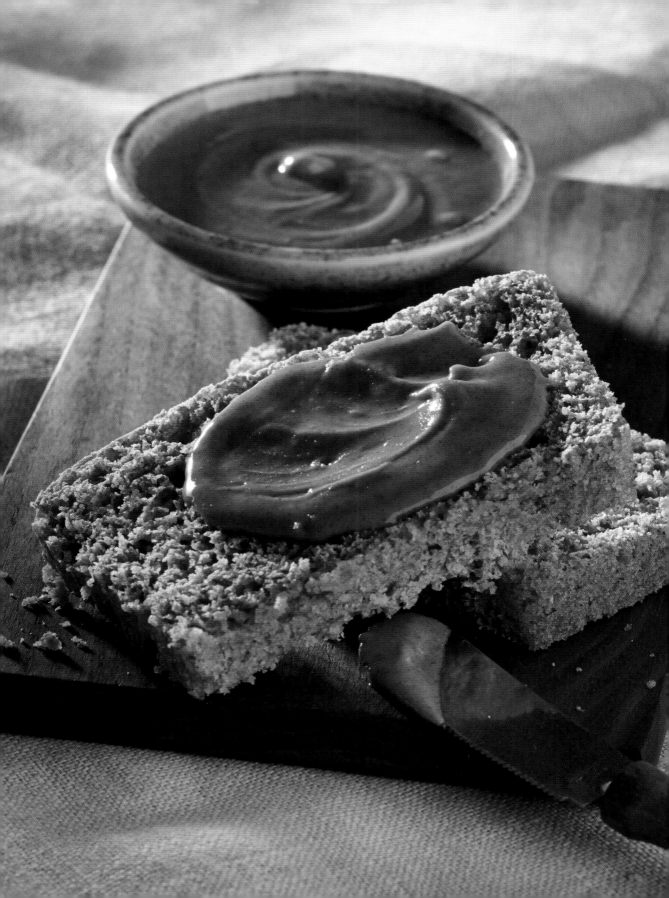

Pecan Peanut Butter

According to the USDA, pecans are the most antioxidant-rich tree nut and rank among the top fifteen foods with the highest levels of antioxidants. Sprinkle toasted pecans on top of your Oat Porridge (page 42), and be sure to make this delicious nut butter, too.

Preparation: **10 minutes**   Processing: **1 minute 25 seconds**   Yield: **360 ml**

220 g lightly salted dry-roasted peanuts

175 g unsalted roasted pecans

1 tablespoon honey

1. Place all the ingredients into the Vitamix container in the order listed and secure the lid. Select Variable 1. Turn the machine on and slowly increase the speed to Variable 10, then to High. Using the tamper, press the ingredients into the blades.

2. In 1 minute you will hear a high-pitched chugging sound. Once the butter begins to flow freely through the blades, the motor sound will change from a high pitch to a low labouring sound. Stop the machine. Then blend for an additional 30 seconds or until it reaches the desired consistency.

AMOUNT PER 35g SERVING: calories 220, total fat 20 g, saturated fat 2 g, cholesterol 0 mg, sodium 60 mg, total carbohydrate 7 g, dietary fibre 3 g, sugars 3 g, protein 7 g

Raisin Almond Breakfast Spread

At once a nut butter and a jam, this spread is a wonderful toast topping or sandwich filling. A little zing from the ginger balances out the savoury nuts and deep sweetness of the honey and dried fruit.

Preparation: **10 minutes**   Processing: **1 minute 30 seconds**   Yield: **360 ml**

2 tablespoons honey or agave nectar

145 g raw almonds

5-cm piece of fresh ginger

2 tablespoons raw sesame seeds

145 g raisins or 70 g raisins plus 4 pitted dates and 4 dried apricots

1. Place all the ingredients into the Vitamix container in the order listed and secure the lid. Select Variable 1. Turn the machine on and slowly increase the speed to Variable 10, then to High. Blend for 40 seconds, using the tamper to press the ingredients into the blades.

2. Stop the machine and remove the lid. Scrape down the sides of the container with a spatula and secure the lid. Select Variable 1. Turn the machine on and slowly increase the speed to Variable 5. Blend for 50 seconds, using the tamper as needed.

AMOUNT PER 30 ML SERVING: calories 140, total fat 7 g, saturated fat 0.5 g, cholesterol 0 mg, sodium 0 mg, total carbohydrate 17 g, dietary fibre 2 g, sugars 13 g, protein 3 g

JANICE SUMMERS

Janice Summers, like many Vitamix owners, heard about the machine from another satisfied Vitamix owner. In 1981, Janice became interested in milling her own fresh flours. 'I wanted to grind my own to have the freshest, and therefore most healthy, grains possible. The taste, smell and texture are far superior to shop-bought flours and meals that have been ageing on the shelf.' Summers went to bookstores in search of information on the process. While she was doing her research, she met a woman who told her how easily she could make flours, among other things, in her Vitamix. 'I called Vitamix's 800 number and, as the saying goes, the rest is history.'

When asked if using a Vitamix has made it easier to eat healthier, Janice says that for her, it absolutely does. 'This is especially the case with vegetables. If I don't have the time to sit and eat a large salad every day, then I drink them. This is great for being on the go. The Vitamix doesn't remove the fibre so I know I'm getting whole vegetables. I just wash the vegetables well, peel those that should be peeled, and throw them in. I use water if [I am] adding fruit, but if I'm only making a vegetable drink I add organic chicken stock to further enhance the taste. Sometimes I choose to add a dash of pepper sauce for a little heat. Pour it over ice, toss in a stick of celery and run out the door.'

Now, in addition to quick vegetable juices, Janice uses her Vitamix to whip up healthy smoothies, make unbeatable coffee frappés and grind flours. Janice has also shared her passion for healthy, home-made foods just as the Barnard family has done. Her niece, daughter and sister all have Vitamix blenders now too, thanks in part to Janice's influence. (And her good cooking too, no doubt!) And when Janice sees a demonstration in progress? If she sees a shopper who seems sceptical that anyone could take whole foods and ice and whip up a delicious drink, she pipes up. 'Seeing their doubt, sometimes I'll mention that I do it all the time. Their eyebrows raise as if the person who just blended the drink in front of them might have had magical powers . . . if an ordinary woman shopping in the store can do it then, maybe it's possible. They always ask if I like it. I let them know that it is my single most used and valued piece of kitchen equipment, that I use for smoothies, sauces, soups, ice cream, slushies and so much more.' As for what is possible, 'Be brave and experiment!' Janice says.

Creating delicious healthy food and then giving people the tools to follow in your lead? A whole-foods–powered legacy to be very proud of!

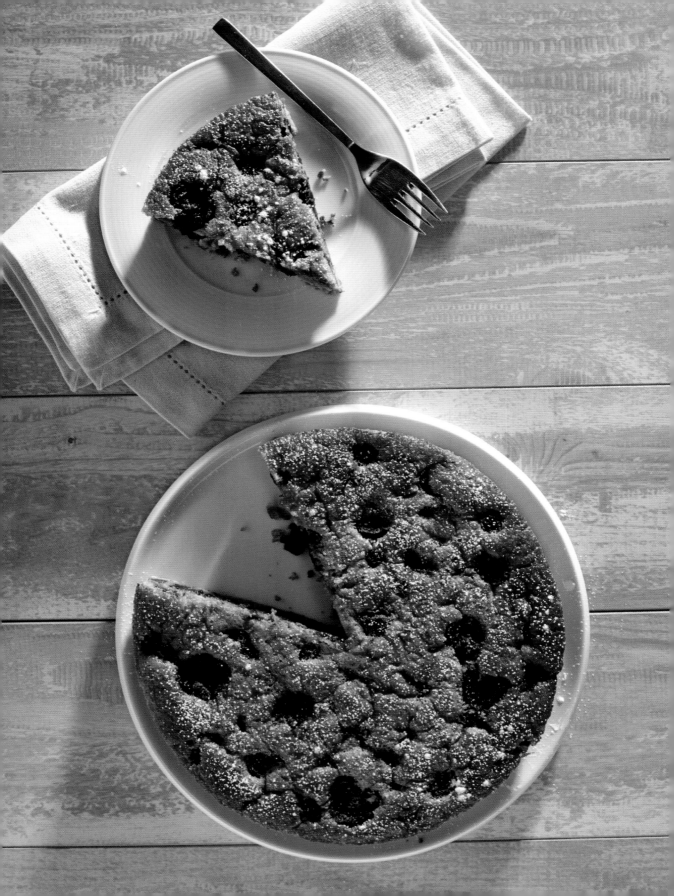

Chapter 7

Desserts

nto every life, some sweetness must fall. Dessert is as right a part of life as sunshine, laughter and hugs, all simple things that can bring us great joy. My grandpa brought sweetness to our lives. He loved to laugh. He was a master of funny faces, jokes and silly stories. Do you remember Mount Tooska Ooska Wooska Choo from the introduction? Fun doesn't have to be complicated. It can be simple and delightfully easy. Grandpa also had more ideas than he knew what to do with, many of which he figured out how to make happen. For example, he decided to get a pilot's licence in his forties and discovered that he loved to fly. My uncle Grove once said that flying 'gave him a freedom that he couldn't justify in his mind otherwise'.

I have a great story that involves both flying and his love of a good joke. When I was looking at colleges, Grandpa offered to fly me out west to look at a school. Before we stopped in Lincoln, Nebraska, to refuel, my ever-mischievous grandpa decided to play a practical joke on the airport staff. When he radioed ahead, he announced that he was about to land with a princess – he made up the country I was from – and asked if the airport staff had the red carpet ready.

There was much confusion among the ground staff, but Grandpa Bill cheerfully insisted that he had called ahead and that not having a red carpet would be a great insult to the princess. A teenager at the time, I cringed and blushed as my grandpa cheerfully chatted on the radio. I wanted to disappear. When we landed, an airport employee rushed to the plane and spread out his coat, the best the staff could come up with on short notice. I emerged, mortified, from the plane, and good old Grandpa had the whole ground crew in stitches, laughing together at his joke.

Just as my grandpa made joy out of the simplest situations, you can use your Vitamix to take simple ingredients and transform them into joyfully delicious desserts. The recipes in this chapter will show you 36 different ways to satisfy your sweet tooth. You will learn about desserts that have little added sugar, lots of whole fruits and other delicious and nutritious ingredients. Some of the treats, particularly the frozen desserts, will come together in minutes. The cakes, cookies, crisps and truffles will take a little longer, but will be worth the wait. Who knew eating whole foods could be so sweet, so satisfying?

Baked Desserts

In Chapter 2 you learned how the Vitamix can help you make delicious quick breads, and here we will show you the cakes and cookies that you can whip up. By mixing up the wet ingredients in the Vitamix, you can use fruit in place of some or all of the refined sugar that you might need otherwise. In Batter Cake with Cherries (page 262), you use pitted dates with a little agave nectar for sweetness. The dates give the cake a deep, satisfying flavour. In Carrot Cake (page 263), a combination of canned pineapple in its own juice and raisins are used in lieu of sugar. Banana Drops (page 269), a homey vegan cookie, get delicious fruit flavour and a moist, tender texture from bananas puréed with a little vanilla, oil and oatmeal.

You can also use the Vitamix to pulse together delicious crisp toppings. In Apple-Ginger Crisp (page 267), corn flakes, whole wheat flour, crystallised ginger and coconut oil are combined to create a crunchy vegan topping for apples. Top this quintessentially autumn dessert with Apple Pie Ice Cream (page 275) or Cashew Crema (page 251) if you like. For Vegan Fruit Crumble (page

268), whole wheat flour, cornmeal, almonds, unsweetened coconut, pitted dates and coconut oil are pulsed with spices and baking powder to form a biscuit-like topping for peaches and blueberries. This crisp is wonderful on its own, yet heavenly when served with Peach Soy Sorbet (page 284).

Frozen Desserts

One of the wonders of the Vitamix is its unique ability to take simple ingredients, some of them frozen, and transform them into delicious, spoonable frozen treats. Seventeen of the desserts in this chapter – including Apple Pie Ice Cream (page 275), Coconut-Pineapple Sherbet (page 279), Pink Grapefruit Granita (page 283) and Strawberry Yoghurt Freeze (page 293) – are all examples of this kind of dessert. Any of these would be delicious topped with fresh fruit, scooped into a cone or capped with Mixed Berry Purée (page 274) or Cashew Crema (page 251) for an over the top – no pun intended – treat. These desserts can be enjoyed right away or packed into a freezer-safe container with a tight-fitting lid for later. Remember to follow the blending instructions carefully to ensure delightfully simple, yummy success every time. Keep in mind that the same machine that can make hot soup can quickly transform a creamy, scoopable treat into a cold smoothie in very little time!

A healthy diet need not be all sacrifice. By making your sweet treats at home and using whole fruits and whole grains, you can satisfy your cravings and get a few more servings of whole food at the same time. Delicious food and peace of mind: What could be sweeter?

Batter Cake with Cherries

Some days, well maybe all days, benefit from a slice of cake eaten in the late afternoon. This delicious cake gets its sweetness from light agave nectar, dates and sweet cherries. Dust with icing sugar before serving.

Preparation: **15 minutes**   Processing: **15 seconds**   Bake time: **35 minutes**   Yield: **8 servings**

1 tablespoon natural 0% Greek yoghurt, stirred

240 ml low-fat (1%) milk

2 tablespoons agave nectar

2 tablespoons chopped pitted dates

1 tablespoon vanilla extract

2 large eggs plus 3 large egg whites

120 g whole grain flour, preferably home-made (page 64)

⅓ teaspoon sea salt

280 g pitted sweet black cherries, fresh (halved and patted dry) or frozen (thawed and well drained)

Icing sugar, for dusting

1. Pre-heat the oven to 220°C. Lightly grease a 23-cm round cake tin.

2. Place the yoghurt, milk, agave, dates, vanilla, whole eggs and egg whites into the Vitamix container in the order listed and secure the lid. Select Variable 1. Turn the machine on and slowly increase the speed to Variable 10, then to High. Blend for 15 seconds until well blended.

3. Combine the flour and salt in a medium bowl. Whisk the yoghurt mixture into the flour mixture until smooth. (The batter will be thin.)

4. Pour the batter into the cake tin, then distribute the cherries evenly over the top. Bake for 15 minutes. Reduce the oven temperature to 200°C. Bake for 20 minutes, or until a toothpick inserted in the centre comes out clean and a golden brown crust has formed on top.

5. Serve warm dusted with icing sugar.

AMOUNT PER SERVING: calories 140, total fat 2 g, saturated fat 0.5 g, cholesterol 50 mg, sodium 90 mg, total carbohydrate 25 g, dietary fibre 2 g, sugars 11 g, protein 6 g

Carrot Cake

This moist, tender carrot cake gets all of its sweetness from whole foods: pineapple in its own juice, raisins and grated carrots. Enjoy in the afternoon with a cup of tea or tuck a square in a school lunchbox for a healthy dessert.

Preparation: **15 minutes**   Processing: **15 seconds**   Bake time: **40–50 minutes**   Yield: **10 servings**

2 large eggs

6 tablespoons vegetable/olive oil blend

1 x 227-g can crushed pineapple in juice

1 teaspoon vanilla extract

120 g raisins

180 g whole grain flour, preferably home-made (page 64)

1 teaspoon ground cinnamon

¼ teaspoon ground allspice

¼ teaspoon ground nutmeg

¼ teaspoon sea salt

1½ teaspoons baking powder

110 g grated carrots (about 2 medium)

1. Pre-heat the oven to 180°C. Coat a 20-cm square baking tin with cooking spray.

2. Place the eggs, oil, pineapple (with juice), vanilla and 50 g of the raisins into the Vitamix container in the order listed and secure the lid. Select Variable 1. Turn the machine on and slowly increase the speed to Variable 10. Blend for 15 seconds.

3. Combine the flour, cinnamon, allspice, nutmeg, salt and baking powder in a medium bowl. Fold in the egg mixture, carrots and remaining raisins by hand.

4. Spread the batter in the tin and bake for 40–50 minutes, or until a toothpick inserted into the centre comes out clean. Cool on wire rack.

AMOUNT PER SERVING: calories 210, total fat 10 g, saturated fat 1 g, cholesterol 35 mg, sodium 160 mg, total carbohydrate 27 g, dietary fibre 3 g, sugars 13 g, protein 4 g

Cornmeal Honey and Date Cake

This homey, cosy cornmeal cake will delight everyone, particularly those who need to avoid gluten. Serve with fresh fruit and whipped cream or simply dust with a little icing sugar.

Preparation: **15 minutes**   Processing: **15 seconds**   Bake time: **30–35 minutes**   Yield: **10 servings**

280 g whole-grain brown rice flour

40 g coarse cornmeal, preferably home-made (page 60)

30 g cornflour

1½ teaspoons bicarbonate of soda

½ teaspoon sea salt

120 ml extra virgin olive oil

2 tablespoons honey

50 g pitted dates

142 g natural 0% Greek yoghurt, stirred

2 teaspoons vanilla extract

1 teaspoon lemon extract

Grated zest of 1 lemon

25 g flax meal

240 ml low-fat (1%) milk

1. Pre-heat the oven to 190°C. Lightly coat a 20-cm square baking tin with cooking spray.

2. Combine the brown rice flour, cornmeal, cornflour, bicarbonate of soda and salt in a medium bowl.

3. Place the olive oil, honey, dates, yoghurt, vanilla, lemon extract, lemon zest, flax meal and milk into the Vitamix container in the order listed and secure the lid. Select Variable 1. Turn the machine on and slowly increase the speed to Variable 10, then to High. Blend for 15 seconds.

4. Pour the oil-yoghurt mixture into the flour mixture and stir lightly by hand to combine.

5. Pour the batter into the tin and bake for 30–35 minutes or until a toothpick inserted in the centre comes out with a few moist crumbs attached. Cool in the pan on a wire rack.

AMOUNT PER SERVING: calories 260, total fat 13 g, saturated fat 2 g, cholesterol 0 mg, sodium 290 mg, total carbohydrate 30 g, dietary fibre 3 g, sugars 8 g, protein 5 g

Mango Flax Cake

Delicious for brunch or for dessert, this wholesome cake is a crowd-pleaser. The cake's nutty flavour comes from whole wheat flour and wheat bran, while dates, mango and just a little brown sugar give it sweetness.

Preparation: **20 minutes**　Processing: **15 seconds**　Bake time: **35–40 minutes**　Yield: **9 servings**

45 g wheat bran

240 ml low-fat (1%) milk

1 large egg

2 tablespoons flax oil

55 g pitted dates

120 g whole grain flour, preferably home-made (page 64)

25 g flax meal

1 tablespoon baking powder

¼ teaspoon salt

1 teaspoon ground cinnamon

2 mangoes, sliced

TOPPING:

55 g dark brown sugar

1 tablespoon whole grain flour, preferably home-made (page 64)

1½ teaspoons ground cinnamon

1 tablespoon flax oil

1. Pre-heat the oven to 190°C. Lightly grease a 20-cm square baking tin.

2. Combine the bran and 180 ml of the milk and let soak for 10 minutes.

3. Place the remaining milk, the egg, flax oil and dates into the Vitamix container in the order listed and secure the lid. Select Variable 1. Turn the machine on and slowly increase the speed to Variable 10, then to High. Blend for 15 seconds, or until the mixture is creamy.

4. Combine the flour, flax meal, baking powder, salt and cinnamon in a medium bowl. Add the milk/egg mixture and soaked bran and stir just until blended.

5. Spread the batter in the baking pan. Place the mango slices over the batter.

6. For the topping: Combine the dark brown sugar, flour, cinnamon and flax oil in a small bowl and mix until the mixture forms crumbs. Sprinkle over the mango slices.

7. Bake for 35–40 minutes, until a toothpick inserted in the centre comes out clean. Serve warm.

AMOUNT PER SERVING: calories 190, total fat 6 g, saturated fat 1 g, cholesterol 20 mg, sodium 220 mg, total carbohydrate 33 g, dietary fibre 6 g, sugars 18 g, protein 5 g

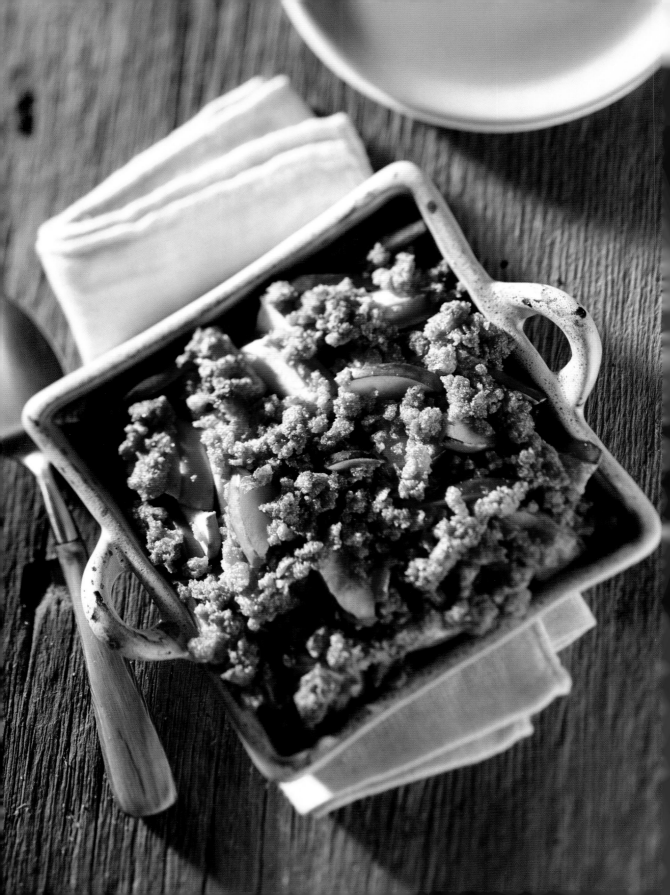

Apple-Ginger Crisp

The perfect dessert to showcase the first delicious apples of autumn, this tasty vegan pudding is made mostly of store cupboard staples. Should you have any leftovers, strongly consider eating the crisp cold with a little soya yoghurt for breakfast.

Preparation: **15 minutes**　　Processing: **10 seconds**　　Bake time: **35–40 minutes**　　Yield: **9 servings**

6 small/medium crisp apples, thinly sliced and slices halved (no more than 1 kg unsliced)

55 g light brown sugar

2 teaspoons fresh lemon juice

30 g cornflakes

3 tablespoons whole grain flour, preferably home-made (page 64)

2 tablespoons crystallised ginger pieces

2 tablespoons coconut oil

1. Pre-heat the oven to 200°C. Coat a 20-cm square baking dish with cooking spray.

2. Place the apples in the baking dish. Add 1 tablespoon of the brown sugar and the lemon juice and toss gently to coat.

3. Place the cornflakes, remaining brown sugar, flour, ginger and coconut oil into the Vitamix container in the order listed and secure the lid. Select Variable 1. Turn the machine on and slowly increase the speed to Variable 5, using the tamper as needed to push ingredients into the blades. Blend for 10 seconds just until blended.

4. Sprinkle the crumb mixture over the apples and press gently. Bake for 35–40 minutes, until the apples are tender and the mixture is bubbling. Serve warm, at room temperature, or chilled.

AMOUNT PER SERVING: calories 140, total fat 3.5 g, saturated fat 2.5 g, cholesterol 0 mg, sodium 25 mg, total carbohydrate 30 g, dietary fibre 3 g, sugars 20 g, protein 1 g

Vegan Fruit Crumble

Coconut, both unsweetened flakes and oil, is a slightly unexpected but totally delightful presence here. The coconut flavour is subtle, but a delicious pairing with the bright blueberries and sweet peaches.

Preparation: **20 minutes**   Processing: **30 seconds**   Bake time: **35–45 minutes**   Yield: **8 servings**

TOPPING:

160 g whole grain flour, preferably home-made (page 64)

40 g cornmeal, preferably home-made (page 60)

1 teaspoon baking powder

½ teaspoon ground cinnamon

55 g slivered almonds

25 g unsweetened coconut flakes

80 g pitted dates

2 tablespoons coconut oil, melted and cooled

½ teaspoon almond extract

FRUIT FILLING:

2 tablespoons water

2 tablespoons cornflour

600 g fresh blueberries

420 g unsweetened frozen peach slices, thawed and drained

1 teaspoon honey

1. Pre-heat the oven to 180°C.

2. For the topping: Place the flour, cornmeal, baking powder and cinnamon in a medium bowl and stir by hand to combine.

3. Place the almonds, coconut flakes and dates into the Vitamix container in the order listed and secure the lid. Select Variable 1. Turn the machine on and slowly increase the speed to Variable 4. Blend for 20 seconds, using the tamper to press the ingredients into the blades. The mixture should form coarse crumbs.

4. Reduce the speed to Variable 1 and remove the lid plug. Drizzle in the coconut oil and almond extract, using the tamper to press the ingredients into the blades. Add the date mixture to the flour mixture and stir well to combine.

5. For the fruit filling: Stir the water into the cornflour in a small bowl to make a paste. Gently combine the blueberries, peach slices, honey and cornflour paste in a large bowl.

6. Transfer the fruit mixture to a large round baking dish with high sides. Crumble the topping mixture evenly over the fruit.

7. Bake for 35–45 minutes, or until the fruit is bubbling and the crumb topping is golden.

AMOUNT PER SERVING: calories 280, total fat 10 g, saturated fat 5 g*, cholesterol 0 mg, sodium 65 mg, total carbohydrate 47 g, dietary fibre 7 g, sugars 20 g, protein 6 g

*Saturated fat is a bit on the high side because of the saturated fat naturally found in coconut oil.

Banana Drops

The batter for these simple, homey vegan biscuits comes together in just 10 minutes. Healthy enough to be eaten for breakfast, these banana drops are wonderful tucked in a lunchbox or as an after-school treat, too.

Preparation: **10 minutes**   Processing: **40 seconds**   Bake time: **20–25 minutes**   Yield: **12 biscuits**

2 ripe bananas, peeled

4 tablespoons vegetable oil

1 teaspoon vanilla extract

160 g rolled oats

165 g raisins

1. Pre-heat the oven to 180°C. Line the baking sheet with foil or a silicone baking mat.

2. Place the bananas, oil, vanilla and 80 g of the oats into the Vitamix container in the order listed and secure the lid. Select Variable 1. Turn the machine on and slowly increase the speed to Variable 10, then to High. Blend for 30 seconds, using the tamper to press the ingredients into the blades.

3. Pour the batter into a bowl. Stir in the raisins and the remaining oats.

4. Form into 12 balls and place on a baking sheet. Press to flatten slightly.

5. Bake for 20–25 minutes or until firm to the touch. Remove and cool in the pan on a wire rack.

AMOUNT PER BISCUIT: calories 150, total fat 6 g, saturated fat 0.5 g, cholesterol 0 mg, sodium 0 mg, total carbohydrate 24 g, dietary fibre 3 g, sugars 12 g, protein 2 g

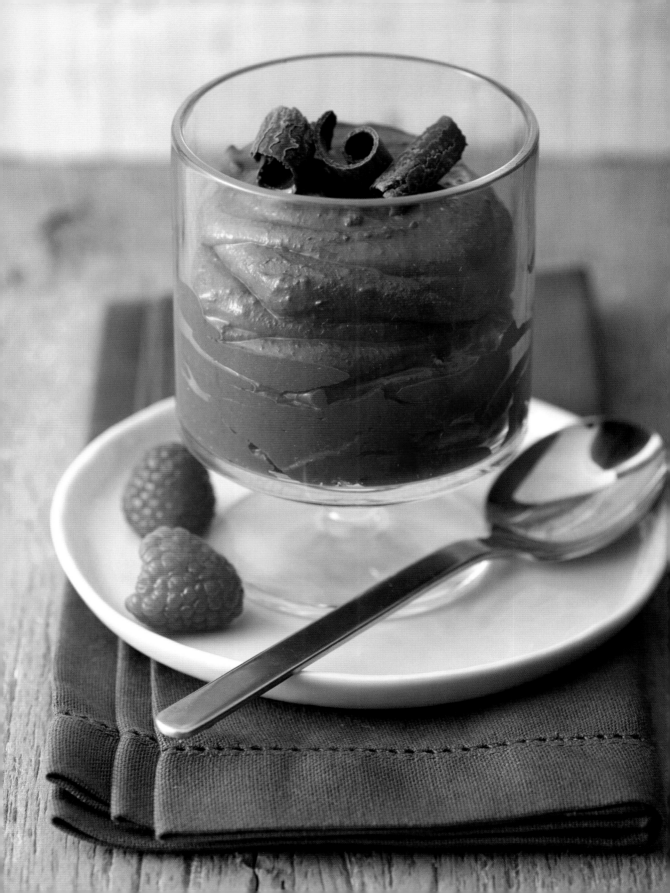

Chocolate Mousse

Who knew chocolate mousse could be so simple and so fast? Once you have the ingredients to hand, you can put this decadent dessert together in a flash.

Preparation: **10 minutes**   Processing: **35–40 seconds**   Yield: **480 ml**

4 tablespoons whole milk

1½ teaspoons vanilla extract

40 g cocoa powder, sifted

15 g milk chocolate, finely chopped

45 g plain chocolate, finely chopped

6 pitted dates

120 ml natural 0% Greek yoghurt, stirred

125 g plus 1 tablespoon reduced-fat ricotta

Fresh seasonal berries, for garnish

1. Place the milk, vanilla, cocoa powder, milk chocolate, plain chocolate, dates, yoghurt and ricotta into the Vitamix container in the order listed and secure the lid. Select Variable 1. Turn the machine on and slowly increase the speed to Variable 10, then to High. Blend for 35–40 seconds, using the tamper to press the ingredients into the blades.

2. Serve immediately, garnished with fresh berries.

AMOUNT PER 120 ML SERVING (WITHOUT BERRIES): calories 200, total fat 10 g, saturated fat 5 g, cholesterol 10 mg, sodium 65 mg, total carbohydrate 25 g, dietary fibre 6 g, sugars 15 g, protein 11 g

Vegan Truffles

A decadent, delicious treat for your next gathering! You can use a melon baller or a 1-tablespoon measuring spoon to shape the truffles if you like. If you use the tablespoon, roll the truffle gently between your palms to create a ball. Dust the finished truffles with extra cocoa powder or icing sugar if desired.

Preparation: **15 minutes**   Processing: **1 minute**   Yield: **24 truffles**

80 ml soya milk

140 g raw almonds

130 g large pitted dates

2 tablespoons agave nectar

1 tablespoon cocoa powder

40 g Coco Wheats cereal

1. Place all the ingredients into the Vitamix container in the order listed and secure the lid. Select Variable 1. Turn the machine on and slowly increase the speed to Variable 10, then to High. Blend for 1 minute, using the tamper to press the ingredient into the blades. The consistency should be thick like dough. If too thick, adjust by adding more milk.

2. Form into 2.5-cm balls and freeze.

AMOUNT PER TRUFFLE: calories 60, total fat 3 g, saturated fat 0 g, cholesterol 0 mg, sodium 0 mg, total carbohydrate 8 g, dietary fibre 1 g, sugars 5 g, protein 2 g

Pumpkin Pudding

This cosy pumpkin pudding has all of the flavours of classic pumpkin pie without the bother of a crust or turning on the oven. The pudding base is heated in the Vitamix – use a thermometer to make sure the mixture has reached 85°C – and then thickened with a paste made with potato starch and water. Delicious served either warm or cold.

Preparation: **15 minutes**   Processing: **7 minutes**   Yield: **1 litre**

240 ml semi-skimmed milk, at room temperature

115 g natural 0% Greek yoghurt, stirred, at room temperature

40 g dark brown sugar

2 pitted dates

2 large eggs

240 ml canned unsweetened pumpkin purée

½ teaspoon ground cinnamon

¼ teaspoon pumpkin pie spice

⅛ teaspoon sea salt

2 teaspoons potato starch

1. Place the milk, yoghurt, brown sugar, dates, eggs, pumpkin purée, cinnamon, pumpkin pie spice and salt into the Vitamix container in the order listed and secure the lid. Select Variable 1. Turn the machine on and slowly increase the speed to Variable 10, then to High. Blend for 6 minutes, or until temperature reaches 85°C.

2. Meanwhile, stir together potato starch and 2 tablespoons water in a small bowl to make a paste.

3. Reduce the speed to Variable 5 and remove the lid plug. Pour the paste in through the lid plug opening. Replace the lid plug. Slowly increase the speed to Variable 10, then to High. Blend an additional 1 minute.

4. Serve warm or chill before serving.

AMOUNT PER 120 ML SERVING: calories 70, total fat 2 g, saturated fat 0.5 g, cholesterol 45 mg, sodium 75 mg, total carbohydrate 11 g, dietary fibre 1 g, sugars 9 g, protein 4 g

Mixed Berry Purée

Frozen fruit, lemon juice, water and a little granulated sugar come together to make a bright, flavourful berry sauce. Spoon it over a frozen dessert such as Coconut-Pineapple Sherbet (page 279) or use it to dress up a simple cake like the gluten-free Cornmeal Honey and Date cake (page 264).

Preparation: **10 minutes** Processing: **3 minutes** Yield: **840 ml**

170 g frozen unsweetened raspberries

210 g frozen unsweetened strawberries

155 g frozen unsweetened blueberries

1 tablespoon fresh lemon juice

50 g granulated sugar

1. Let the berries sit at room temperature for 10 minutes to partially thaw.

2. Place the lemon juice, berries and sugar with 240 ml water into the Vitamix container in the order listed and secure the lid. Select Variable 1. Turn the machine on and slowly increase the speed to Variable 10, then to High. Blend for 3 minutes, using the tamper to press ingredients into the blades.

AMOUNT PER 60 ML SERVING: calories 30, total fat 0 g, saturated fat 0 g, cholesterol 0 mg, sodium 0 mg, total carbohydrate 8 g, dietary fibre 1 g, sugars 6 g, protein 0 g

Apple Pie Ice Cream

This simple, delicious dessert is apple pie à la mode in ice-cream form! Real apple pie should be this easy.

Prep time: **10 minutes**   Processing: **30 seconds**   Yield: **720 ml**

90 ml frozen apple juice concentrate

60 g low-fat vanilla yoghurt

½ medium apple, cored and quartered

1 tablespoon vanilla extract

¼ teaspoon ground cinnamon

½ ripe banana

720 ml ice cubes

Place all the ingredients into the Vitamix container in the order listed and secure the lid. Select Variable 1. Turn the machine on and slowly increase the speed to Variable 10, then to High. Use the tamper to press the ingredients into the blades. In about 30 seconds, the sound of the motor will change and 4 mounds should form in the mixture. Stop the machine. Do not overmix or melting will occur. Serve immediately.

AMOUNT PER 120 ML SERVING: calories 60, total fat 0 g, saturated fat 0 g, cholesterol 0 mg, sodium 10 mg, total carbohydrate 12 g, dietary fibre 1 g, sugars 10 g, protein 1 g

Papaya Tropical Dessert

Curious about papaya and guava but not sure how to serve them? Use one or a combination of both to make this delicious frozen dessert. Greek yoghurt and banana give the dessert a creamy texture while the papaya or guava add a tropical flavour.

Preparation: **10 minutes**   Processing: **30–45 seconds**   Yield: **1 litre**

120 ml natural 0% Greek yoghurt, stirred

250 g fresh papaya or guava chunks

1 banana, peeled, quartered and frozen

1 orange, peeled and halved

½ lemon, peeled

1 tablespoon honey or agave nectar

720 ml ice cubes

Place all the ingredients into the Vitamix container in the order listed and secure the lid. Select Variable 1. Turn the machine on and slowly increase the speed to Variable 10, then to High, using the tamper to press the ingredients into the blades. In 30–45 seconds, the sound of the motor will change and 4 mounds should form in the mixture. Stop the machine. Do not overmix or melting will occur. Serve immediately.

AMOUNT PER 120 ML SERVING: calories 45, total fat 0 g, saturated fat 0 g, cholesterol 0 mg, sodium 10 mg, total carbohydrate 10 g, dietary fibre 1 g, sugars 7 g, protein 2 g

Frozen Bananas Foster

All of the deliciousness of traditional Bananas Foster without making caramel or setting rum ablaze. Both the cinnamon and the pecans balance the sweetness in this decadent dessert.

Preparation: **15 minutes**   Processing: **45–55 seconds**   Yield: **1 litre**

5 large bananas, peeled, halved and frozen

320 g natural low-fat yoghurt

2 teaspoons rum extract (optional)

2 tablespoons caramel sauce

1 teaspoon honey

1 teaspoon ground cinnamon

50 g unsalted roasted pecans

1. Let the bananas sit at room temperature for 15 minutes to soften.

2. Place the yoghurt, bananas, rum extract (if using), caramel sauce, honey, cinnamon and pecans into the Vitamix container in the order listed and secure the lid. Select Variable 1. Turn the machine on and slowly increase the speed to Variable 10, then to High, using the tamper to press the ingredients into the blades. In about 45–55 seconds, the sound of the motor will change and 4 mounds should form in the mixture. Stop the machine. Do not overmix or melting will occur. Serve immediately.

AMOUNT PER 120 ML SERVING: calories 140, total fat 5 g, saturated fat 1 g, cholesterol 0 mg, sodium 35 mg, total carbohydrate 22 g, dietary fibre 2 g, sugars 13 g, protein 3 g

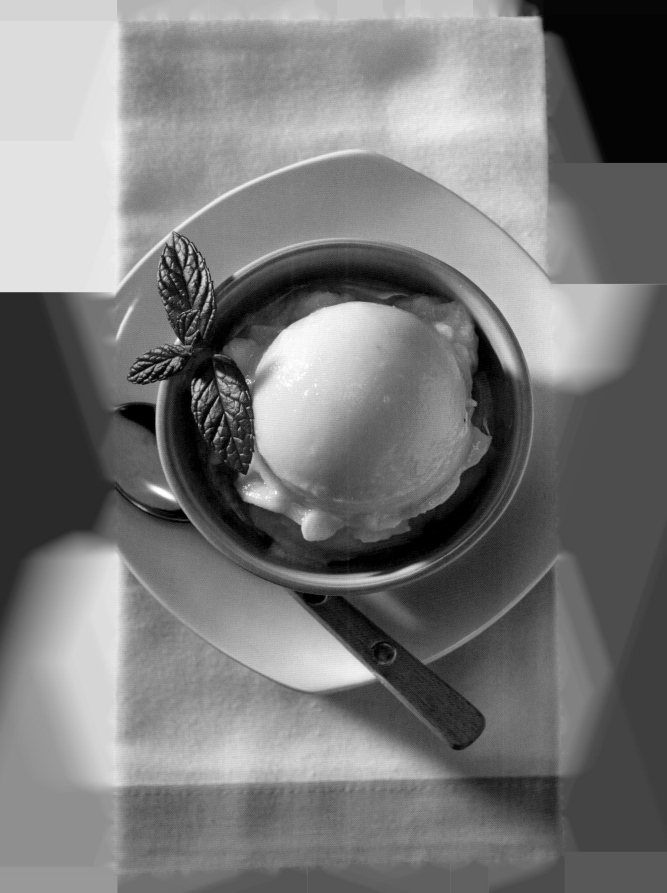

Coconut-Pineapple Sherbet

Simple ingredients – light coconut milk, agave nectar, vanilla and frozen pineapple – are quickly transformed into something quite special. Garnish with fresh fruit or a sprinkle of toasted unsweetened coconut if desired.

Preparation: **10 minutes**   Processing: **35–45 seconds**   Yield: **840 ml**

240 ml canned light coconut milk

1 teaspoon agave nectar

¼ teaspoon vanilla extract

1450 g frozen unsweetened pineapple chunks

Place all the ingredients into the Vitamix container in the order listed and secure the lid. Select Variable 1. Turn the machine on and slowly increase the speed to Variable 10, then to High, using the tamper to press the ingredients into the blades. In 35–45 seconds, the sound of the motor will change and 4 mounds should form in the mixture. Stop the machine. Do not overmix or melting will occur. Serve immediately.

AMOUNT PER 120 ML SERVING: calories 60, total fat 2.5 g, saturated fat 2 g, cholesterol 0 mg, sodium 5 mg, total carbohydrate 10 g, dietary fibre 1 g, sugars 2 g, protein 0 g

Berry Sorbet with Mixed Spices

Adding aromatic spices – cinnamon, cloves, allspice, nutmeg and vanilla – to this sublime sorbet makes it taste like a baked dessert, almost cookie-like, but without masking the bright fruit flavour. The gentle spice of the fresh ginger keeps the fruits' sweetness from being cloying.

Preparation: **25 minutes**   Processing: **1 minute 5 seconds**   Yield: **1.1 litres**

150 g frozen unsweetened strawberries

140 g frozen unsweetened blueberries

140 g frozen unsweetened blackberries

140 g frozen unsweetened raspberries

300 g frozen pitted cherries

15 g fresh ginger, peeled

50 g granulated sugar

13 g fresh mint leaves

½ teaspoon ground cinnamon

¼ teaspoon ground nutmeg

⅛ teaspoon ground allspice

⅛ teaspoon ground cloves

1 teaspoon vanilla extract

1. Let the frozen fruit sit at room temperature for 20 minutes to partially thaw.

2. Place the ginger, sugar and 240 ml cold water into the Vitamix container and secure the lid. Select Variable 1. Turn the machine on and slowly increase the speed to Variable 8. Blend for 20 seconds, or until the ginger is finely chopped.

3. Stop the machine and remove the lid. Add the fruit, mint, spices and vanilla to the container and secure the lid. Select Variable 1. Turn the machine on and slowly increase the speed to Variable 10, then to High, using the tamper to press the ingredients into the blades. In about 45–55 seconds, the sound of the motor will change and 4 mounds should form in the mixture. Stop the machine. Do not overmix or melting will occur. Serve immediately.

AMOUNT PER 120 ML SERVING: calories 70, total fat 0 g, saturated fat 0 g, cholesterol 0 mg, sodium 0 mg, total carbohydrate 19 g, dietary fibre 3 g, sugars 14 g, protein 1 g

Orange Sorbet

A wonderful whole-fruit dessert bursting with flavour! Drizzle it with Mixed Berry Purée (page 274) or serve a scoop alongside Batter Cake with Cherries (page 262).

Preparation: **10 minutes**   Processing: **30–40 seconds**   Yield: **840 ml**

2 medium oranges, peeled and halved

2 tablespoons honey

1 tablespoon frozen orange juice concentrate

1 teaspoon grated orange zest

1.2 litres ice cubes

Place all the ingredients into the Vitamix container in the order listed and secure the lid. Select Variable 1. Turn the machine on and slowly increase the speed to Variable 10, then to High, using the tamper to press the ingredients into the blades. In 30–40 seconds, the sound of the motor will change and 4 mounds should form in the mixture. Stop the machine. Do not overmix or melting will occur. Serve immediately.

AMOUNT PER 120 ML SERVING: calories 40, total fat 0 g, saturated fat 0 g, cholesterol 0 mg, sodium 0 mg, total carbohydrate 10 g, dietary fibre 1 g, sugars 9 g, protein 0 g

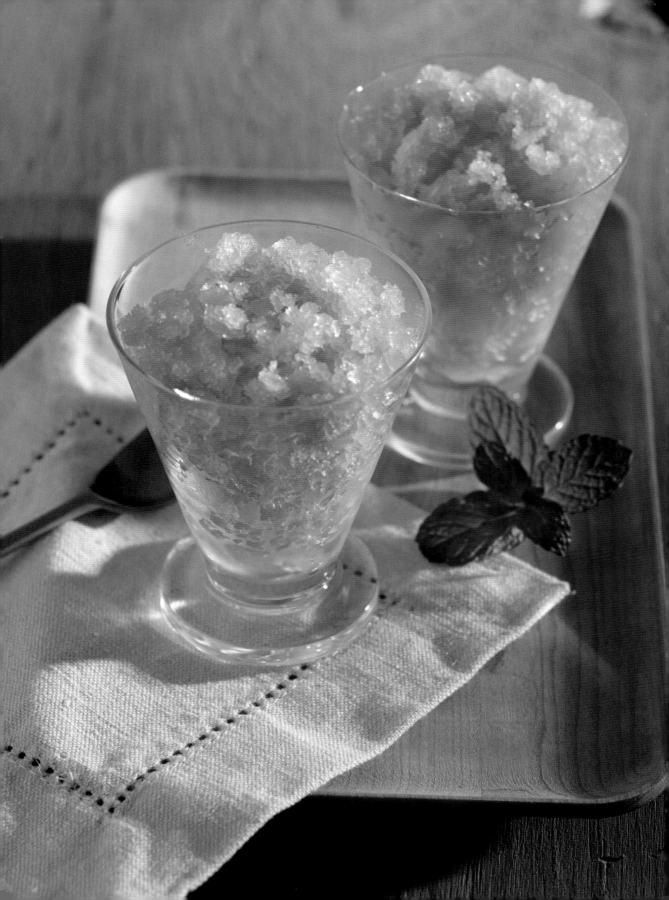

Pink Grapefruit Granita

Most granita recipes instruct you to freeze the combined ingredients and then stir every 30 minutes or so to create a flaky texture. In our recipe, you freeze this no-sugar-added mixture until it is hard and then quickly pulse it in the Vitamix to create the finished dessert.

Preparation: **3–4 hours**   Processing: **pulsing**   Yield: **720 ml**

600 ml fresh pink grapefruit juice

4 teaspoons stevia blend

1. Combine the juice and stevia with 240 ml water in a bowl and whisk until the stevia has dissolved. Pour the liquid into a baking tin and freeze until hard, 3–4 hours.

2. With a fork, break the granita into large chunks. Transfer the chunks to the Vitamix container and secure the lid. Select Variable 4. Use the On/Off switch to quickly pulse the mixture while using the tamper to press the ingredients into the blades. Continue pulsing until the mixture is smooth. Do not overmix or melting will occur.

3. Serve immediately.

AMOUNT PER 120 ML SERVING: calories 45, total fat 0 g, saturated fat 0 g, cholesterol 0 mg, sodium 0 mg, total carbohydrate 11 g, dietary fibre 1 g, sugars 7 g, protein 1 g

Peach Soy Sorbet

A creamy, dairy-free sorbet for a hot summer day or a midwinter ice-cream craving. Scoop this sweet treat into a cone or serve in a dish with sliced fruit and toasted sliced almonds.

Preparation: **10 minutes**   Processing: **45 seconds**   Yield: **1.2 litres**

450 g frozen unsweetened peach slices

340 g natural soya yoghurt

1 teaspoon vanilla extract

1½ tablespoons honey

1. Let the peaches sit at room temperature for 15 minutes to soften slightly.

2. Place the yoghurt, vanilla, peaches and honey into the Vitamix container in the order listed and secure the lid. Select Variable 1. Turn the machine on and slowly increase the speed to Variable 10, then to High, using the tamper to press ingredients into the blades. In about 45 seconds, the sound of the motor will change and 4 mounds should form in the mixture. Stop the machine. Do not overmix or melting will occur. Serve immediately.

AMOUNT PER 120 ML SERVING: calories 70, total fat 1 g, saturated fat 0 g, cholesterol 0 mg, sodium 0 mg, total carbohydrate 13 g, dietary fibre 1 g, sugars 11 g, protein 2 g

A Burst of Fruit Frozen Dessert

With six varieties of fruit, yoghurt, wheatgerm, flax seeds and herbs, you may be tempted to eat this delicious frozen dessert for breakfast as well as after dinner.

Preparation: **10 minutes**   Processing: **45–60 seconds**   Yield: **1.2 litres**

240 ml coconut water

120 ml vanilla 0% Greek yoghurt, stirred

½ medium banana, peeled and frozen

6 pitted dates

1 teaspoon flax seeds

1 teaspoon toasted wheatgerm

2 fresh basil leaves

3 fresh mint leaves

100 g frozen mixed berries (strawberries, blackberries, blueberries, raspberries)

240 ml ice cubes

Place all the ingredients into the Vitamix container in the order listed and secure the lid. Select Variable 1. Turn the machine on and slowly increase the speed to Variable 10, then to High, using the tamper to press the ingredients into the blades. In about 45–60 seconds the sound of the motor will change and 4 mounds should form in the mixture. Stop the machine. Do not overmix or melting will occur. Serve immediately.

AMOUNT PER 120 ML SERVING: calories 40, total fat 0 g, saturated fat 0 g, cholesterol 0 mg, sodium 5 mg, total carbohydrate 9 g, dietary fibre 1 g, sugars 6 g, protein 1 g

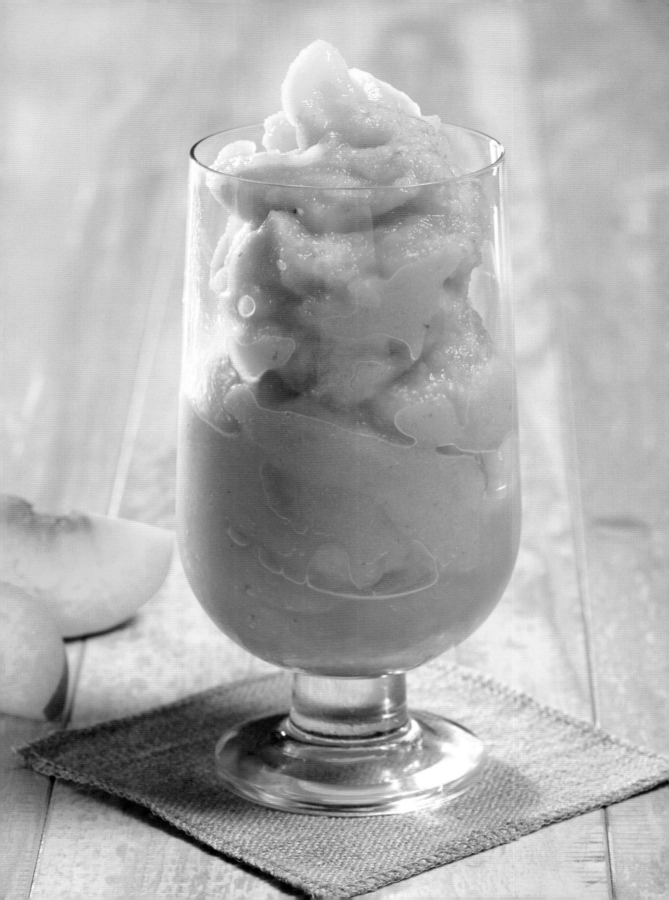

Ginger Peach Tea Ice

The perfect dessert for a sweltering summer afternoon when you hanker for a tall glass of sweet tea. Cold green tea and fresh ginger pair wonderfully with the peaches and honey in this refreshing dessert.

Preparation: **10 minutes**   Processing: **1 minute 45 seconds**   Yield: **1 litre**

450 g frozen unsweetened peach slices

240 ml brewed green tea, cold

1 teaspoon honey

¾ teaspoon vanilla extract

1 teaspoon grated fresh ginger

480–600 ml ice cubes

1. Let the peaches sit at room temperature for 10 minutes to soften slightly.

2. Place the tea, honey, vanilla, ginger, peaches and ice cubes into the Vitamix container in the order listed and secure the lid. Select Variable 1. Turn the machine on and slowly increase the speed to Variable 10, then to High, using the tamper to press the ingredients into the blades. In about 1 minute 45 seconds, the sound of the motor will change and 4 mounds should form in the mixture. Stop the machine. Do not overmix or melting will occur. Serve immediately.

AMOUNT PER 120 ML SERVING: calories 20, total fat 0 g, saturated fat 0 g, cholesterol 0 mg, sodium 0 mg, total carbohydrate 6 g, dietary fibre 1 g, sugars 5 g, protein 0 g

Green Tea Fruit Freeze

Drinking a lot of sweetened beverages has been shown to have a negative impact on health, in part because it is easy to consume a lot of calories quickly. If you like sweetened green tea, consider making this dessert when you get a craving. Full of whole fruits, it has a wonderful tea flavour, sweetness without refined sugar, and fibre, too.

Preparation: **10 minutes**   Processing: **45 seconds**   Yield: **600 ml**

120 ml cold brewed green tea or ½ teaspoon matcha green tea powder stirred into 120 ml water

60 g natural or vanilla low-fat yoghurt

2 tablespoons honey or agave nectar

1 banana, peeled and frozen

55 g frozen cranberries

160 g frozen pineapple chunks

75 g frozen unsweetened strawberries

Place all the ingredients into the Vitamix container in the order listed and secure the lid. Select Variable 1. Turn the machine on and slowly increase the speed to Variable 10, then to High, using the tamper to press the ingredients into the blades. In about 45 seconds, the sound of the motor will change and 4 mounds should form in the mixture. Stop the machine. Do not overmix or melting will occur. Serve immediately.

AMOUNT PER 120 ML SERVING: calories 80, total fat 0 g, saturated fat 0 g, cholesterol 0 mg, sodium 10 mg, total carbohydrate 19 g, dietary fibre 2 g, sugars 14 g, protein 1 g

Goji and Strawberry Frozen Dessert

If you are struggling to get your five servings of fruits and vegetables every day, consider adding this dessert to your repertoire. Frozen strawberries, fresh spinach, pitted dates and dried goji berries pack nutrients into a cold, sweet, spoonable treat that you will find yourself making again and again.

Preparation: **10 minutes**   Processing: **30–60 seconds**   Yield: **720 ml**

300 ml unsweetened almond milk

2 teaspoons fresh lemon juice

1 teaspoon vanilla extract

22 g dried goji berries

6 large pitted dates

40 g baby or regular spinach

350 g frozen unsweetened strawberries

Place all the ingredients into the Vitamix container in the order listed and secure the lid. Select Variable 1. Turn the machine on and slowly increase the speed to Variable 10, then to High, using the tamper to press the ingredients into the blades. In 30–60 seconds, the sound of the motor will change and 4 mounds should form in the mixture. Stop the machine. Do not overmix or melting will occur. Serve immediately.

AMOUNT PER 120 ML SERVING: calories 50, total fat 0.5 g, saturated fat 0 g, cholesterol 0 mg, sodium 55 mg, total carbohydrate 11 g, dietary fibre 2 g, sugars 6 g, protein 1 g

Banana Freeze

Bananas have a wonderfully creamy texture when frozen and blended that is very similar to ice cream. This delicious banana freeze comes together in under 10 minutes and is the perfect dessert for a hot summer's day or whenever the ice-cream craving strikes.

Preparation: **5 minutes**   Processing: **30 seconds**   Yield: **1.2 litres**

240 ml skimmed milk

3 ripe bananas, peeled

1 tablespoon granulated sugar

1.2 litres ice cubes

Place all the ingredients into the Vitamix container in the order listed and secure the lid. Select Variable 1. Turn the machine on and slowly increase the speed to Variable 10, then to High. Use the tamper to press ingredients into the blades. In about 30 seconds, the sound of the motor will change and 4 mounds should form in the mixture. Stop the machine. Do not overmix or melting will occur. Serve immediately.

AMOUNT PER 120 ML SERVING: calories 45, total fat 0 g, saturated fat 0 g, cholesterol 0 mg, sodium 10 mg, total carbohydrate 11 g, dietary fibre 1 g, sugars 7 g, protein 1 g

Strawberry Tofu Freeze

A delicious, creamy vegan dessert! A teaspoon of vanilla extract takes this deeply fruity treat and makes it taste much like old-fashioned strawberry ice cream.

Preparation: **15 minutes**   Processing: **1 minute**   Yield: **1.2 litres**

680 g frozen unsweetened strawberries

340 g extra-firm silken tofu

4 tablespoons fresh orange juice (page 303)

½ orange, peeled and halved

1 teaspoon vanilla extract

1. Let the strawberries sit at room temperature for 10 minutes to soften slightly.

2. Place the tofu, orange juice, orange, vanilla and strawberries into the Vitamix container in the order listed and secure the lid. Select Variable 1. Turn the machine on and slowly increase the speed to Variable 10, then to High, using the tamper to press the ingredients into the blades. In about 1 minute, the sound of the motor will change and 4 mounds should form in the mixture. Stop the machine. Do not overmix or melting will occur. Serve immediately.

AMOUNT PER 120 ML SERVING: calories 40, total fat 0 g, saturated fat 0 g, cholesterol 0 mg, sodium 35 mg, total carbohydrate 8 g, dietary fibre 2 g, sugars 4 g, protein 3 g

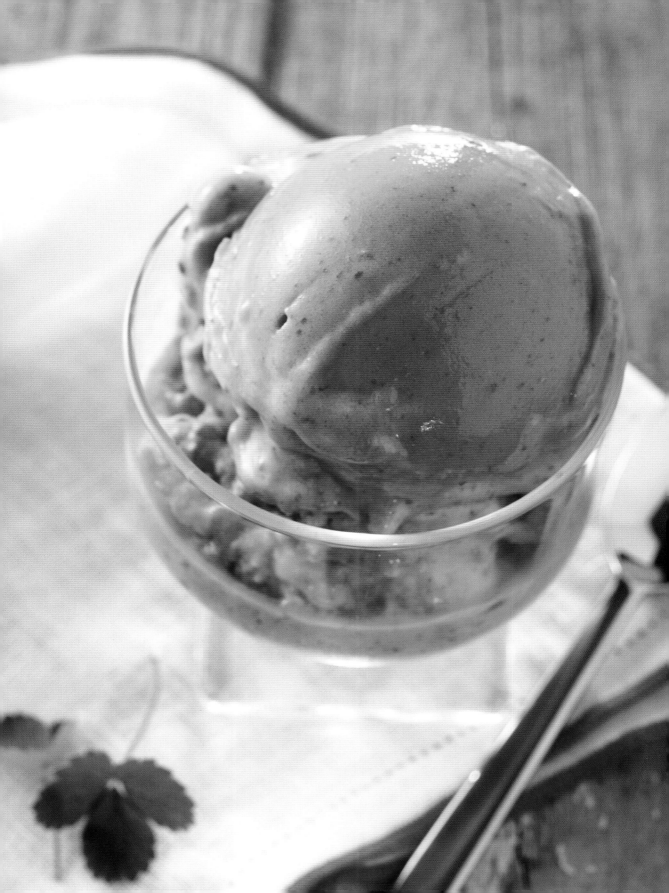

Strawberry Yoghurt Freeze

This delightful, 2-ingredient dessert can be whipped up in under 10 minutes. And since it is just yoghurt and strawberries, you could even serve it for breakfast!

Preparation: **10 minutes**   Processing: **30–60 seconds**   Yield: **780 ml**

240 g vanilla low-fat yoghurt

450 g frozen unsweetened strawberries

Place all the ingredients into the Vitamix container in the order listed and secure the lid. Select Variable 1. Turn the machine on and slowly increase the speed to Variable 10, then to High, using the tamper to press the ingredients into the blades. In 30–60 seconds, the sound of the motor will change and 4 mounds should form in the mixture. Stop the machine. Do not overmix or melting will occur. Serve immediately.

AMOUNT PER 120 ML SERVING: calories 60, total fat 0.5 g, saturated fat 0 g, cholesterol 0 mg, sodium 25 mg, total carbohydrate 13 g, dietary fibre 2 g, sugars 9 g, protein 3 g

Pineapple Freeze

If you have the three ingredients for this dessert on hand, you can go from an empty dish to a sweet treat in just 5 minutes. The soft tofu gives this freeze a creamy full flavour without any dairy.

Preparation: **5 minutes**   Processing: **30 seconds**   Yield: **480 ml**

160 g soft tofu

260 g frozen pineapple chunks

½ teaspoon fresh lime juice

Place all the ingredients into the Vitamix container in the order listed and secure the lid. Select Variable 1. Turn the machine on and slowly increase the speed to Variable 10, then to High, using the tamper to press the ingredients into the blades. In about 30 seconds, the sound of the motor will change and 4 mounds should form in the mixture. Stop the machine. Do not overmix or melting will occur. Serve immediately.

AMOUNT PER 120 ML SERVING: calories 70, total fat 1.5 g, saturated fat 0 g, cholesterol 0 mg, sodium 0 mg, total carbohydrate 11 g, dietary fibre 1 g, sugars 2 g, protein 4 g

Tropical Freeze

This tasty tropical dessert is perfect for serving after a meal of Fish Tacos with Slaw (page 203) or Spicy Jerk Chicken (page 220). Cool, creamy and tangy, this frozen dessert can be garnished with extra fresh fruit or scooped into ice-cream cones.

Preparation: **10 minutes**   Processing: **35–40 seconds**   Yield: **840 ml**

190 g frozen mango pieces

240 ml pineapple juice

1 medium banana, peeled

120 ml natural 0% Greek yoghurt, stirred

½ teaspoon grated lemon zest

3 fresh mint leaves

180 ml ice cubes

1. Let the mango sit at room temperature for 5 minutes to soften slightly.

2. Place the pineapple juice, banana, yoghurt, lemon zest, mint, mango and ice cubes into the Vitamix container in the order listed and secure the lid. Select Variable 1. Turn the machine on and slowly increase the speed to Variable 10, then to High, using the tamper to press the ingredients into the blades. In 35–40 seconds the sound of the motor will change and 4 mounds should form in the mixture. Stop the machine. Do not overmix or melting will occur. Serve immediately.

AMOUNT PER 120 ML SERVING: calories 60, total fat 0 g, saturated fat 0 g, cholesterol 0 mg, sodium 10 mg, total carbohydrate 13 g, dietary fibre 1 g, sugars 10 g, protein 2 g

Tropical Mango Freeze

Once you get the hang of making this and other delicious frozen desserts in your Vitamix, you may hesitate to buy ice cream or frozen yoghurt at the supermarket. The key is to not overmix the ingredients, or you will end up with a very cold smoothie instead of a spoonable dessert.

Preparation: **10 minutes**   Processing: **1 minute**   Yield: **720 ml**

225 g frozen unsweetened mango chunks

225 g frozen unsweetened pineapple chunks

225 g natural 0% Greek yoghurt, stirred

1 teaspoon vanilla extract

1. Let the frozen fruit sit at room temperature for 10 minutes to soften slightly.

2. Place the yoghurt, vanilla and fruit into the Vitamix container in the order listed and secure the lid. Select Variable 1. Turn the machine on and slowly increase the speed to Variable 10, then to High, using the tamper to press the ingredients into the blades. In about 1 minute, the sound of the motor will change and 4 mounds should form in the mixture. Stop the machine. Do not overmix or melting will occur. Serve immediately.

AMOUNT PER 120 ML SERVING: calories 70, total fat 0 g, saturated fat 0 g, cholesterol 0 mg, sodium 15 mg, total carbohydrate 13 g, dietary fibre 1 g, sugars 8 g, protein 4 g

PAMELA FLEMING

Grandma and Grandpa Barnard's children learned about the importance of health and good nutrition around their own kitchen table and through their work with the Vitamix business. As the years went by, subsequent generations of Barnards inherited and expanded this legacy of health. Out on the East Coast and in an entirely different family, Pamela Fleming was learning about good nutrition from a beloved aunt.

As a child, Pamela would travel from her home in Brooklyn, New York, to spend her summers in the Poconos in Pennsylvania with her Aunt Wini. Wini had had rheumatic fever as a child, and as a young adult had been plagued by health problems. By chance she wandered into a health food store – a relative rarity in the 1950s – and the proprietor told her about the Vitamix and the ways she could address her health problems through her diet. Wini bought a Vitamix and began blending fruit, vegetables and nuts into healthy drinks. Wini's subsequent transformation, Pamela recalls, was apparent. '[Our] family remarked that she was an ugly duckling that had become a swan.'

Convinced by her own success, Wini became the manager of a health food store and, later, a holistic nutritionist. When Pamela visited her aunt in the Poconos, nutrition and health often came up in conversation. When they picked produce in Wini's organic garden for their smoothies, Wini would talk to young Pamela about the importance of good nutrition and avoiding pesticides. Back in

Brooklyn, Pamela remembers, 'I would try and lecture all of my friends and family [about] holistic health, but it was a strange concept back then.'

Flash forward to 2009. Inspired by years of gentle encouragement from Wini, Pamela purchased a Vitamix. Pamela says she has actively used the machine ever since. Pamela enjoys whipping up 'health drinks, smoothies, soups – even healthy frozen yoghurt for my grandkids.' Pamela also carries on Aunt Wini's legacy, teaching friends and family about good nutrition and health. 'Nearly every day of my life, I find myself quoting my Aunt Wini, or silently thanking her for her wisdom and generosity in sharing her knowledge. I consider myself an advocate of good nutrition, and feel I am indeed carrying Aunt Wini's torch. Both my daughters are nutritionally aware, and are raising their children to be so.'

When Pamela sees a Vitamix demonstration, she likes to offer her encouragement to the crowd. Pamela says her friends often say that she works for Vitamix, and she says, 'In a way, I do. It's a product I truly believe in.' We call this 'spreading the health!' If every one of us spread the health to a dozen other people, the world would be a healthier place in no time.

Not unlike the Barnards, Pamela's family now has a strong legacy of achieving better health and wellness by using their Vitamix machines to eat more whole foods. What sort of healthy life legacy do you hope to share with your friends and family?

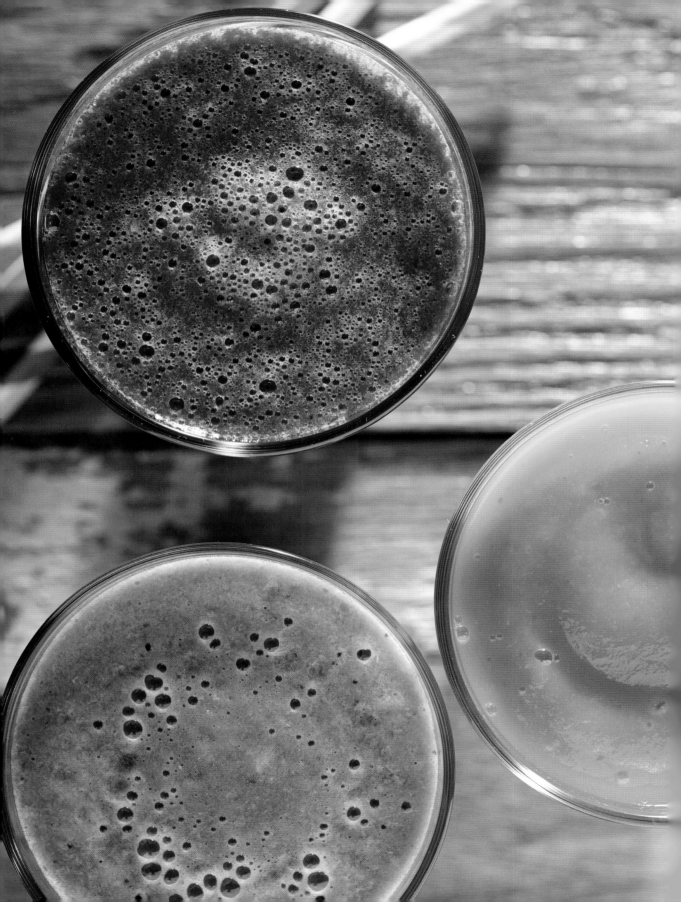

Chapter 8

Drinks

As you can imagine, I learned the breadth of uses for the Vitamix very early on. It was the family business, after all! Some I learned probably sooner than I should have. When I was growing up my parent's favourite party drink was the blended whiskey sour. I will admit that we kids would hide under the table and when the party moved to the other room; we would sneak out and share the few drops that remained in the Vitamix container. This may be how I came up with the idea of serving my husband smoothies with a shot of vodka after a long day at the office. I quickly weaned him off the vodka and it took a while before he thought to even ask. Now it is straight smoothie – no chaser!

Spiked or not, smoothies are now a part of the culinary landscape. Perhaps because smoothies are quick to prepare and easy to drink in the flurry of our morning routine, lunch or workout routine, Americans drink a lot of them. Our research team at Vitamix tells us that, between July 2013 and June 2014, Americans whipped up 3.42 billion home-made smoothies, a jaw-dropping number.

Blended drinks involve a much wider range of drinks than smoothies, of course. Blended tea and coffee drinks pop up more and more and in an expanding range of flavours. Juice, also a blended drink depending on how it is produced, has come to encompass a staggering range of ingredients, too. We can now buy or make a wide range of juices with fruits, vegetables and other healthy ingredients. And nut milks? A quick Internet search shows that lots of us are interested in drinking, and making, non-dairy milks, too, and we are using our Vitamix to do it.

Does this explosion of interest in blended drinks translate into a healthier America? While there is never a silver bullet, we can hope for positive change. If, by drinking smoothies and whipping up nut milks and fresh juices we are eating more whole foods, then we are on the right track. If by making these drinks and snacks at home we are consuming less sodium and sugar, then that is also good, even if the transformation is not yet dramatic.

Small simple steps towards increasing your health and vitality are absolutely worth taking. In this chapter we will look at the different ways you can use your Vitamix to make drinks that contain whole foods and avoid lots of extra salt and sugar. Let's raise a glass to our health!

Smoothies

According to research that we mentioned above, 25 per cent of Vitamix owners add kale to their smoothies. We love our green smoothies here at Vitamix! Several of the recipes in this chapter – Basil Romaine Boost (page 318), Fresh Mint with Sprouts Beverage (page 347), Kale-Flax Smoothie with Pear (page 337), Going Green Smoothie (page 328) and Greens Juice Blend (page 309) to name just a few – give you new and creative ways to add fruits and leafy green vegetables to your diet.

Of course, whole vegetable juices and drinks aren't just about greens. Salsa in a Glass (page 334) and Digestive Juice Drink (page 310) offer two ways to enjoy whole-food tomato juice with much less sodium than many packaged varieties. Nourishing Beetroot (page 339) pairs deeply purple and naturally sweet beetroot and apples with chilli pepper, garlic, celery and ginger for a delicious and slightly unconventional whole-vegetable drink. Spinach Sparkler (page 333) combines greens, celery, cucumber, a whole lemon, a splash of pineapple juice and sparkling water for a fresh, effervescent drink that would delight Popeye and Olive Oyl alike.

Many smoothies, even vegetable-based ones, benefit from fresh, dried or frozen fruit to add a little sweetness. Banana Boost (page 319), Cherry Red

Smoothie (page 323), Fig Smoothie with Goji Berries and Chia Seeds (page 324), Purple Fruit Smoothie (page 317) and Tofu Tropic Smoothie (page 341) will give you new and delicious ways to work more fruits into your breakfasts and afternoon snacks.

Whole Food Juicing

What, you might ask, is the difference between whole-food smoothies and whole-food juices? Here at Vitamix, our chef and manager of recipe development, Bev Shaffer, says smoothies have a silky smooth texture of varying thicknesses while juices tend to be thinner and could retain some of the texture of the fruits and vegetables.

Whole-food juices, like smoothies, contain all of the fibre and nutrients that you would get from eating the fruit or vegetable on its own. Whole-food juices can be made quite thin, but because of the fibre, they will tend to have a thicker texture than a drink made with a juicer/juice extractor. If you want your drink to be more like the liquid produced by a juicer, you can strain the liquid through a fine-mesh sieve before you drink it.

You can make delicious juices with both fruits and vegetables. Recipes for Apple Juice (page 304), Berry Veggie Juice Blend (page 309), Cherry Anise Juice Blend (page 312), Greens Juice Blend (page 309) and Tart Citrus Juice Blend (page 311), among others, will show you how. You can also make your own Orange Juice (page 303) and either drink it on its own or use it in a smoothie or as part of a juice blend.

Non-dairy Milks

If you want milk but are avoiding dairy, your options are increasing quickly these days. Milks made from hemp seeds, soy, rice and a wide variety of nuts abound. However, packaged non-dairy milks often contain thickeners, sweeteners and additives. Thankfully these milks are easy to make at home with a few simple ingredients and the amazing Vitamix. Not only can you adjust the sweetness and the texture to your own preferences, the fresh flavour is pretty unbeatable. Explore the do-it-yourself non-dairy milk options with recipes such as Almond Milk (page 352), Sweet Almond Cinnamon Milk (page 355) and Soya milk (page 351). Once made, these milks will keep in the fridge for about a week.

Caffeinated Drinks

A green smoothie may give you a boost, but few things can compete with the eye-opening powers of coffee or green tea. Heavily sweetened blended coffee and tea drinks are widely available, but they are easier, cheaper, and often healthier to make at home. Try a Mocha Cooler (page 359), a Tea of Green Smoothie (page 360) or an Espresso Banana Drink (page 357) the next time you need a caffeine boost. Loyal Vitamix owner Janice Summers (read more about her on page 257) says she started blending her own coffee drinks because she wanted an all-organic drink, and now she prefers her home-blended coffees. 'Now that I make my own, they are so much better than what I get when out, that even if I could get organic I wouldn't choose to since I like the creaminess and taste of mine better!'

Techniques for the Best Results

Here are a couple of quick tips to ensure that you make the best smoothies, juices and other blended drinks.

- Put the ingredients in the Vitamix in the order that they are listed. In general, liquids go in first, then dry goods, leafy greens, fruits and veggies and, last, any frozen ingredients. Why, you might ask? Because the heavier frozen ingredients help push everything into the blades.

- Start the machine slowly – this helps the blades 'grab' the ingredients – but then quickly switch to a higher speed. Using the top speeds is actually easier on the motor, so increase the speed as directed.

- If needed, add a little more liquid or use the tamper to help the ingredients circulate fully and blend more completely.

- As we say in our *Personal Blending* book, 'Perfection cannot be rushed. Blend for the full processing time suggested in the recipe at least the first time you make it.' If you prefer to shorten the blend time in the future, your drink may not be quite as smooth, but it is all about preference.

Cheers!

Orange Juice

You are just minutes away from fresh, delicious orange juice! Enjoy this drink on its own or add it to any recipe in this book that calls for orange juice.

Preparation: **10 minutes**   Processing: **1 minute**   Yield: **960 ml**

4 large oranges, peeled and halved

120 ml ice cubes

Place all the ingredients and 120 ml water into the Vitamix container in the order listed and secure the lid. Select Variable 1. Turn the machine on and slowly increase the speed to Variable 10, then to High. Blend for 1 minute, or until the desired consistency is reached.

AMOUNT PER 120 ML SERVING: calories 45, total fat 0 g, saturated fat 0 g, cholesterol 0 mg, sodium 0 mg, total carbohydrate 11 g, dietary fibre 2 g, sugars 9 g, protein 1 g

Apple Juice

This refreshing cider-like drink tastes wonderfully and simply of apples. It is sure to be a hit with young and old alike!

Preparation: **10 minutes**   Processing: **45 seconds**   Yield: **2 servings**

680 g apples, quartered and cored

1. Place 60 ml water into the Vitamix container, add the apples and secure the lid. Select Variable 1. Turn the machine on and slowly increase the speed to Variable 10, then to High. Blend for 45 seconds, using the tamper to press the ingredients into the blades.

2. Transfer the purée to a bowl lined with 4 layers of muslin and twist until the juice is extracted.

AMOUNT PER SERVING: calories 60, total fat 0 g, saturated fat 0 g, cholesterol 0 mg, sodium 15 mg, total carbohydrate 15 g, dietary fibre 0 g, sugars 13 g, protein 0 g

Apple Pear Fruit Juice

Save a little of the home-made apple juice (page 304) and make this flavour-packed whole fruit juice. Fresh ginger and a little cinnamon balance out the natural sweetness of the apples, pears and green grapes.

Preparation: **10 minutes**   Processing: **1 minute**   Yield: **4–5 servings**

180 ml unsweetened apple juice

75 g green grapes

2 apples (380 g), halved and cored

2 pears (450 g), halved and cored

1-cm piece of fresh ginger, peeled

½ teaspoon ground cinnamon

Place all the ingredients into the Vitamix container in the order listed and secure the lid. Select Variable 1. Turn the machine on and slowly increase the speed to Variable 10, then to High. Blend for 1 minute, or until the desired consistency is reached, using the tamper to press the ingredients into the blades.

AMOUNT PER 240 ML SERVING: calories 140, total fat 0 g, saturated fat 0 g, cholesterol 0 mg, sodium 5 mg, total carbohydrate 38 g, dietary fibre 6 g, sugars 27 g, protein 1 g

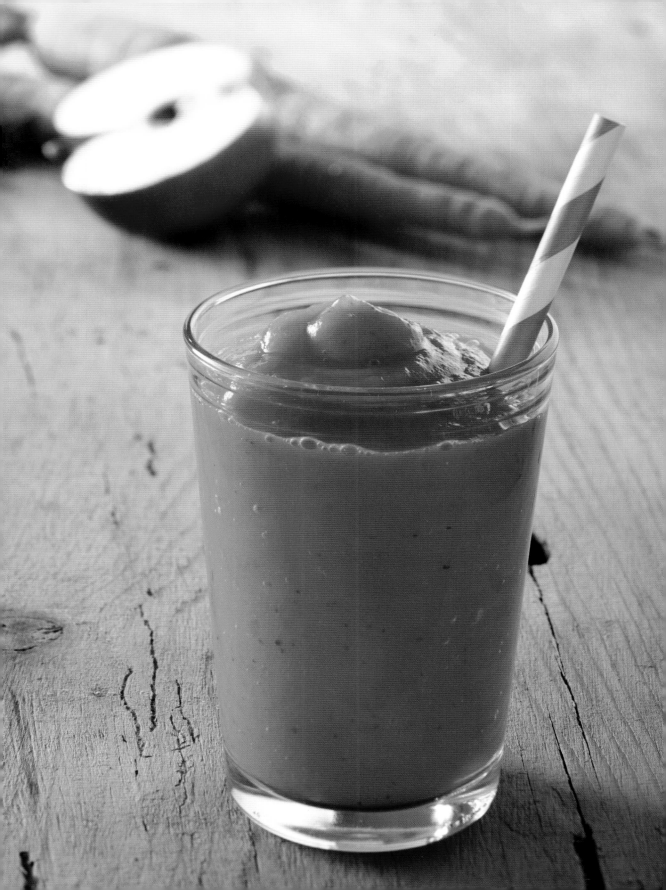

Carrot-Apple Juice Blend

This lip-smacking juice blend takes a little more planning than some of the other drinks. Carrots, steamed and cooled before blending, give this drink a delightfully smooth texture. The basil might seem out of place but don't skip it. The herby, anise flavour balances the sweetness of the apple, apple juice and the carrots.

Preparation: **15 minutes**   Processing: **1 minute**   Yield: **2–3 servings**

120 ml unsweetened apple juice

4 medium carrots (225 g), peeled, cut into pieces, steamed until tender and cooled

1 tablespoon chopped fresh basil

1 small apple, halved and seeded

120 ml ice cubes

Place all the ingredients and 120 ml water into the Vitamix container in the order listed and secure the lid. Select Variable 1. Turn the machine on and slowly increase the speed to Variable 10, then to High. Blend for 1 minute, or until the desired consistency is reached, using the tamper to press the ingredients into the blades.

AMOUNT PER 240 ML SERVING: calories 80, total fat 0 g, saturated fat 0 g, cholesterol 0 mg, sodium 55 mg, total carbohydrate 20 g, dietary fibre 4 g, sugars 13 g, protein 1 g

Mango Carrot Juice Blend

Marigold-hued and bursting with flavour, this mango carrot blend may replace plain orange juice as your morning beverage. There is still some naturally occurring sugar in this whole-foods juice (19 grams versus 22 grams for a cup of orange juice), but along with that sugar, you get 4 grams of fibre. You also get a greater variety of fruits and veggies in a cup of this juice blend. And is variety not the spice of life?

Preparation: **15 minutes**   Processing: **1 minute**   Yield: **4 servings**

120 ml no-sugar-added mango nectar

1 teaspoon grated orange zest

1 orange, peeled and halved

1 small apple, halved and cored

3 carrots (170 g), quartered

190 g frozen mango chunks

240 ml ice cubes

Place 180 ml water into the Vitamix container, then add all the ingredients in the order listed and secure the lid. Select Variable 1. Turn the machine on and slowly increase the speed to Variable 10, then to High. Blend for 1 minute, or until the desired consistency is reached, using the tamper to press the ingredients into the blades.

AMOUNT PER 240 ML SERVING: calories 90, total fat 0 g, saturated fat 0 g, cholesterol 0 mg, sodium 35 mg, total carbohydrate 24 g, dietary fibre 4 g, sugars 19 g, protein 1 g

Spicy Tomato Drink

Make this bright, zippy drink when tomatoes are in season for the best flavour. Consider serving it with a cheese sandwich on wholegrain bread for a summertime twist on the classic tomato soup and grilled cheese pairing.

Preparation: **10 minutes**   Processing: **20 seconds**   Yield: **3–4 servings**

680 g tomatoes, quartered

1 lemon, peeled and halved

2 tablespoons chopped onion

6 dashes of hot sauce

120 ml ice cubes

Place all the ingredients into the Vitamix container in the order listed and secure the lid. Select Variable 1. Turn the machine on and slowly increase the speed to Variable 10, then to High. Blend for 20 seconds, or until the desired consistency is reached.

AMOUNT PER 240 ML SERVING: calories 40, total fat 0 g, saturated fat 0 g, cholesterol 0 mg, sodium 15 mg, total carbohydrate 10 g, dietary fibre 3 g, sugars 6 g, protein 2 g

Greens Juice Blend

Juicing whole foods allows you to keep the fibre and nutrients that the ingredients contain, but the resulting drink is thicker, more smoothie-like. Here we use equal parts water and ice to give this juice blend a thinner, more juice-like quality without sacrificing any of its nutritional benefits.

Preparation: **15 minutes**   Processing: **35 seconds**   Yield: **3–4 servings**

70 g broccoli florets

85 g fresh pineapple chunks

½ apple, halved and cored

½ banana

28 g baby spinach

15 g chopped kale leaves

15 g fresh flatleaf parsley leaves

2 fresh basil leaves

240 ml ice cubes

Place all the ingredients and 240 ml water into the Vitamix container in the order listed and secure the lid. Select Variable 1. Turn the machine on and slowly increase the speed to Variable 10, then to High. Blend for 35 seconds, or until the desired consistency is reached, using the tamper to press the ingredients into the blades.

AMOUNT PER 240 ML SERVING: calories 60, total fat 0 g, saturated fat 0 g, cholesterol 0 mg, sodium 30 mg, total carbohydrate 14 g, dietary fibre 3 g, sugars 7 g, protein 2 g

Berry Veggie Juice Blend

Pairing naturally sweet, nutrient-rich vegetables like sweetcorn, carrots and roasted beetroot with frozen berries creates a delicious, flavourful smoothie. If you are trying to add (or sneak!) more veggies into your daily diet, this tasty drink is great way to do it.

Preparation: **10 minutes plus roasting**   Processing: **1 minute**   Yield: **4–5 servings**

50 g fresh or thawed frozen strawberries

115 g frozen raspberries

1 medium red beetroot, roasted, peeled and quartered

2 carrots, quartered

145 g corn kernels

240 ml ice cubes

Place all the ingredients and 300 ml water into the Vitamix container in the order listed and secure the lid. Select Variable 1. Turn the machine on and slowly increase the speed to Variable 10, then to High. Blend for 1 minute, or until the desired consistency is reached, using the tamper to press the ingredients into the blades.

AMOUNT PER 240 ML SERVING: calories 60, total fat 0.5 g, saturated fat 0 g, cholesterol 0 mg, sodium 40 mg, total carbohydrate 15 g, dietary fibre 3 g, sugars 7 g, protein 2 g

Digestive Juice Drink

Move over, salty vegetable juices, there is a new, healthier drink in town! A great way to get your veggies on the go, this whole-foods juice is packed with tomatoes, carrots, fennel, beetroot, celery, garlic, herbs and spices. Pack in a Thermos for a healthy lunch or snack.

Preparation: **15 minutes**   Processing: **1 minute**   Yield: **4–5 servings**

2 medium tomatoes, quartered

2 carrots, cut into pieces

¼ fennel bulb, cut into chunks

1 garlic clove, peeled

4 fresh basil leaves

1 tablespoon dill sprigs

½ teaspoon fresh thyme leaves

2 celery sticks

1 small/medium red beetroot, quartered

¼ teaspoon ground turmeric

¼ teaspoon dry mustard

¼ teaspoon ground cumin

240 ml ice cubes

Place 120 ml water, then all the ingredients into the Vitamix container in the order listed and secure the lid. Select Variable 1. Turn the machine on and slowly increase the speed to Variable 10, then to High. Blend for 1 minute, or until the desired consistency is reached, using the tamper to press the ingredients into the blades.

AMOUNT PER 240 ML SERVING: calories 45, total fat 0 g, saturated fat 0 g, cholesterol 0 mg, sodium 65 mg, total carbohydrate 10 g, dietary fibre 3 g, sugars 5 g, protein 2 g

Tart Citrus Juice Blend

This zippy, bright juice blend will really get your eyes open in the morning! Full of whole citrus fruits, this drink has a little honey for sweetness as well whole cranberries for colour and extra pucker. Cut the juice with sparkling water for a bubbly treat or use as a base for a whole fruit margarita.

Preparation: **10 minutes**   Processing: **1 minute**   Yield: **3–4 servings**

2 oranges, peeled and halved

1 grapefruit, peeled and halved

1 lime, peeled

65 g cranberries, fresh or frozen

1 teaspoon honey

120 ml ice cubes

Place all the ingredients and 120 ml water into the Vitamix container in the order listed and secure the lid. Select Variable 1. Turn the machine on and slowly increase the speed to Variable 10, then to High. Blend for 1 minute, or until the desired consistency is reached, using the tamper to press the ingredients into the blades.

AMOUNT PER 240 ML SERVING: calories 80, total fat 0 g, saturated fat 0 g, cholesterol 0 mg, sodium 0 mg, total carbohydrate 21 g, dietary fibre 4 g, sugars 10 g, protein 1 g

Cherry Anise Juice Blend

The subtle liquorice flavour of fennel complements the sweetness of the cherries in this drink. Don't worry if you are not ordinarily a liquorice fan, the taste of fennel is more vegetable and less assertive than your average black liquorice whip. Adding this delicious vegetable and a whole peeled lime gives this whole juice bright flavour and fibre without adding a lot of extra calories.

Preparation: **15 minutes**   Processing: **40 seconds**   Yield: **2 servings**

150 g green grapes

½ lime, peeled

¼ fennel bulb, cut into pieces

140 g frozen pitted dark cherries

Place all the ingredients and 120 ml water into the Vitamix container in the order listed and secure the lid. Select Variable 1. Turn the machine on and slowly increase the speed to Variable 10, then to High. Blend for 40 seconds, or until the desired consistency is reached, using the tamper to press the ingredients into the blades.

AMOUNT PER SERVING: calories 110, total fat 0 g, saturated fat 0 g, cholesterol 0 mg, sodium 20 mg, total carbohydrate 29 g, dietary fibre 4 g, sugars 21 g, protein 2 g

Breakfast Shake

The King of Shake (Rattle and Roll, that is) Elvis Presley may have preferred his banana and peanut butter fried in a sandwich with bacon, but perhaps he would have enjoyed his favourite flavours in this breakfast drink, too. Easily put together with store cupboard staples, it is a crowd – and specifically a kid – pleaser!

Preparation: **10 minutes**   Processing: **15–20 seconds**   Yield: **2 servings**

80 ml skimmed milk

180 ml natural 0% Greek yoghurt

1 teaspoon vanilla extract

1 teaspoon honey

1 medium banana

1 tablespoon peanut butter

1. Place all the ingredients into the Vitamix container in the order listed and secure the lid.

2. Select Variable 1. Turn the machine on and slowly increase the speed to Variable 10, then to High. Blend for 15 to 20 seconds, until the desired consistency is reached.

AMOUNT PER 240 ML SERVING: calories 190, total fat 6 g, saturated fat 1.5 g, cholesterol 5 mg, sodium 110 mg, total carbohydrate 27 g, dietary fibre 2 g, sugars 19 g, protein 9 g

Wake Up Breakfast Smoothie

Need to dash out the door but still want a healthy breakfast? Take traditional breakfast ingredients – milk, yoghurt, strawberries, banana, wheatgerm and maple syrup – and blend them into a tasty, nutritious and entirely portable meal. Really pressed for time? Whip this smoothie up the night before for a truly grab-and-go breakfast.

Preparation: **15 minutes**   Processing: **30 seconds**   Yield: **5 servings**

120 ml skimmed milk

360 ml plain 0% Greek yoghurt

½ teaspoon vanilla extract

330 g sliced fresh strawberries

1 small banana, peeled and halved

2 tablespoons wheatgerm

1 tablespoon pure maple syrup

360 ml ice cubes

Place all the ingredients into the Vitamix container in the order listed and secure the lid. Select Variable 1. Turn the machine on and slowly increase the speed to Variable 10, then to High. Blend for 30 seconds, or until the desired consistency is reached, using the tamper to press the ingredients into the blades.

AMOUNT PER 240 ML SERVING: calories 110, total fat 0.5 g, saturated fat 0 g, cholesterol 0 mg, sodium 65 mg, total carbohydrate 20 g, dietary fibre 2 g, sugars 15 g, protein 6 g

Banana Apple Oatmeal Smoothie

Vanilla yoghurt, banana, apple and two tablespoons of quick-cook oats work together to give this smoothie a thick, creamy texture. Dried cranberries add a bit of tartness to balance out the sweet, and cinnamon adds the gentlest bit of spice. A wonderful drink to start your day or give you a late-afternoon boost!

Preparation: **10 minutes**   Processing: **45 seconds**   Yield: **2 servings**

60 g vanilla low-fat yoghurt

½ banana

2 tablespoons quick-cook oats

½ medium apple, halved and cored

30 g dried unsweetened cranberries

⅛ teaspoon ground cinnamon

Place all the ingredients and 240 ml water into the Vitamix container in the order listed and secure the lid. Select Variable 1. Turn the machine on and slowly increase the speed to Variable 10, then to High. Blend for 45 seconds, or until the desired consistency is reached.

AMOUNT PER 240 ML SERVING: calories 140, total fat 1 g, saturated fat 0 g, cholesterol 0 mg, sodium 30 mg, total carbohydrate 32 g, dietary fibre 3 g, sugars 24 g, protein 3 g

Raspberry Oatmeal Smoothie

The most delicious and drinkable oatmeal you have ever had! This smoothie is full of fibre, protein and a gentle sweetness from the raspberries and the honey. Feel free to try this smoothie with other fruits and berries, too, adjusting the honey depending on the sweetness of the fruit.

Preparation: **10 minutes**   Processing: **20 seconds**   Yield: **1 serving**

1½ tablespoons quick-cook oats

125 g fresh or frozen raspberries, partially thawed if frozen

1 teaspoon honey

3 tablespoons natural 0% Greek yoghurt, stirred

1. Soak oats in 120 ml boiling water for 10 minutes.

2. Place 60 ml water, the oat mixture with any remaining liquid, the raspberries, honey and yoghurt into the Vitamix container in that order and secure the lid. Select Variable 1. Turn the machine on and slowly increase the speed to Variable 10, then to High. Blend for 20 seconds.

AMOUNT PER SERVING: calories 130, total fat 0.5 g, saturated fat 0 g, cholesterol 0 mg, sodium 25 mg, total carbohydrate 30 g, dietary fibre 9 g, sugars 7 g, protein 6 g

Almond Milk Banana Smoothie

This delicious smoothie, perfect for breakfast or an afternoon pick-me-up, is a great way to use home-made almond milk. A portion of flaked almonds adds an extra nutty flavour, and the vanilla extract makes the drink taste almost dessert-like.

Preparation: **10 minutes**   Processing: **25 seconds**   Yield: **3–4 servings**

480 ml unsweetened almond milk, preferably home-made (page 352), cold

55 g flaked almonds

2 ripe small bananas, peeled and halved

1½ teaspoons vanilla extract

120 ml ice cubes

Place all the ingredients into the Vitamix container in the order listed and secure the lid. Select Variable 1. Turn the machine on and slowly increase the speed to Variable 10. Blend for 25 seconds or until the desired consistency is reached.

AMOUNT PER 240 ML SERVING: calories 160, total fat 9 g, saturated fat 0.5 g, cholesterol 0 mg, sodium 95 mg, total carbohydrate 17 g, dietary fibre 4 g, sugars 7 g, protein 5 g

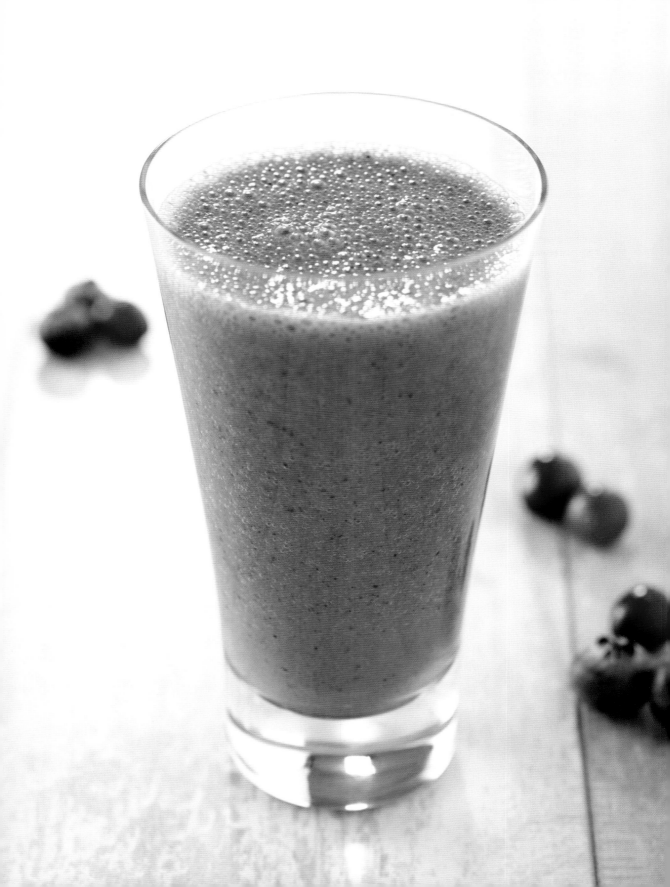

Purple Fruit Smoothie

Unsweetened cranberry juice contains 13 micrograms of vitamin K (14% of the daily vitamins for women, 10% for men), but many of us find it too tart to drink on its own. Blend it with a non-dairy milk, blueberries, cherries and a banana, however, and you get all of the nutrition in a sweeter, purple-hued drink that is much less tart.

Preparation: **10 minutes**   Processing: **30 seconds**   Yield: **2 servings**

60 ml unsweetened cranberry juice

120 ml unsweetened soya milk or nut milk

75 g fresh or frozen blueberries

70 g fresh or frozen pitted cherries

1 banana, peeled and halved

120 ml ice cubes

Place all the ingredients into the Vitamix container in the order listed and secure the lid. Select Variable 1. Turn the machine on and slowly increase the speed to Variable 10, then to High. Blend for 30 seconds.

AMOUNT PER 240 ML SERVING: calories 140, total fat 2 g, saturated fat 0 g, cholesterol 0 mg, sodium 0 mg, total carbohydrate 30 g, dietary fibre 3 g, sugars 19 g, protein 4 g

Basil Romaine Boost

Vibrantly green and lightly sweet, greens in the morning (or the afternoon or the evening) have never tasted so good! Make this smoothie the night before you want to drink it, if you like. Simply stir the smoothie to re-emulsify it before you enjoy it.

Preparation: **10 minutes**   Processing: **45 seconds**   Yield: **3–4 servings**

1 pear, quartered and cored

1 orange, peeled and halved

45 g chopped broccoli

85 g baby romaine lettuce mix

16 g fresh basil leaves

240 ml ice cubes

Place all the ingredients and 240 ml water into the Vitamix container in the order listed and secure the lid. Select Variable 1. Turn the machine on and slowly increase the speed to Variable 10, then to High. Blend for 45 seconds, or until the desired consistency is reached, using the tamper to press the ingredients into the blades.

AMOUNT PER 240 ML SERVING: calories 45, total fat 0 g, saturated fat 0 g, cholesterol 0 mg, sodium 20 mg, total carbohydrate 11 g, dietary fibre 3 g, sugars 7 g, protein 1 g

Banana Boost

We all love bananas: We eat more bananas than apples and oranges combined. Why not boost the creamy sweet flavour of the banana with other whole fruits? Here a peeled and halved lemon, pitted dates and half a pineapple, core and all, are blended with banana and soya milk for a tasty drink that is sure to give your day a lift!

Preparation: **10 minutes**   Processing: **30 seconds**   Yield: **4 servings**

300 ml unsweetened soya milk, cold

1 lemon, peeled and halved

1 small ripe banana, peeled

4–5 pitted dates

½ pineapple (500 g), cut into pieces, core included

Place all the ingredients into the Vitamix container in the order listed and secure the lid. Select Variable 1. Turn the machine on and slowly increase the speed to Variable 10, then to High. Blend for 30 seconds, or until the desired consistency is reached.

AMOUNT PER 240 ML SERVING: calories 230, total fat 2 g, saturated fat 0 g, cholesterol 0 mg, sodium 0 mg, total carbohydrate 54 g, dietary fibre 4 g, sugars 41 g, protein 6 g

Berry Beetroot Blast

A half-cup of roasted beetroot, deeply purple and with an earthy sweetness, blends beautifully with orange and lemon juices, a little honey and mixed berries to create a delicious juice. The beetroot combines so seamlessly with the berries; you may forget you are drinking a vegetable!

Preparation: **10 minutes**   Processing: **45 seconds**   Yield: **420 ml**

1 tablespoon fresh lemon juice

120 ml fresh orange juice (page 303)

1 teaspoon honey

90 g roasted beetroot chunks

80 g frozen mixed berries

120 ml ice cubes

Place all the ingredients and 60 ml water into the Vitamix container in the order listed and secure the lid. Select Variable 1. Turn the machine on and slowly increase the speed to Variable 10, then to High. Blend for 45 seconds, or until desired consistency is reached, using the tamper to press the ingredients into the blades.

AMOUNT PER 240 ML SERVING: calories 90, total fat 0 g, saturated fat 0 g, cholesterol 0 mg, sodium 40 mg, total carbohydrate 22 g, dietary fibre 3 g, sugars 17 g, protein 2 g

Fruit Nut Shake

Adding protein, healthy fats and fibre to your shakes can help them keep you full longer. Here pecans, skimmed milk and Greek yoghurt give a protein boost to blueberries and peaches and create a drink that will help power you through your busiest days.

Preparation: **10 minutes**   Processing: **30 seconds**   Yield: **2 servings**

140 g frozen unsweetened peach slices

120 ml skimmed milk

240 ml natural 0% Greek yoghurt, stirred

1 tablespoon pecan pieces

½ teaspoon vanilla extract

40 g fresh or frozen blueberries

1. Let the peaches sit at room temperature for 15 minutes to thaw slightly.

2. Place the milk, yoghurt, pecans, vanilla, peaches and blueberries into the Vitamix container in the order listed and secure the lid. Select Variable 1. Turn the machine on and slowly increase the speed to Variable 10, then to High. Blend for 30 seconds, or until the desired consistency is reached.

AMOUNT PER 240 ML SERVING: calories 140, total fat 3 g, saturated fat 0 g, cholesterol 0 mg, sodium 70 mg, total carbohydrate 17 g, dietary fibre 2 g, sugars 15 g, protein 13 g

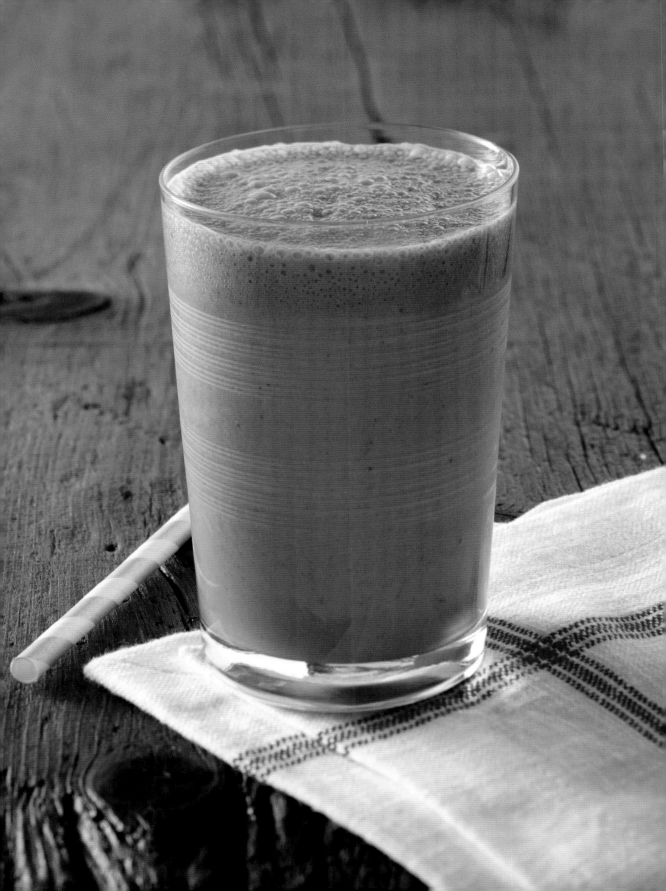

Cherry Red Smoothie

Combining unsweetened cherry juice – made from tart cherries – and frozen sweet cherries gives you a bright, sweet taste without refined sugar. Vanilla extract and 0% Greek yoghurt lend a creamy, almost ice-cream-like flavour.

Preparation: **10 minutes**   Processing: **45 seconds**   Yield: **3–4 servings**

240 ml unsweetened cherry juice

400 ml natural 0% Greek yoghurt, stirred

1 teaspoon vanilla extract

165 g frozen pitted sweet cherries

120 ml ice cubes

Place all the ingredients into the Vitamix container in the order listed and secure the lid. Select Variable 1. Turn the machine on and slowly increase the speed to Variable 10, then to High. Blend for 45 seconds, or until the desired consistency is reached, using the tamper to press the ingredients into the blades.

AMOUNT PER 240 ML SERVING: calories 120, total fat 0 g, saturated fat 0 g, cholesterol 0 mg, sodium 45 mg, total carbohydrate 20 g, dietary fibre 1 g, sugars 16 g, protein 10 g

Fig Smoothie with Goji Berries and Chia Seeds

This super-tasting, superfood-packed smoothie has a lot going on: a whopping 7 grams of fibre, 90% of the DV for vitamin A, 15% of the DV for iron and calcium. You get two kinds of greens, chia seeds, walnuts and dried goji berries and figs, too. Thanks to the power of the Vitamix, all of these hearty ingredients can be blended into a smooth, delicious drink. Raise a glass to your health!

Preparation: **10 minutes**   Processing: **1 minute**   Yield: **4–5 servings**

240 ml pomegranate juice

100 g dried figs

65 g kale, torn

28 g spinach leaves

42 g chia seeds

25 g walnuts

45 g dried goji berries

120 ml ice cubes

Place all the ingredients and 480 ml water into the Vitamix container in the order listed and secure the lid. Select Variable 1. Turn the machine on and slowly increase the speed to Variable 10, then to High. Blend for 1 minute, or until the desired consistency is reached, using the tamper to press the ingredients into the blades.

AMOUNT PER 240 ML SERVING: calories 220, total fat 7 g, saturated fat 0.5 g, cholesterol 0 mg, sodium 30 mg, total carbohydrate 37 g, dietary fibre 7 g, sugars 26 g, protein 4 g

Ginger Smoothie

Used in Ayurvedic and traditional Chinese medicines for hundreds of years, ginger has been the subject of more modern research, some of which suggests it may have anti-inflammatory properties. Regardless of what the scientists conclude about its benefits, we can confidently say that ginger is delicious! Paired with pears, cucumbers and kale, ginger lends a bright, slightly spicy flavour to this delicious drink.

Preparation: **10 minutes**   Processing: **1 minute**   Yield: **5 servings**

½ **cucumber (115 g), cut into large pieces**

2 pears, quartered and cored

4-cm piece of fresh ginger, peeled

6 Tuscan (black) kale leaves

120 ml ice cubes

Place 480 ml water into the Vitamix container, then add all the ingredients in the order listed and secure the lid. Select Variable 1. Turn the machine on and slowly increase the speed to Variable 10, then to High. Blend for 1 minute, or until the desired consistency is reached, using the tamper to press the ingredients into the blades.

AMOUNT PER 240 ML SERVING: calories 50, total fat 0 g, saturated fat 0 g, cholesterol 0 mg, sodium 10 mg, total carbohydrate 13 g, dietary fibre 3 g, sugars 7 g, protein 1 g

Blackberry-Pear Smoothie

If you like something sweet in the morning, even if it is a glass of orange juice or a cup of sweetened yoghurt, consider whipping up this flavourful drink instead. Lightly sweet and packed with naturally occurring nutrients and fibre, this creamy smoothie is sure to please!

Preparation: **10 minutes**   Processing: **45 seconds**   Yield: **4–5 servings**

250 g natural low-fat yoghurt

2 bananas, peeled and halved

1 pear, halved and cored

1 apple, halved and cored

280 g frozen blackberries

Place 160 ml water into the Vitamix container, then add all the ingredients in the order listed and secure the lid. Select Variable 1. Turn the machine on and slowly increase the speed to Variable 10, then to High. Blend for 45 seconds, or until the desired consistency is reached, using the tamper to press the ingredients into the blades.

AMOUNT PER 240 ML SERVING: calories 140, total fat 2 g, saturated fat 1 g, cholesterol 5 mg, sodium 25 mg, total carbohydrate 31 g, dietary fibre 6 g, sugars 21 g, protein 3 g

Cinnapeach Smoothie

Trying to convert a spinach-sceptic into a Popeye-esqe enthusiast? This tasty drink has 60 g of nutrient-packed spinach, but the flavours of peaches, rice or almond milk, vanilla and cinnamon dominate. A quick, delicious way to add greens to anyone's diet!

Preparation: **10 minutes**   Processing: **25 seconds**   Yield: **2–3 servings**

240 ml unsweetened almond or rice milk

140 g peach slices, fresh or thawed if frozen

½ teaspoon ground cinnamon

½ teaspoon vanilla extract

60 g spinach leaves

3 mint leaves

120 ml ice cubes

Place all the ingredients into the Vitamix container in the order listed and secure the lid. Select Variable 1. Turn the machine on and slowly increase the speed to Variable 10, then to High. Blend for 25 seconds, or until the desired consistency is reached, using the tamper to press the ingredients into the blades.

AMOUNT PER 240 ML SERVING: calories 60, total fat 1 g, saturated fat 0 g, cholesterol 0 mg, sodium 105 mg, total carbohydrate 13 g, dietary fibre 3 g, sugars 8 g, protein 2 g

Going Green Smoothie

A pretty pale green and full of delicious fruit flavour, this smoothie is a terrific place to start if you are new to green smoothies. Fresh spinach blends with fruit, ice and water to create a refreshing smoothie that even the most vegetable-wary kid can enjoy.

Preparation: **10 minutes**   Processing: **30 seconds**   Yield: **600 ml**

150 g green grapes

75 g fresh pineapple chunks

½ medium banana

60 g spinach

120 ml ice cubes

Place all the ingredients and 120 ml water into the Vitamix container in the order listed and secure the lid. Select Variable 1. Turn the machine on and slowly increase the speed to Variable 10, then to High. Blend for 30 seconds, or until the desired consistency is reached.

AMOUNT PER 240 ML SERVING: calories 90, total fat 0 g, saturated fat 0 g, cholesterol 0 mg, sodium 40 mg, total carbohydrate 23 g, dietary fibre 2 g, sugars 15 g, protein 1 g

Silky Green Smoothie

Avocados, a fruit botanically speaking, have a mild, creamy texture that blends as easily into a smoothie as a banana. Here vanilla almond milk and non-fat natural yoghurt play up the avocado's creamy side, while the spinach highlights its savoury qualities. Dates, lemon juice and a splash of vanilla transform this diverse group of ingredients into something truly delicious and nutritious.

Preparation: **15 minutes**   Processing: **35 seconds**   Yield: **2 servings**

240 ml unsweetened vanilla almond milk, preferably home-made (page 352)

2 teaspoons fresh lemon juice

120 ml natural 0% yoghurt

½ teaspoon vanilla extract

6 pitted dates

½ avocado, pitted and peeled

85 g spinach

120 ml ice cubes

Place all the ingredients into the Vitamix container in the order listed and secure the lid. Select Variable 1. Turn the machine on and slowly increase the speed to Variable 10, then to High. Blend for 35 seconds, or until the desired consistency is reached.

AMOUNT PER 240 ML SERVING: calories 190, total fat 7 g, saturated fat 0.5 g, cholesterol 0 mg, sodium 180 mg, total carbohydrate 33 g, dietary fibre 6 g, sugars 24 g, protein 5 g

Very Citrus Slushy

Better than lemonade, this vibrantly flavourful slushy will help you cool down on the very hottest afternoon. Drink through a curly straw if you like.

Preparation: **15 minutes**   Processing: **1–2 minutes**   Yield: **1.4 litres**

680 g pink grapefruit, peeled and quartered

1 tablespoon grated orange zest

1 orange, peeled and quartered

1 lime, peeled and halved

1 tablespoon honey

720–960 ml ice cubes, more for a slushier consistency

Place all the ingredients into the Vitamix container in the order listed and secure the lid. Select Variable 1. Turn the machine on and slowly increase the speed to Variable 10, then to High. Blend for 1–2 minutes, using the tamper to press the ingredients into the blades, until desired consistency is reached.

AMOUNT PER 120 ML SERVING: calories 60, total fat 0 g, saturated fat 0 g, cholesterol 0 mg, sodium 0 mg, total carbohydrate 15 g, dietary fibre 2 g, sugars 5 g, protein 1 g

Green Goodness

Green smoothies often contain leafy greens, but some, like this one, can make delicious use of green fruits. Complete with fibre and vitamin C, green Bartlett pears are delicious and widely available. Blend, skin and all, with green grapes, soya milk, wheatgerm and a pinch of nutmeg for a tasty and nutritious drink.

Preparation: **10 minutes**   Processing: **30 seconds**   Yield: **2 servings**

60 ml unsweetened soya milk

190 g green grapes

1 tablespoon wheatgerm

¼ teaspoon ground nutmeg

1 large Bartlett pear, quartered and cored

180 ml ice cubes

Place all the ingredients into the Vitamix container in the order listed and secure the lid. Select Variable 1. Turn the machine on and slowly increase the speed to Variable 10, then to High. Blend for 30 seconds, or until the desired consistency is reached, using the tamper to press the ingredients into the blades.

AMOUNT PER 240 ML SERVING: calories 160, total fat 1.5 g, saturated fat 0 g, cholesterol 0 mg, sodium 5 mg, total carbohydrate 37 g, dietary fibre 5 g, sugars 27 g, protein 4 g

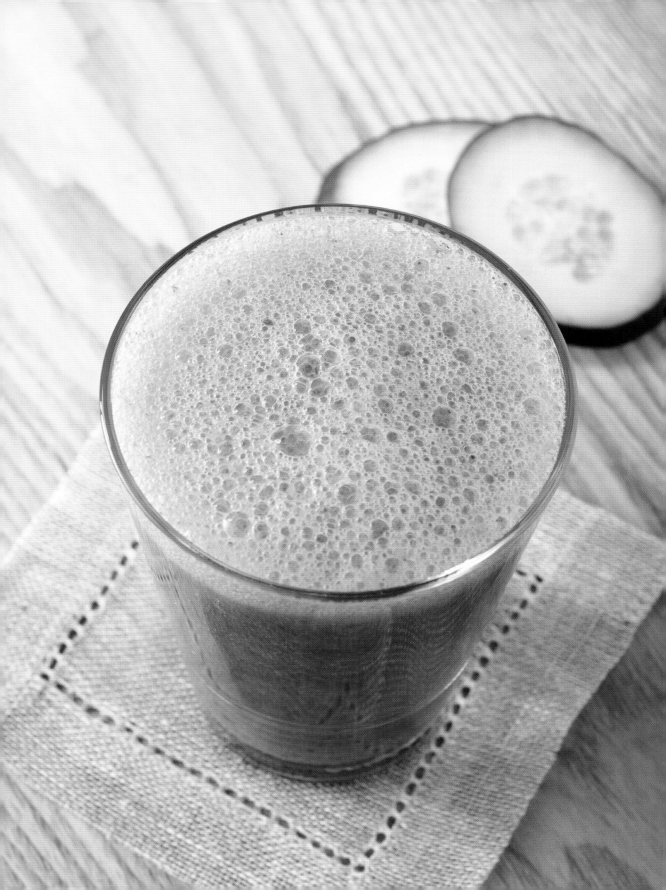

Spinach Sparkler

Bright green and delightfully bubbly, this sparkler gives you a new and enchanting way to drink your vegetables. Using almost all of a lemon here – the zest and the fruit, but not the bitter pith – gives you bright citrus flavour.

Preparation: **15 minutes**   Processing: **45 seconds**   Yield: **3 servings**

1 medium cucumber, cut into pieces

1 celery stick, halved

70 g spinach leaves

2 tablespoons fresh flatleaf parsley leaves

Grated zest of 1 lemon

1 lemon, peeled and halved

1 tablespoon pineapple juice

120 ml ice cubes

80–160 ml sparkling water

1. Place 60 ml water into the Vitamix container, then add the cucumber, celery, spinach, parsley, lemon, pineapple juice and ice cubes in the order listed and secure lid. Select Variable 1. Turn the machine on and slowly increase the speed to Variable 10, then to High. Blend for 45 seconds, using the tamper to press the ingredients into the blades.

2. Divide into 3 glasses and top with sparkling water.

AMOUNT PER 240 ML SERVING: calories 35, total fat 0 g, saturated fat 0 g, cholesterol 0 mg, sodium 55 mg, total carbohydrate 10 g, dietary fibre 3 g, sugars 3 g, protein 2 g

Salsa in a Glass

Bright, spicy and full of fresh vegetable flavour, this juice really ought to be garnished with a celery stick or wedge of lime. The perfect on-the-go, veggie-packed snack! Having friends over for brunch? Add vodka and transform this drink into a whole-food Bloody Mary.

Preparation: **15 minutes**   Processing: **40 seconds**   Yield: **3–4 servings**

450 g tomatoes, quartered

1 jalapeño pepper, seeded

2 tablespoons chopped onion

6 fresh coriander sprigs

½ lime, peeled

120 ml ice cubes

Place all the ingredients into the Vitamix container in the order listed and secure the lid. Select Variable 1. Turn the machine on and slowly increase the speed to Variable 10, then to High. Blend for 1–2 minutes, using the tamper to press the ingredients into the blades, until desired consistency is reached.

AMOUNT PER 120 ML SERVING: calories 60, total fat 0 g, saturated fat 0 g, cholesterol 0 mg, sodium 0 mg, total carbohydrate 15 g, dietary fibre 2 g, sugars 5 g, protein 1 g

Velvet Smoothie

Part of the value of a Vitamix is its ability to create silky smooth purées. Naturally smooth ingredients like avocado and banana can create an extra velvety smoothie, even when chewy dates and crunchy sunflower seeds are added.

Preparation: **10 minutes**   Processing: **25 seconds**   Yield: **3–4 servings**

360 ml unsweetened rice milk, preferably home-made (page 353)

½ avocado, peeled and pitted

½ banana

¼ teaspoon grated lemon zest

¼ lemon, peeled

1 tablespoon chopped pitted dates

1 teaspoon clover honey

1 tablespoon sunflower seeds

240 ml ice cubes

Place all the ingredients into the Vitamix container in the order listed and secure the lid. Select Variable 1. Turn the machine on and slowly increase the speed to Variable 10, then to High. Blend for 25 seconds, or until the desired consistency is reached.

AMOUNT PER 240 ML SERVING: calories 120, total fat 6 g, saturated fat 0.5 g, cholesterol 0 mg, sodium 60 mg, total carbohydrate 17 g, dietary fibre 3 g, sugars 6 g, protein 1 g

Banana Chia Smoothie

You might not want a bowl of kale, chia seeds and almond butter for breakfast. But if you buzz these nutritious ingredients in a Vitamix with dates, fresh blueberries and frozen bananas, you will have a drink that you will want to make again and again. With 7 grams of fibre, 6 grams of protein and healthy fats from the almond butter and chia seeds, this drink will really stick to your ribs too.

Preparation: **15 minutes**   Processing: **1 minute**   Yield: **4 servings**

65 g almond butter

2 tablespoons chia seeds

5 large pitted dates

75 g fresh blueberries

6 kale leaves

2 large bananas, peeled and frozen

Place all the ingredients and 420 ml water into the Vitamix container in the order listed and secure the lid. Select Variable 1. Turn the machine on and slowly increase the speed to Variable 10, then to High. Blend for 1 minute, or until the desired consistency is reached, using the tamper to press the ingredients into the blades.

AMOUNT PER 240 ML SERVING: calories 230, total fat 11 g, saturated fat 1.5 g, cholesterol 0 mg, sodium 45 mg, total carbohydrate 31 g, dietary fibre 7 g, sugars 17 g, protein 6 g

Kale-Flax Smoothie with Pear

Grinding flax seeds makes their nutritional benefits – including omega-3 fatty acids and fibre – more accessible. (Whole flax seeds may pass through your body, more or less undigested.) Thanks to the Vitamix, you can add ground flax seed to this tasty smoothie. Like many of the recipes in this chapter, fresh vegetables like kale are blended with whole fruits to create delicious results. Encouraging people to improve their vitality is central to Vitamix's mission, and if adding pears and half a banana to a drink helps you eat more greens, we are all for it!

Preparation: **15 minutes**   Processing: **30 seconds**   Yield: **3–4 servings**

240 ml no-sugar-added pear nectar

120 ml vanilla rice milk or soya milk

2 Bartlett or Forelle pears, cut into large chunks and cored

½ medium banana

2 tablespoons flax seeds

2 fresh mint leaves

150 g torn kale leaves

120 ml ice cubes

Place all the ingredients into the Vitamix container in the order listed and secure the lid. Select Variable 1. Turn the machine on and slowly increase the speed to Variable 10, then to High. Blend for 30 seconds, or until the desired consistency is reached.

AMOUNT PER 240 ML SERVING: calories 200, total fat 3 g, saturated fat 0 g, cholesterol 0 mg, sodium 45 mg, total carbohydrate 42 g, dietary fibre 7 g, sugars 15 g, protein 5 g

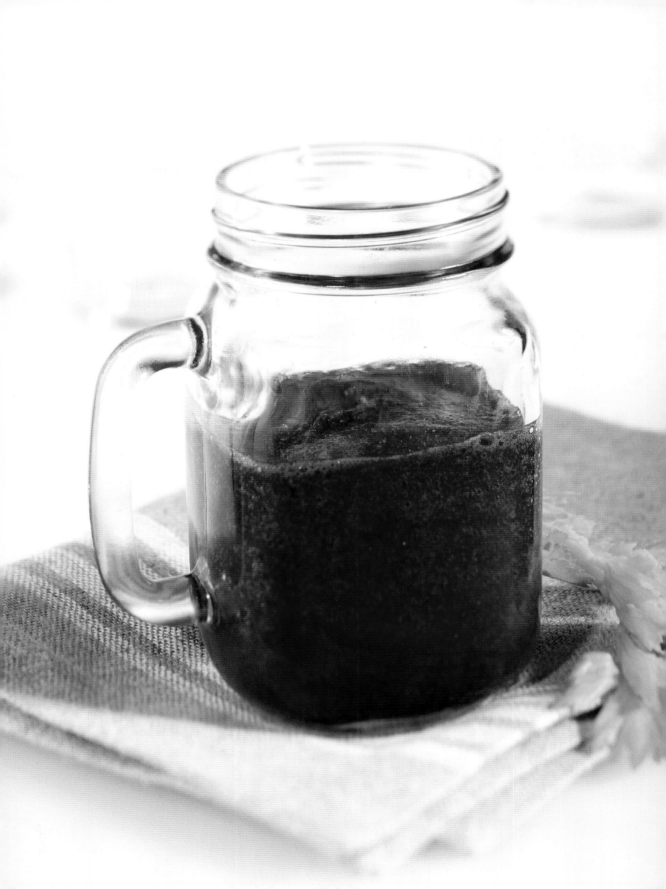

Nourishing Beetroot

Many purchased vegetable juices feature tomatoes, but when you make your own, you can move purple-hued, nutrient-packed beetroot to centre stage. (And unlike many of its bottled counterparts, this drink has no added salt.) Apples complement the beetroot's natural sweetness, while the fresh chilli, a chunk of fresh ginger and garlic lend spice. The vegetal flavour of celery keeps the overall taste more savoury than sweet.

Preparation: **15 minutes**   Processing: **2 minutes**   Yield: **7 servings**

3 small/medium beetroots (680 g), tops intact, cut into pieces

1-cm piece of fresh ginger, peeled

1 fresh chilli pepper

2 small apples, quartered

1 garlic clove, peeled

2 celery sticks, cut into pieces

240 ml ice cubes

1. Place 240 ml water into the Vitamix container, then add the beetroot, ginger, chilli, apples, garlic and celery and secure the lid. Select Variable 1. Turn the machine on and slowly increase the speed to Variable 10, then to High. Blend for 1 minute 30 seconds, using the tamper to press the ingredients into the blades.

2. Stop the machine and remove the lid. Add 240 ml water and the ice cubes to the Vitamix container and secure the lid. Select Variable 1. Turn the machine on and slowly increase the speed to Variable 10, then to High. Blend for 30 additional seconds.

AMOUNT PER 240 ML SERVING: calories 60, total fat 0 g, saturated fat 0 g, cholesterol 0 mg, sodium 75 mg, total carbohydrate 15 g, dietary fibre 4 g, sugars 10 g, protein 2 g

Liquid Apple Pie

Why drink plain old apple juice when you can sip apple pie instead? Cinnamon, nutmeg, vanilla and maple syrup pack classic apple pie flavours into a delicious, slushy drink.

Preparation: **10 minutes**   Processing: **15–20 seconds**   Yield: **1 serving**

120 ml unsweetened apple juice

60 ml unsweetened soya milk

1 teaspoon pure maple syrup

¼ teaspoon vanilla extract

⅛ teaspoon ground cinnamon

⅛ teaspoon ground nutmeg

120 ml ice cubes

Place all the ingredients and 60 ml water into the Vitamix container in the order listed and secure the lid. Select Variable 1. Turn the machine on and slowly increase the speed to Variable 10. Blend for 15–20 seconds, leaving a little slushy consistency. Serve immediately.

AMOUNT PER SERVING: calories 110, total fat 2 g, saturated fat 0 g, cholesterol 0 mg, sodium 10 mg, total carbohydrate 20 g, dietary fibre 1 g, sugars 17 g, protein 3 g

Tofu Tropic Smoothie

Soft, silken tofu has a rich, creamy texture that blends beautifully into this tropical-flavoured smoothie. Partially defrosted fruit seems to have a fuller flavour, which is why we suggest that you thaw the mango for 10 minutes before blending.

Preparation: **10 minutes**   Processing: **45 seconds**   Yield: **4 servings**

375 g frozen mango chunks

300 ml pineapple juice

170 g soft silken tofu

Grated zest of 1 lime

1 lime, peeled and halved

1. Let the mango sit at room temperature for 10 minutes to thaw slightly.

2. Place 120 ml water into the Vitamix container, then add the pineapple juice, tofu, lime zest, lime and mango and secure the lid. Select Variable 1. Turn the machine on and slowly increase the speed to Variable 10, then to High. Blend for 45 seconds, or until the desired consistency is reached, using the tamper to press the ingredients into the blades.

AMOUNT PER 240 ML SERVING: calories 140, total fat 1.5 g, saturated fat 0 g, cholesterol 0 mg, sodium 25 mg, total carbohydrate 29 g, dietary fibre 3 g, sugars 22 g, protein 4 g

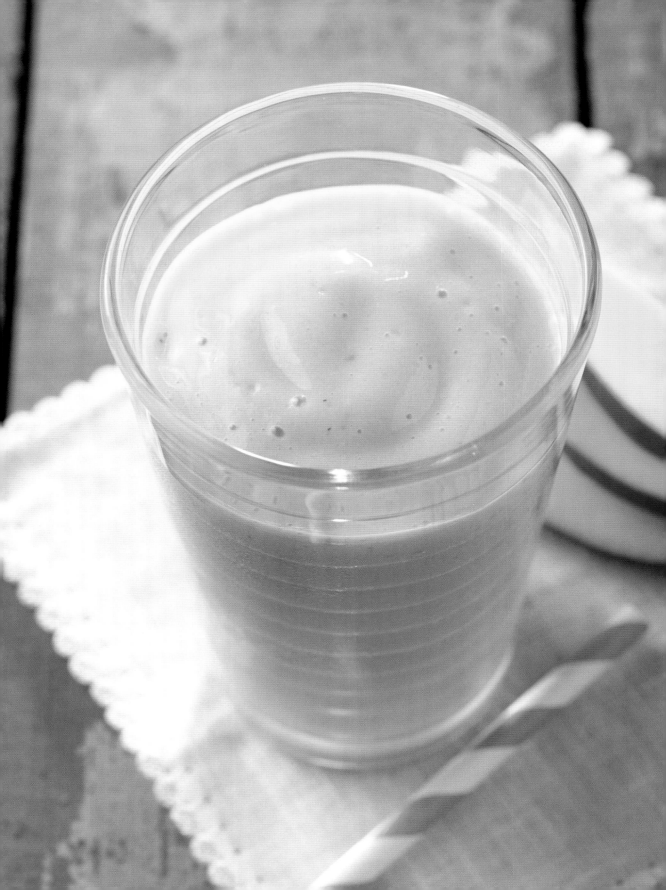

Tropical Shake

Kids (and the kid in all of us) love slurping up a sweet shake through a straw. Vegan and busting with zippy fresh fruit flavour, this shake will be a hit with young and old alike.

Preparation: **15 minutes**   Processing: **40 seconds**   Yield: **780 ml**

240 ml pineapple juice

180 ml soya milk

½ lemon, peeled

1 banana, peeled and frozen

190 g frozen mango chunks

Place all the ingredients into the Vitamix container in the order listed and secure the lid. Select Variable 1. Turn the machine on and slowly increase the speed to Variable 10, then to High. Blend for 40 seconds.

AMOUNT PER 240 ML SERVING: calories 150, total fat 1 g, saturated fat 0 g, cholesterol 0 mg, sodium 35 mg, total carbohydrate 35 g, dietary fibre 3 g, protein 3 g

Mango Freeze Drink

Cultivated since about 2000 BC, mangoes give us vitamins A and C as well as fibre, magnesium and potassium. Blend this healthy fruit with a little peach nectar and ice on a hot summer's day for a refreshing treat. Garnish with a lime wedge if you like.

Preparation: **15 minutes**   Processing: **1 minute**   Yield: **5–6 servings**

360 ml no-sugar-added peach nectar, chilled

3 medium mangoes, peeled, pitted and cut into chunks

600 ml ice cubes

Place all the ingredients into the Vitamix container in the order listed and secure the lid. Select Variable 1. Turn the machine on and slowly increase the speed to Variable 10, then to High. Blend for 1 minute, or until the desired consistency is reached, using the tamper to press the ingredients into the blades.

AMOUNT PER 240 ML SERVING: calories 190, total fat 1 g, saturated fat 0 g, cholesterol 0 mg, sodium 5 mg, total carbohydrate 47 g, dietary fibre 3 g, sugars 3 g, protein 0 g

Melon Madness

Our tasty Melon Madness is the perfect drink to whip up when the shops and markets are full of ripe melons. Skimmed milk and Greek yoghurt add calcium and protein to this wonderfully fruit-filled drink.

Preparation: **15 minutes**   Processing: **25 seconds**   Yield: **4–5 servings**

140 g frozen peach slices

240 ml skimmed milk

180 ml peach 0% Greek yoghurt, stirred

½ teaspoon vanilla extract

80 g cantaloupe pieces

85 g honeydew melon pieces

70 g watermelon pieces

80 ml ice cubes

1. Let the frozen peaches sit at room temperature for 10 minutes to thaw slightly.

2. Place the milk, yoghurt, vanilla, melon pieces, peaches, ice cubes and 60 ml water into the Vitamix container in the order listed and secure the lid. Select Variable 1. Turn the machine on and slowly increase the speed to Variable 10, then to High. Blend for 25 seconds, or until the desired consistency is reached.

AMOUNT PER 240 ML SERVING: calories 80, total fat 0 g, saturated fat 0 g, cholesterol 0 mg, sodium 45 mg, total carbohydrate 15 g, dietary fibre 1 g, sugars 14 g, protein 6 g

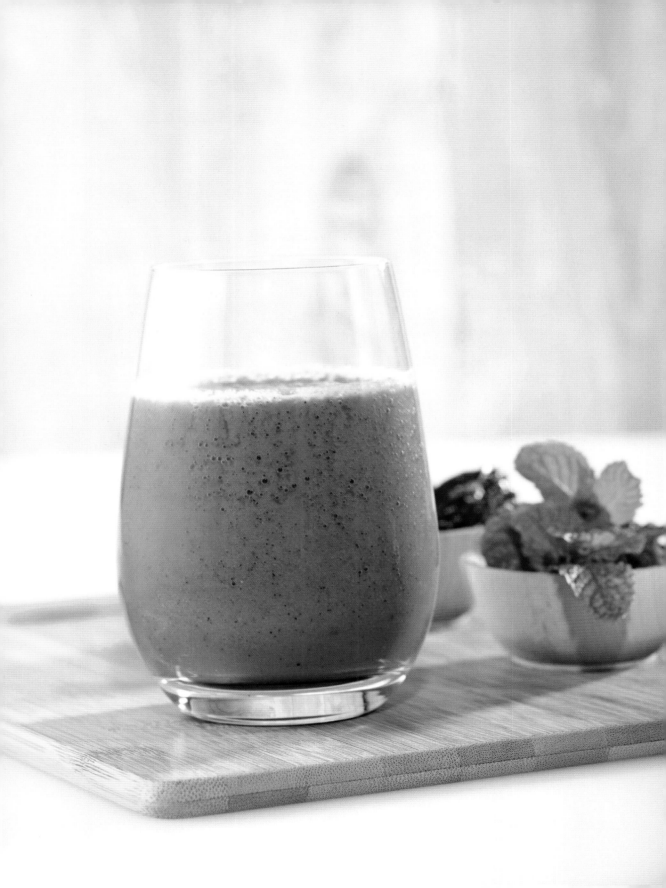

Fresh Mint with Sprouts Beverage

You may eat your greens most days, but sometimes you may want or need to drink them, too! This vibrant, minty drink combines the green goodness of kiwi fruit, broccoli, kale, mint and sprouts with almond milk, dates and a little vanilla. Sweet enough to be totally slurpable but not so sweet that the flavour of the greens is hidden.

Preparation: **15 minutes**   Processing: **40 seconds**   Yield: **2–3 servings**

240 ml unsweetened almond milk

2 kiwi fruit, peeled and halved

25 g chopped broccoli florets

2 pitted dates

20 g torn kale leaves

13 g fresh mint leaves

16 g alfalfa sprouts or broccoli sprouts, rinsed and patted dry

1 teaspoon vanilla extract

120 ml ice cubes

Place all the ingredients into the Vitamix container in the order listed and secure the lid. Select Variable 1. Turn the machine on and slowly increase the speed to Variable 10, then to High. Blend for 40 seconds, or until the desired consistency is reached, using the tamper to press the ingredients into the blades.

AMOUNT PER 240 ML SERVING: calories 80, total fat 1.5 g, saturated fat 0 g, cholesterol 0 mg, sodium 80 mg, total carbohydrate 15 g, dietary fibre 3 g, sugars 9 g, protein 2 g

Nuts and Seeds Smoothie

Not just for the birds anymore, nuts and seeds can be a good way to add protein, omega-3 fatty acids, fibre, calcium and iron to your diet. While absolutely nutrient-dense and a source of healthy fats, nuts and seeds also pack a bigger calorific-punch, so enjoy them in moderation.

Preparation: **15 minutes**   Processing: **1 minute**   Yield: **3 servings**

45 g unsalted sunflower seeds

48 g blanched almonds

1 tablespoon chia seeds, soaked in 3 tablespoons water until a gel is formed

60 g dried apricots

½ avocado, pitted and peeled

85 g spring greens mix

½ teaspoon ground cinnamon

¼ teaspoon ground nutmeg

1 teaspoon vanilla extract

420 ml ice cubes

Place all the ingredients and 360 ml water into the Vitamix container in the order listed and secure the lid. Select Variable 1. Turn the machine on and slowly increase the speed to Variable 10, then to High. Blend for 1 minute, or until the desired consistency is reached, using the tamper to press the ingredients into the blades.

AMOUNT PER 240 ML SERVING: calories 300, total fat 20 g, saturated fat 2 g, cholesterol 0 mg, sodium 40 mg, total carbohydrate 26 g, dietary fibre 9 g, sugars 9 g, protein 8 g

Soy Fruit Splendour

Not only do dried figs lend a caramel-like sweetness to this vegan drink, they also add calcium. Eighty grams of dried figs contains about the same amount of calcium as a 120 ml of low-fat (1%) milk: 133 milligrams versus 142 milligrams.

Preparation: **10 minutes**   Processing: **1 minute**   Yield: **3–4 servings**

200 ml fresh orange juice (page 303)

4 tablespoons unsweetened soya milk

1½ apples (400 g), quartered and cored

5 dried figs

240 ml ice cubes

Place all the ingredients into the Vitamix container in the order listed and secure the lid. Select Variable 1. Turn the machine on and slowly increase the speed to Variable 10, then to High. Blend for 1 minute, or until the desired consistency is reached, using the tamper to press the ingredients into the blades.

AMOUNT PER 240 ML SERVING: calories 130, total fat 1 g, saturated fat 0 g, cholesterol 0 mg, sodium 5 mg, total carbohydrate 33 g, dietary fibre 4 g, sugars 24 g, protein 2 g

B-Smoothie

This simple smoothie gives you a delicious way to add the nutrient-packed goodness of wheatgerm, flax seed and hemp seeds into your diet. Chia seeds contain omega-3 fatty acids, fibre (10 grams per two tablespoons), iron, calcium and more. Hemp seeds contribute omega-3 and omega-6 fatty acids, magnesium, fibre (2 grams per three tablespoons) and protein (10 grams per three tablespoons) to your diet. Good old wheatgerm gives this drink an extra boost of magnesium, fibre and vitamins B5 and E. This smoothie is delicious and nutritious. What could be better?

Preparation: **10 minutes**   Processing: **40 seconds**   Yield: **2–3 servings**

120 ml pineapple juice

4 tablespoons unsweetened almond milk

1 small ripe banana

165 g pineapple chunks, fresh or frozen

1 tablespoon wheatgerm

2 teaspoons flax seeds

½ teaspoon hemp seeds

120 ml ice cubes

Place all the ingredients into the Vitamix container in the order listed and secure the lid. Select Variable 1. Turn the machine on and slowly increase the speed to Variable 10, then to High. Blend for 40 seconds, or until the desired consistency is reached.

AMOUNT PER 240 ML SERVING: calories 120, total fat 2 g, saturated fat 0 g, cholesterol 0 mg, sodium 20 mg, total carbohydrate 26 g, dietary fibre 2 g, sugars 16 g, protein 2 g

Soya Milk

Once your dried soybeans are soaked and steamed, this preservative and additive-free fresh soya milk comes together in a flash. If you are going to use the milk in smoothies, don't worry about straining it. If you want to stir it into your coffee or pour it over cereal, you might want to use a fine mesh strainer to get an end product that is even creamier.

Preparation: **8 hours**   Processing: **1 minute**   Cook time: **15 minutes**
Yield: **960 ml unstrained or 720 ml strained**

200 g dried soybeans

1 tablespoon granulated sugar

1. Rinse dried soybeans and pick over for debris. Place in a bowl and add water to cover by 8 cm for 4–8 hours.

2. Steam for about 15 minutes. Remove the soybeans to a bowl and let cool. Measure out 260 g cooked beans. Reserve any leftover soybeans in the fridge for another use.

3. Place 840 ml water in the Vitamix container, then add the cooked beans and sugar and secure the lid. Select Variable 1. Turn the machine on and slowly increase the speed to Variable 10, then to High. Blend for 1 minute, or until your desired consistency – thin, thick or coarse – is reached.

4. To obtain commercial-style soya milk, strain the milk through a fine-mesh sieve.

For a refreshing flavour, add a 2.5-cm piece of ginger before blending.

AMOUNT PER 240 ML SERVING: calories 120, total fat 6 g, saturated fat 1 g, cholesterol 0 mg, sodium 10 mg, total carbohydrate 10 g, dietary fibre 4 g, sugars 5 g, protein 11 g

Almond Milk

You can purchase almond milk, but you will often be buying stabilisers, added sugar and preservatives along with the convenience. Once you have a Vitamix, you can blend your own almond milk and add as much or as little sweetness as you like. (A few pitted dates can be added in lieu of sugar.) The resulting nut milk is fresh and delicious, and it will keep in the fridge for 3–4 days.

Preparation: **8 hours**   Processing: **45 seconds**   Yield: **1 litre or 660 ml strained**

140 g raw almonds, soaked at least 8 hours, drained

Granulated sugar or sweetener, to taste (optional)

1. Place the almonds in a bowl. Cover with 2.5 cm water and let sit for 8 hours to soak. Drain well.

2. Place 720 ml water in the Vitamix container in the order listed, then add the almonds and secure the lid. Select Variable 1. Turn the machine on and slowly increase the speed to Variable 10, then to High. Blend for 45 seconds. Add sugar to taste, if desired.

3. To obtain commercial-style almond milk, strain the milk through a fine-mesh sieve.

AMOUNT PER 240 ML SERVING: calories 180, total fat 16 g, saturated fat 1 g, cholesterol 0 mg, sodium 5 mg, total carbohydrate 7 g, dietary fibre 4 g, sugars 1 g, protein 7 g

Rice Milk

Purchased rice milk, just like most non-dairy milks, can contain a lot of preservatives, thickeners and sweeteners. By blending your own fresh rice milk, you skip the additives and focus on the flavour, adding sweeteners and vanilla to taste.

Preparation: **10 minutes**   Processing: **1 minute**   Yield: **540 ml**

100 g cooked brown rice, cooled

½ tablespoon brown sugar or other sweetener, or more, to taste

½ teaspoon vanilla extract (optional)

Place the rice and 480 ml water into the Vitamix container, then add the sugar and vanilla (if using) and secure the lid. Select Variable 1. Turn the machine on and slowly increase the speed to Variable 10, then to High. Blend for 1 minute, or until the desired consistency is reached.

AMOUNT PER 240 ML SERVING: calories 60, total fat 0 g, saturated fat 0 g, cholesterol 0 mg, sodium 10 mg, total carbohydrate 13 g, dietary fibre 1 g, sugars 3 g, protein 1 g

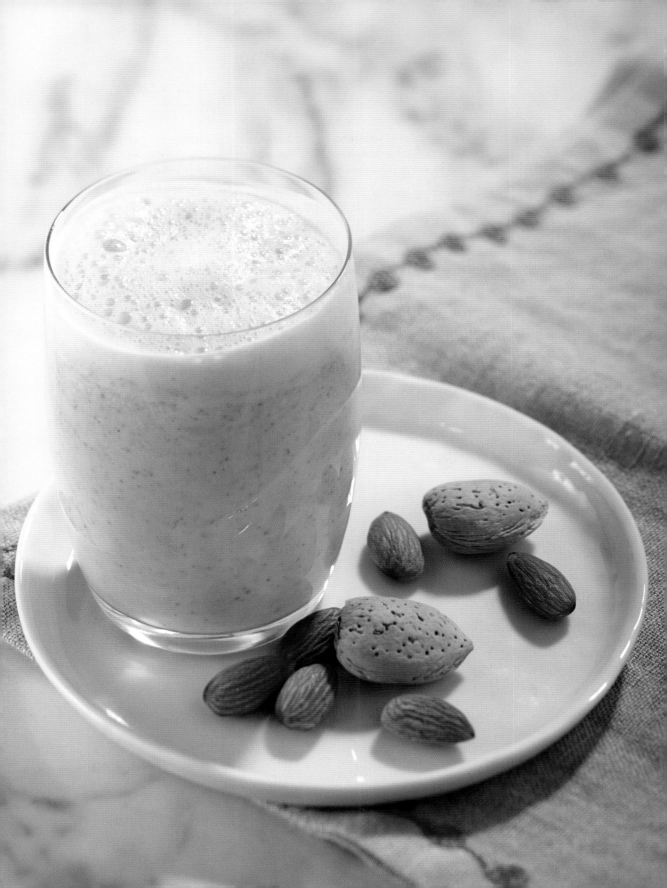

Sweet Almond Cinnamon Milk

Purchased almond milk's flavour pales in comparison to the fresh, nutty flavour of the real deal. Dates give the nut milk a rich, almost brown-sugar-like sweetness and the cinnamon complements this taste. Our sweet almond milk tastes amazing plain, blended into a smoothie or poured over cereal.

Preparation: **10 minutes**   Processing: **45 seconds**   Yield: **1 litre**

150 g raw almonds, soaked at least 8 hours, drained

½ teaspoon ground cinnamon

4 pitted dates

1. Place the almonds in a bowl with water to cover by 10 cm and let soak for at least 8 hours. Drain.

2. Place 720 ml water into the Vitamix container, then add the drained almonds, cinnamon and dates and secure the lid. Select Variable 1. Turn the machine on and slowly increase the speed to Variable 10, then to High. Blend for 45 seconds. To obtain commercial-style almond milk, strain the milk through a fine-mesh sieve.

AMOUNT PER 240 ML SERVING: calories 200, total fat 16 g, saturated fat 1 g, cholesterol 0 mg, sodium 10 mg, total carbohydrate 12 g, dietary fibre 5 g, sugars 6 g, protein 7 g

Iced Frappé

Coffee and chocolate, a great combination or the greatest combination? Regardless of your answer, this iced frappé will help you power through your day and for much less than the usual coffee-shop prices.

Preparation: **10 minutes**   Processing: **15 seconds**   Yield: **3–4 servings**

240 ml strong brewed coffee, cold

120 ml skimmed milk

1 teaspoon honey

2 pitted dates

2 tablespoons chopped plain chocolate

120 ml ice cubes

Place all the ingredients into the Vitamix container in the order listed and secure the lid. Select Variable 1. Turn the machine on and slowly increase the speed to Variable 8. Blend for 15 seconds. Serve immediately.

AMOUNT PER 240 ML SERVING: calories 60, total fat 2 g, saturated fat 1 g, cholesterol 0 mg, sodium 25 mg, total carbohydrate 10 g, dietary fibre 1 g, sugars 8 g, protein 2 g

Espresso Banana Drink

Do you love the icy cold blended coffee drinks sold at coffee shops but wish they were healthier? Our espresso banana drink will remind you of your favourite sweet, smooth iced coffee, but with only 7 grams of sugar per serving. Sweet, creamy bananas, eye-opening espresso, soya milk and ice whirl together to make a treat that can start the morning or perk up the most sluggish afternoon.

Preparation: **10 minutes**   Processing: **20 seconds**   Yield: **1 serving**

60 ml brewed espresso, cold

½ small ripe banana

120 ml unsweetened soya milk

120 ml ice cubes

Place all the ingredients into the Vitamix container in the order listed and secure the lid. Select Variable 1. Turn the machine on and slowly increase the speed to Variable 10, then to High. Blend for 20 seconds, or until the desired consistency is reached.

AMOUNT PER SERVING: calories 110, total fat 3.5 g, saturated fat 0.5 g, cholesterol 0 mg, sodium 15 mg, total carbohydrate 15 g, dietary fibre 2 g, sugars 7 g, protein 7 g

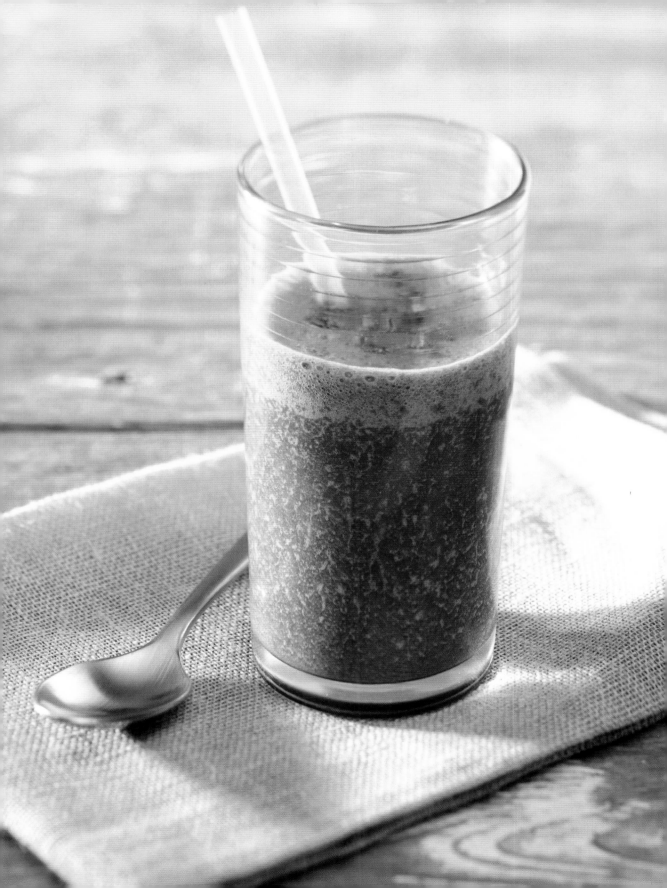

Mocha Cooler

The mellow, creamy flavour of banana and the deeper and more caramel-like sweetness of dates pair beautifully with the natural bitterness of espresso and cocoa powder. Together with ice, some fat-free milk and a splash of vanilla, these ingredients make a refreshing and indulgent-tasting mocha.

Preparation: **10 minutes**   Processing: **15 seconds**   Yield: **2 servings**

240 ml skimmed milk

1 medium banana, peeled

1 large pitted date

2 teaspoons cocoa powder

1 teaspoon instant espresso powder

½ teaspoon vanilla extract

120 ml ice cubes

Place all the ingredients into the Vitamix container in the order listed and secure the lid. Select Variable 1. Turn the machine on and slowly increase the speed to Variable 10, then to High. Blend for 15 seconds, or until the desired consistency is reached.

AMOUNT PER 240 ML SERVING: calories 160, total fat 0 g, saturated fat 0 g, cholesterol 0 mg, sodium 55 mg, total carbohydrate 36 g, dietary fibre 3 g, sugars 27 g, protein 6 g

Tea of Green Smoothie

Brewing your own green tea delivers far more of the naturally occurring antioxidants than purchased iced tea. In some cases, you would have to drink almost twenty bottles of the bought stuff to get the same benefits present in one home-made cup. Here, home-made iced green tea is blended with four different fruits to create a refreshing smoothie without any refined sugar.

Preparation: **10 minutes**   Processing: **40 seconds**   Yield: **3 servings**

240 ml freshly brewed green tea, chilled

1 small banana, peeled

340 g honeydew melon chunks

2 pitted dates

1 kiwi fruit, peeled and sliced

Place all the ingredients into the Vitamix container in the order listed and secure the lid. Select Variable 1. Turn the machine on and slowly increase the speed to Variable 10. Blend for 40 seconds, or until the desired consistency is reached.

AMOUNT PER 240 ML SERVING: calories 100, total fat 0 g, saturated fat 0 g, cholesterol 0 mg, sodium 20 mg, total carbohydrate 25 g, dietary fibre 3 g, sugars 18 g, protein 1 g

Thai Eye Opener

A splash of creamy coconut milk, fresh pineapple, carrots, apple and fresh ginger are blended together to create a vibrant, Thai-inspired juice. When you are cutting up your pineapple, just cut away the thinnest layer of the skin. The 'eyes' of the pineapple and the fibrous core will be puréed to silky perfection in your Vitamix!

Preparation: **20 minutes**   Processing: **1 minute**   Yield: **2–3 servings**

60 ml coconut milk

40 g fresh pineapple chunks

2 carrots, halved

1 medium apple, quartered and cored

¼ teaspoon chopped fresh ginger

240 ml ice cubes

Place all the ingredients into the Vitamix container in the order listed and secure the lid. Select Variable 1. Turn the machine on and slowly increase the speed to Variable 10, then to High. Blend for 1 minute, or until the desired consistency is reached, using the tamper to press the ingredients into the blades.

AMOUNT PER 240 ML SERVING: calories 100, total fat 4 g, saturated fat 3.5 g, cholesterol 0 mg, sodium 40 mg, total carbohydrate 17 g, dietary fibre 3 g, sugars 12 g, protein 1 g

BRAD AND ALLYSON SHEDD

Countless articles have been devoted to getting wary children to eat their vegetables. Scanning the literature, several trends emerge. First, you have to set a good example. Not making many healthy choices yourself? It's a challenge to get kids to eat their veggies if the adults around them don't. Another frequently heard theme is the importance of including your children in preparing food. Kids, in theory, are often more apt to enjoy a salad that they helped prepare. But think of it this way. Most adults eat the same foods they were exposed to as a child. So the key may be as simple as exposing them to the flavours of fruits and vegetables in a way that is delicious as early as you can. Put a green smoothie in a sippy cup, and most kids will cry for more.

For parents that did not start their kids out young, persuading one or maybe two children to eat vegetables can be a seemingly impossible task. But ten? It is a challenge that Brad and Alyson Shedd handle with great grace. And, perhaps, with a little help from their Vitamix, a gift for Alyson's birthday in 2010. Do they set a good example? Yes! 'We have lots of fruit and vegetables throughout the day – usually a huge salad each evening – but the Vitamix helps our day get started right with fruits and vegetables at the very beginning of the day! We all have started craving it', says Brad. They created a delicious Shedd-family formula for their morning smoothies – yoghurt, spinach, frozen fruit and apple juice – that they enjoy right along with their kids. 'We are able to mix up the smoothie mix for all ten of us (we just about go over-capacity on the machine!) each morning!' Brad says. Brad and Alyson use kid-friendly ingredients like yoghurt and fruit to make it nutritious and delicious.

And do they involve their kids? Yes! Brad says his daughter Laura, now eight years old, is his primary smoothie assistant. In fact, Laura, who has been helping Brad for the past two years, can assemble all of the ingredients herself and just needs help operating the machine.

Getting your kids to enjoy their veggies every day? The Shedd family is definitely a whole foods success story. When asked if he had any advice for someone considering buying a Vitamix, Brad had this to say, 'The Vitamix is such a powerful, versatile kitchen tool. It can be overwhelming when you first pull it out of the box. But start with some of the simple recipes included with the package, and begin to experiment and branch out from there. There's no rush. You're going to be using this tool pretty much the rest of your life!'

UNIVERSAL CONVERSION CHART

OVEN TEMPERATURE EQUIVALENTS

120 ˚C = 250 ˚F

135 ˚C = 275 ˚F

150 ˚C = 300 ˚F

160 ˚C = 325 ˚F

180 ˚C = 350 ˚F

190 ˚C = 375 ˚F

200 ˚C = 400 ˚F

220 ˚C = 425 ˚F

230 ˚C = 450 ˚F

240 ˚C = 475 ˚F

260 ˚C = 500 ˚F

MEASUREMENT EQUIVALENTS
Measurements should always be level unless directed otherwise.

⅛ teaspoon = 0.5 ml

¼ teaspoon = 1 ml

½ teaspoon = 2 ml

1 teaspoon = 5 ml

1 tablespoon = 3 teaspoons = ½ fluid ounce = 15 ml

2 tablespoons = ⅛ cup = 1 fluid ounce = 30 ml

4 tablespoons = ¼ cup = 2 fluid ounces = 60 ml

5 tablespoons = ⅓ cup = 3 fluid ounces = 80 ml

8 tablespoons = ½ cup = 4 fluid ounces = 120 ml

10 tablespoons = 223 cup = 5 fluid ounces = 160 ml

12 tablespoons = ¾ cup = 6 fluid ounces = 180 ml

16 tablespoons = 1 cup = 8 fluid ounces = 240 ml

Acknowledgements

This book started as a desire to share the story of my ancestors and how their commitment to whole food blending and health created a legacy that I have the honor of stewarding for the next generation. The number of people, and the work they did to take it from a desire to a reality, is impressive. I want to thank our friends at Falls Communications and the numerous Vitamix employees, with a special call out to our talented chefs that developed the delicious recipes; Bev Shaffer, Anne Thacker and Adam Wilson.

Thank you to all of my family who made our story possible and especially to those that helped tell the story and verify the details, it was truly a multi-generational project - my father John Barnard, my cousin Loree Connors, my sister Beth McBride and my niece Robin Dieterich. Thank you Heather Gaynor for keeping the project on track and for Beth McBride for bringing our family story to life.

Index